Artificial Intelligence (AI) in Forensic Sciences

Published and forthcoming titles in the Forensic Science in Focus series

Published

The Global Practice of Forensic Science
Douglas H. Ubelaker (Editor)

Forensic Chemistry: Fundamentals and Applications
Jay A. Siegel (Editor)

Forensic Microbiology
David O. Carter, Jeffrey K. Tomberlin, M. Eric Benbow and
Jessica L. Metcalf (Editors)

Forensic Anthropology: Theoretical Framework and Scientific Basis
Clifford Boyd and Donna Boyd (Editors)

The Future of Forensic Science
Daniel A. Martell (Editor)

Forensic Anthropology and the U.S. Judicial System
Laura C. Fulginiti, Alison Galloway and Kristen Hartnett-McCann
(Editors)

*Forensic Science and Humanitarian Action: Interacting with the Dead
and the Living*
Roberto C. Parra, Sara C. Zapico and Douglas H. Ubelaker (Editors)

Disaster Victim Identification in the 21st Century: A US Perspective
John Williams and Victor Weedn (Editors)

The Forensic Evaluation of Burnt Human Remains
Sarah Ellingham, Joe Adserias Garriga, Sara C. Zapico and Douglas H. Ubelaker (Editors)

Anthropology of Violent Death: Theoretical Foundations for Forensic Humanitarian Action
Roberto C. Parra and Douglas H. Ubelaker (Editors)

AI In Forensic Science
Zeno Geradts and Karin Franke (Editors)

Forthcoming

An Illustrated Guide to Forensic Skeletal Trauma Analysis
Donna Boyd

Artificial Intelligence (AI) in Forensic Sciences

EDITED BY

Zeno Geradts

Netherlands Forensic Institute, Ministry of Justice and Security, The Hague, The Netherlands

Katrin Franke

Norwegian University of Science and Technology, Gjøvik, Norway

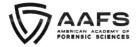 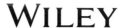

Registered Office(s)
John Wiley & Sons, Inc., 111 River Street, Hoboken, NJ 07030, USA
John Wiley & Sons Ltd, The Atrium, Southern Gate, Chichester, West Sussex, PO19 8SQ, UK

For details of our global editorial offices, customer services, and more information about Wiley products visit us at www.wiley.com.

Wiley also publishes its books in a variety of electronic formats and by print-on-demand. Some content that appears in standard print versions of this book may not be available in other formats.

Library of Congress Cataloging-in-Publication Data
Names: Geradts, Zeno J., editor. | Franke, Katrin, editor. | John Wiley & Sons, publisher.
Title: Artificial intelligence (AI) in forensic sciences / edited by Zeno Geradts, Katrin Franke.
Other titles: Forensic science in focus.
Description: Hoboken, NJ : JW-Wiley, 2024. | Series: Forensic science in focus | Includes bibliographical references and index. | Summary: "This book is in the AAFS Reference Series Library and serves a guide on using AI in forensic science. In Zeno's year of Presidency of the AAFS, one of the topics was Artificial Intelligence and the impact it can have on forensic science. In many forensic products Artificial Intelligence and Deep Learning is already included without the user being aware of it. Examples are software for facial and speaker comparison, many digital forensic packages for searching on for instance firearms. Furthermore, it is upcoming in chemometrics and many other fields. Also, the use of AI can impact forensic science, for instance on easier to make deepfakes, so spoofing evidence becomes easier. Different jurisdictions will handle the use of AI differently, depending on the laws. Examples are provided of good use of artificial intelligence, where the expert should be in the loop. The expert as well as the courts also needs to know the limitations of the approach. The book is composed out of chapters which can be used in a course, and will finalize with the newest research in developing approaches with graph neural networks. The book first does an introduction in the field as such, then it will go deeper in the legal issues with AI and the need for developing standard. Many examples of using AI are discussed and presented, such as smart cities, IoT in Hansken and at the end Also, the use of AI for making deepfakes will be discussed as well as how to detect it. The field develops rapidly, and much awareness is also being made by the European Commission on regulation of AI in practical use. In the United States NIST is working on standards on using Artificial Intelligence. New legislation is expected in many states, for example Colorado has legislation on use of facial recognition services and Vermont has legislation enacted on ethical use of artificial intelligence. One of the most significant applications of AI in forensic science is in the analysis of DNA evidence. DNA sequencing technology has advanced significantly in recent years, allowing scientists to analyze large amounts of genetic data quickly and accurately. However, the sheer volume of data generated by these techniques can be overwhelming for human analysts. AI algorithms can be used to quickly and accurately identify genetic markers that are associated with specific individuals or groups, making it easier for forensic scientists to identify suspects or eliminate suspects from an investigation"-- Provided by publisher.
Identifiers: LCCN 2023021269 (print) | LCCN 2023021270 (ebook) | ISBN 9781119813323 (hardback) | ISBN 9781119813330 (pdf) | ISBN 9781119813347 (epub)
Subjects: LCSH: Digital forensic science. | Forensic sciences--Data processing. | Electronic evidence. | Artificial intelligence.
Classification: LCC HV8078.7 .A77 2024 (print) | LCC HV8078.7 (ebook) | DDC 363.250285/63--dc23/eng/20230601
LC record available at https://lccn.loc.gov/2023021269
LC ebook record available at https://lccn.loc.gov/2023021270

Cover image: © Olga Tsyvinska/Getty Images
Cover design by Wiley

Set in 10.5/13.5pt Meridien by Integra Software Services Pvt. Ltd, Pondicherry, India
Printed and bound by CPI Group (UK) Ltd, Croydon, CR0 4YY

C9781119813323_240724

Contents

About the editors

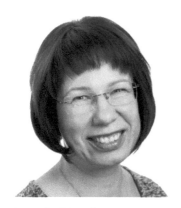

Katrin Franke

Katrin Franke is a professor in computer science within the information security environment at NTNU in Gjøvik. In 2007 she joined the Norwegian Information Security Lab (NISlab) with the mission to establish research and education in digital and computational forensics. In this context she was instrumental in setting up the partnership with the Norwegian police organizations as part of the Center for Cyber and information Security (CCIS). Dr. Franke is now associate director SFI NORCICS and also leading the NTNU Digital Forensics group. Dr. Franke has 25+ years experiences in basic and applied research for financial services and law enforcement agencies (LEAs) working closely with banks and LEAs in Europe, North America and Asia.

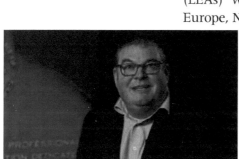

Zeno Geradts

Dr Zeno Geradts is a senior forensic scientist in the digital and biometric traces section of the Netherlands Forensic Institute. Since 1991, over 800 forensic reports and testimony have been given in several high profile cases. He is Past President of the American Academy of Forensic Sciences, and is a full professor of Forensic Data Science at the University of Amsterdam. Furthermore, he is Chief Editor of the *Journal of Forensic Science International Digital Investigation*. He has received several awards, including the Distinguished Forensic Scientist award from the European Network of Forensic Science (ENFSI).

List of Contributors

Timothy Bollee
Ecole des Sciences Criminelles
Police Scientifique
UNIL Lausanne, Switzerland

Eoghan Casey
Ecole des Sciences Criminelles
Police Scientifique
UNIL Lausanne, Switzerland

Katrin Franke
NTNU Teknologivegen
Gjøvik, Norway

Zeno Geradts
Netherlands Forensic Institute
Ministry of Justice and Security
The Hague, The Netherlands

Hans Henseler
Netherlands Forensic Institute
Den Haag, The Netherlands

Neminath Hubballi
Indian Institute of Technology Indore
Simrol, Indore, India

Meike Kombrink
Netherlands Forensic Institute
Ministry of Justice and Security
The Hague, The Netherlands

Pratibha Khandait
Indian Institute of Technology
Indore
Simrol, Indore, India

Didier Meuwly
Netherlands Forensic Institute
Den Haag, The Netherlands

Jeanne Mifsud Bonnici
NTNU Teknologivegen
Gjøvik, Norway

Kyle Porter
NTNU Teknologivegen
Gjøvik, Norway

Daniel Ramos
AUDIAS Lab. Universidad Autonoma
de Madrid, Madrid, Spain

Bente Skattor
NTNU Teknologivegen
Gjøvik, Norway

Radina Stoykova
NTNU Teknologivegen
Gjøvik, Norway

Harm van Beek
Netherlands Forensic Institute
Den Haag, The Netherlands

Marcel Worring
University of Amsterdam
Amsterdam, The Netherlands

Jan William Johnsen
NTNU Teknologivegen
Gjøvik, Norway

Rolf Ypma
Netherlands Forensic Institute
Den Haag, The Netherlands

Series Preface

The forensic sciences represent diverse, dynamic fields that seek to utilize the very best techniques available to address legal issues. Fueled by advances in technology, research and methodology, as well as new case applications, the forensic sciences continue to evolve. Forensic scientists strive to improve their analyses and interpretations of evidence and to remain cognizant of the latest advancements. This series results from a collaborative effort between the American Academy of Forensic Sciences (AAFS) and Wiley to publish a select number of books that relate closely to the activities and Objectives of the AAFS. The book series reflects the goals of the AAFS to encourage quality scholarship and publication in the forensic sciences. Proposals for publication in the series are reviewed by a committee established for that purpose by the AAFS and also reviewed by Wiley. The AAFS was founded in 1948 and represents a multidisciplinary professional organization that provides leadership to advance science and its application to the legal system. The 11 sections of the AAFS consist of Criminalistics, Digital and Multimedia Sciences, Engineering Sciences, General, Pathology/Biology, Questioned Documents, Jurisprudence, Anthropology, Toxicology, Odontology, and Psychiatry and Behavioral Science. There are over 7000 members of the AAFS, originating from all 50 States of the United States and many countries beyond. This series reflects global AAFS membership interest in new research, scholarship, and publication in the forensic sciences.

Zeno Geradts
Senior forensic scientist at the
Netherlands Forensic Institute of the
Ministry of Justice.
Netherlands
Series Editor

Preface Book

The idea for this book on AI in Forensic Science, was conceived in 2020, when Katrin Franke and Zeno Geradts regularly met to discuss this topic, and also since the many developments that have occurred in this area. The use of artificial intelligence in forensic science might seem somewhat contradictory, since often deep learning is not well explainable in court. This is one of the reasons that in 2020 Zeno Geradts, as president of the American Academy of Forensic Sciences, presented this topic, as many products already use deep learning, such as software for faces, handwriting, fingerprints, DNA, bullets, and many more. This book provides greater insight into how to use artificial intelligence properly in forensic science. New developments in law, such as the AI Act, are discussed. Also, many examples are provided of real-world implementations. The adversarial use of AI in deepfakes and anti-forensics is also presented.

Acknowledgements

We would like to thank all of the contributors to this book; their hard work and dedication have made this project possible.

We are also grateful to the AAFS and Wiley for their support. The AAFS provided us with a forum to share our research, and Wiley helped us to bring this book to publication.

Finally, we would like to thank our families and friends for their support. They have been there for us throughout this project, and their encouragement has meant the world.

This book would not have been possible without the help of all of these people. We are truly grateful.

Thank you.

CHAPTER 1

Introduction

Zeno Geradts[1] and Katrin Franke[2]

[1] Netherlands Forensic Institute, Laan van Ypenburg 6, GB Den Haag, Netherlands
[2] Norwegian Univ of Science & Technology, Høgskoleringen 1, Trondheim, Norway

This book is in the AAFS Reference Series Library and serves a guide on using artificial intelligence (AI) in forensic science. In Zeno's year of Presidency of the AAFS, one of the topics was AI and the impact it can have on forensic science. In many forensic products AI and deep learning is already included without the user being aware of it. Examples are software for facial and speaker comparison, and in many digital forensic software packages one can serch for images, for instance of firearms. Furthermore, its use is increasing in chemometrics and many other fields. Also, the use of AI can impact forensic science, for instance on easier to make deepfakes, so spoofing evidence becomes easier. Different jurisdictions will handle the use of AI differently, depending on their laws.

Examples are provided of good use of AI, where the expert should be in the loop. Experts as well as the courts also need to know the limitations of the approach.

The book is comprised of chapters which can be used as a reference for lectures, and ends with the newest research in developing approaches with graph neural networks. The book first provides an introduction to the field, it then goes deeper into the legal issues associated with AI and the need for developing a standard. Many examples of using AI are discussed and presented, such as smart cities, IoT in Hansken and finally, the use of AI for making deepfakes will be discussed as well as how to detect them.

The field is developing rapidly, and increasing awareness is also being created by the European Commission on the regulation of AI in practical use. In the United States NIST is working on standards for using AI. New legislation is expected in many states, for example Colorado has legislation on the use of facial recognition services and Vermont has legislation enacted on the ethical use of AI.

One of the most significant applications of AI in forensic science is in the analysis of DNA evidence. DNA sequencing technology has advanced significantly in recent years, allowing scientists to analyze large amounts of genetic data quickly and accurately. However, the sheer volume of data generated by these techniques can be overwhelming for human analysts. AI algorithms can be used to quickly and accurately identify genetic markers that are associated with specific individuals or groups, making it easier for forensic scientists to identify suspects or eliminate suspects from an investigation.

AI is also being used in the field of fingerprint analysis. Fingerprint analysis is a crucial aspect of forensic science, as fingerprints are unique to each individual and can be used to identify suspects. However, the process of manually analyzing fingerprints can be time-consuming and is prone to human error. AI algorithms can be used to quickly and accurately analyze fingerprints, reducing the time and resources required for this task.

Another area where AI is being used in forensic science is in the analysis of video and audio evidence. Video and audio recordings are often used as evidence in criminal investigations, but the process of analyzing these recordings can be labor-intensive and time-consuming. AI algorithms can be used to quickly identify and analyze key features in video and audio recordings, such as faces, voices, and other relevant details, making it easier for forensic scientists to identify suspects or gather important evidence.

In conclusion, AI is rapidly becoming an essential tool in the field of forensic science. It enables forensic scientists to analyze large amounts of data quickly and accurately, making it easier to identify suspects, establish facts, and gather evidence in criminal and civil legal matters. As technology continues to advance (such as we have seen with ChatGPT), it is likely that we will see even more applications in the near future.

Additionally, AI is also being used in the field of digital forensics. Digital forensics is the process of identifying, collecting, analyzing, and preserving electronic evidence in order to establish facts in criminal and civil legal matters. The increasing amount of digital data and the rapid pace of technological change make it difficult for human analysts to keep up with the volume and complexity of digital evidence. AI algorithms can be used to quickly and accurately identify and analyze digital evidence, such as email, text messages, and other forms of electronic communication.

This book aims to provide a foundation for using AI in forensic science, and describes issues, risks, and solutions.

CHAPTER 2

AI-based Forensic Evaluation in Court: The Desirability of Explanation and the Necessity of Validation

Rolf J.F. Ypma[1], Daniel Ramos[2], and Didier Meuwly[1,3]

[1] *Netherlands Forensic Institute, Netherlands*
[2] *AUDIAS Lab. Universidad Autonoma de Madrid, Madrid, Spain*
[3] *University of Twente, Enschede, Netherlands*

2.1 Introduction

Artificial intelligence (AI) is based on complex algorithms, methods using them, and systems. In this chapter, we understand *algorithms* as the core technology (e.g., a deep neural network (DNN)), the *methods* as the application of that core technology to a particular problem (e.g., the use of a DNN to evaluate fingerprint evidence), and the system as the software tool(s) that implement that method and algorithm (e.g., the GUI software package, or API, that is commercialized). The core technology typically includes pattern recognition and machine learning algorithms, whose complexity and performance has increased dramatically over the last years. These algorithms are often explainable in their inputs and their outputs, but the rationale that governs their internal mechanisms can be very difficult to explain. A prime example is DNNs, a family of algorithms forming the so-called deep learning field (LeCun et al. 2015). A DNN is a dense and very complex grid of connections between units called *neurons*. These connections can even be recurrent, or complemented with filters that interrelate different regions in the input features. Originally, a neural network aimed at mimicking the topology of the human brain, hence its name. The input of a DNN is typically a list of numbers representing some textual or sensory raw data (e.g., a fingermark image or an audio file). The output of a DNN consists of continuous or discrete outputs, depending on the task (e.g., a probability for each of a set of classes in a classification task or a magnitude of interest to predict in a regression task). Thus, the inputs and outputs are well defined, and even explainable in many cases. However, it is

---

very difficult to know or explain what the activation of any single neuron, or a group of them, means. Although some intuitions exist, interpreting those intermediate outcomes is extremely difficult in general. Indeed, the explainability of machine learning algorithms is a field in itself, named explainable AI (XAI), (Doshi-Velez and Kim 2017; Guidotti et al. 2018; LeCun et al. 2015; Molnar 2020) covering explainable algorithms for machine learning and AI. XAI is closely related to more philosophical areas such as ethics, fairness, and the risk of applicability of AI to real-world problems.

In the context of forensic evaluation using algorithms, we consider that to interpret means providing a forensic meaning to the results of the computation (e.g., a set of features or a score obtained or extracted from the evidence), and modelling them probabilistically in the form of a likelihood ratio. The likelihood ratio is a numerical expression of the probative value that is meaningful in the judicial context, where the defence and the prosecution alternative propositions are disputed (Evett et al. 2000; Jackson et al. 2013). However, the interpretation by humans in understandable terms of the inner components of the "black box" that forms many machine learning algorithms (such as DNNs) is still an issue, particularly for high-impact decisions as in forensic science. At this point it is worth highlighting that we distinguish between the interpretation of the inner components and workings of an AI algorithm, and the interpretation of its results (e.g., outputs such as the strength of evidence expressed as a likelihood ratio (LR) computed by an algorithm, or a class probability of a classifier). In the XAI literature these are often referred to as "global" and "local" explanations. The likelihood ratio framework is considered as a logical approach for the forensic interpretation of results of evidence evaluation, in this case in the context of a Bayesian decision scenario. But we can also think about the interpretation of the rationale of the methods themselves, i.e., *how do they work* internally.

Machine learning algorithms, when training has finished, are completely deterministic and thus reproducible and repeatable. This is good news when trying to characterize the performance and the behavior of a given algorithm in a given experimental set-up. Indeed, as it is described below, this repeatability and reproducibility makes the system testable, which is at the basis of a rigorous empirical validation process. However, in recent years the size and complexity of DNNs has steadily increased. As a consequence, creating explanations to provide insight into the rationale of the algorithm has become more challenging. We can, therefore, state that machine learning and pattern recognition algorithms in AI systems can be validated, but their rationale remains hard to explain.

As an example in the context of forensic science, it is common to use complex analytical chemistry methods for forensic examination. We can think about the use of laser ablation with inductively coupled plasma mass spectrometry (LA-ICP-MS) for glass comparative analysis. In court, it is extremely difficult to explain the process of extraction of information from glass with a LA-ICP-MS analytical device. As a result, explainability of the technical details of the method is not helpful in general, with lawyers generally lacking the competence to understand such an explanation. However, the results of the method are typically trusted and assumed to be reliable: courts generally accept forensic examination based on these chemical profiles as valuable evidence, as we think it should be. We believe that an important reason for this is the fact that the process of producing and comparing analytical results in forensic glass examination with LA-ICP-MS has been tested and validated according to international quality standards and accredited by a national accreditation body. This proves the method's reliability in court, more than any explanations that the forensic scientist could give to the judge or jury. In this case, explainability is welcome if it makes the whole process more understandable and transparent, but is not essential.

Explainability problems pile up if we consider a typical operational scenario, where the data have not been seen before, and may not have been well represented in the controlled dataset that was used to train the algorithms. It is very difficult to predict the behavior of a system trained on a controlled dataset in all situations. This is due to the complexity of the algorithm, but also to the diversity and variability of the possible scenarios. Even in controlled conditions, the complexity of the feature and parameter spaces of modern machine learning algorithms is huge. If the scenario in which the machine learning algorithm is going to operate is not very well characterized and targeted, the results might be unpredictable. The bad news is that, when this degradation of performance happens, it is very difficult to scrutinize the inner behavior of the algorithm in order to solve, or even explain, this lack of performance.

One recent problem that can help to understand this situation is the sensitivity of DNNs to adversarial noise. Lately, it was discovered that DNNs, although presenting extremely competitive performance in a wide variety of tasks, are also highly sensitive to so-called adversarial examples. Goodfellow et al. (2014) present a simple scenario in an image classification task, where a DNN is used to classify input images in classes (e.g., written digits, or type of objects in the image). The performance of the DNN was excellent in those tasks, where the conditions of the training and the testing datasets were similar. However, by adding so-called *adversarial noise*, i.e., a controlled degradation in the input image, the performance of the DNN dramatically dropped. The most intriguing fact about the experiment is that the adversarial noise could not be perceived by a human observer: the original and the noisy image looked exactly the same to the human eye. Also, this ability of adversarial noise to fool a DNN seems to manifest in different datasets and DNN architectures, revealing a vulnerability of DNNs for image classification in general. Of course, in forensic science it is difficult to manipulate data in order to add this kind of perturbation. However, the adversarial noise is a good example of potential unknown unknowns resulting in unexpected results from an AI-based system, illustrating our lack of understanding of such systems. The main message for forensic examiners is important: even if an algorithm such as a DNN has been tested in controlled conditions, it can fail in unexpected ways when dataset conditions are different.

Unfortunately, forensic conditions are always very variable, uncontrolled, and uncertain. This is a very challenging and unfavorable situation for any machine learning algorithm, but in particular it threatens the reliability of complex AI algorithms such as DNNs. Under such circumstances, the machine learning field has to continue to improve in order to generate solutions to a variety of scenarios where the operational data can be very variable and different to the training data. This includes strategies such as uncertainty incorporation to models, probabilistic calibration, domain adaptation, or transfer learning. All these approaches are aimed at making the system more robust to variation between datasets and data scarcity. Yet, safeguards at the operational level, such as a knowledgeable forensic examiner operating the method, and case-by-case validation are needed.

We believe that it is essential to realize that there is always a possibility that machine learning algorithms can fail. There is nothing in life that never fails. We will not generate trust by claiming that our system will never fail, because this is simply impossible. Failures like the voiceprint method (Gruber and Poza 1995), the Brandon Mayfield or Shirley McKie fingermark cases (Campbell 2011; the Inspector General 2006) are sad examples of what may happen if a forensic method is claimed to be error-free. Conversely, we have to explain and characterize *in which circumstances* a method fails, and *by how much*. We believe that trust can be achieved when we perform a transparent exercise where we test our systems and report the testing results. This is what we want to achieve with the validation of machine learning and AI in forensic science.

Once validation is conducted, the final decision is whether we will use that technology in a specific court case. This decision is now informed. Then, we will assume the risk of using the technology under the knowledge of the quantified performance, as it happens in many other aspects of our lives.

2.1.1 AI for Forensic Evaluation

We will restrict our discussion to the use of machine learning in forensic science, where DNNs are a typical example of a black-box complex algorithm. Moreover, among all machine learning algorithms, the rate of improvement is the largest in deep neural networks, showing outstanding performance in a constantly increasing number of tasks (LeCun et al. 2015). Machine learning has been increasingly proposed in forensic science both for investigation and evaluation. For instance, database searches of fingerprints and marks by means of automated fingerprint identification systems (AFIS) are particularly relevant. Also, biometric technology, in general, is prone to the use of score-based architectures that make its use for evaluative purposes easier (Meuwly 2022). This can be seen in successful approaches on the use of this technology for evaluative purposes in the field of forensic voice comparison, see (J. Gonzalez-Rodriguez et al. 2007; Morrison et al. 2020). The use of such AFIS systems has been also explored in the past for forensic evaluation (Egli et al. 2007; Haraksim et al. 2017; Leegwater et al. 2017; Ramos et al. 2017). More recently, machine learning methods have also been used in broader forensic fields, e.g., for chemical (Matzen et al. 2022; Ramos et al. 2021), digital (Bosma et al. 2020), and biological (Ypma et al. 2021) traces.

2.2 The Desirability for Explanation and the Necessity of Validation

In general, we would prefer methods for evidence evaluation to be explainable. The question is whether explainability is merely desirable, or a necessity (Quattrocolo et al. 2020). In our view, it is validation that is necessary, not explainability. We will argue our case using two example methods: forensic DNA analysis and infectious disease vaccines.

The largest and arguably most well-known subfield of forensic science is forensic DNA analysis. This is an established field of forensic science which is accepted in courts. In modern evaluation of forensic DNA traces, complex statistical models play a major role by supplying an LR for a pair of propositions. We distinguish three groups of users, which can and should understand these statistical models to different degrees:
1. those consuming the output of the models (lawyers and lay people)
2. those deciding on application of the models (forensic DNA scientists)
3. those designing the models (forensic statisticians)

The medical domain is arguably the best example of an applied scientific field studying a complex system (the human body) where high-impact decisions are continuously made. One important field in medical research is the development of vaccines, which prime the body's immune system to fight future infections. The recent COVID-19 pandemic showed how our ability to design, produce, and administer vaccines to a novel virus can save countless lives. But, as in the forensic DNA case, the working of these vaccines can and should be understood at different levels for different relevant groups:
1. those consuming the vaccines (lay people)
2. those deciding on application of the vaccines (e.g., medical doctors)
3. those designing the vaccines (scientists and engineers)

In both domains, the consumers (1) understand the general concepts behind the models/vaccines. A decision on consumption is taken mainly on the trust consumers have in (2). This trust derives from professional authority, e.g., from experience or certification of the person, and quality control systems such as peer review of methods. Additional explanations on how models/vaccines work can be given to increase transparency and improve the consumers' trust, although these are necessarily simplifications.

In both domains, those deciding on application (2) have a more thorough, but not complete, understanding of the models/vaccines. Medical doctors know when the vaccines can or cannot be used, how to apply them, and how to monitor potential side effects. Their main source of knowledge on how the models/vaccines work is those designing them (3). Trust for group 2 thus derives both from their (incomplete) understanding of the model/vaccine, and their trust in (3) and the quality control systems they put in place. In the same way, forensic DNA scientists know when the model can or cannot be used, how to apply it and how its output should be interpreted.

In the two domains, there is a strong difference in the level of understanding of those designing the model/vaccine. In forensic DNA analysis, the forensic statisticians that constructed the model fully understand it. They can explain what the various parameters of the model represent and why they were included, and argue under what assumptions the model is correct. The importance of explainability of models used in forensic evidence evaluation is often stressed (Bollé et al. 2020; Hall et al. 2021; L. Kelly et al. 2020; Phillips and Przybocki 2020), possibly with forensic DNA examination in mind.

In contrast, scientists and engineers do not fully understand (i.e., cannot fully predict) what effect various choices in the vaccine development process have on the final efficacy and side-effects. They understand enough that they can make informed decisions, and efficiently search the vast space of possible biochemical compounds for promising vaccine candidates. Ultimately, however, the decision if and to whom vaccines will be administered is based on large scale tests of their performance. These tests, named "clinical trials", involve administering the vaccine to tens of thousands of volunteers and measuring infection rates. In the forensic context, we call this validation.

We set these two domains side-by-side to stress the roles and usage of explanation and validation. Explanations are desirable as they increase trust in a system for all involved, may uncover errors in the model and allow designers of complex systems to improve their solutions more efficiently. The next section focuses on different methods that exist and that are being developed for explaining AI-based forensic evaluation systems. However, particularly for systems that are too complex to fully understand, validation is a necessity as it allows us to make informed decisions on if and when to apply them. We set out the various steps in the validation process in the final part of this chapter.

2.3 Explainability (and its Validity)

In this section we give a brief introduction to the developing field of explainable AI (XAI). We discuss reasons to pursue explanations, common techniques used and pitfalls. We do not aim to rigorously define what constitutes a (good) explanation, still a topic of academic debate, but merely assert the intuition that an explanation seeks to instill the subjective feeling of better understanding, while being scientifically substantiated. What form such an explanation should take, and to what extent it can be an approximation of the model's working, depends on the intended audience.

2.3.1 Reasons to Pursue Explanations

In the context of determining fitness for use in court, the main reason to pursue explanations is to garner trust (see Chapter 3 for additional reasons). AI-based evidence evaluation methods output a single number, e.g., an LR to express the strength of evidence. The extent to which the court will weigh this number in their decision depends on how much they trust the method. This trust can increase with explanations. For example, trust would increase if the method selects features that we expect to contain relevant information (e.g., the shape of the eyes in facial comparisons), but not features we know to be irrelevant (e.g., the color of the background). This reason for explanation is most relevant for consumers, e.g., lawyers and lay people.

Another related use of explanations is determining if a method can be applied in a certain case. For example, if we know that a facial comparison method mainly compares eye shapes, we know it should not be used for photos where eyes are covered. This use of explanations is most relevant for the forensic examiners that apply the methods in case work. A more extreme version is if we find a face recognition method that mainly considers items of clothing; it should never be applied in case work.

Lastly, understanding the functioning of a method is important in efforts to improve it. For example, discovering that a facial comparison method performs more poorly under low light conditions can help engineers to improve it. If a method is understood well, improving a method may be achieved by tweaking the rules and equations that form the method. For deep learning based methods such understanding is usually not feasible, and engineers improve the method by extending the training database with images reflecting the scenario of bright light conditions. This use of explanations is most relevant to those designing the methods.

2.3.2 Types of Explanations

A useful distinction is whether we want to explain a whole method ("general explanation") or an individual output of the method ("local explanation"). A good general explanation is more desirable but in practice is only feasible for relatively simple models. This is a good reason to use simple models in practice, provided their performance approaches that of more complex methods. A simple technique for global understanding often used in method development is error analysis. This technique comprises manually assessing examples of errors made by the method, to find patterns that provide an understanding of how the method works (and how it can be improved).

Explanations of a single output, e.g., a LR as expression of the strength of evidence, are very relevant in the evidence evaluation context. The types of methods commonly used for such local explanations are feature importance methods (Ribeiro et al. 2016). These methods explain the output by showing what features of the evidence were most relevant in reaching this output.

Examples of feature importance methods are shown for image (Figure 2.1) and tabular data (Figure 2.2). Figure 2.1 visualizes what part of an image was used by a deep neural network that predicts the manufacturer of the firearm used to fire a cartridge, using an image of the cartridge case bottom. The explanation consists of a heatmap that indicates what part of the image was most important for the method to reach its output (Selvaraju et al. 2017). For tabular data, Shapley values (Shapley 1951) can be visualized using the SHAP package (Lundberg and Lee 2017). This is done in Figure 2.2 for a random-forest based LR method evaluating the presence of vaginal mucosa from a measurement on mRNA (Ypma et al. 2021).

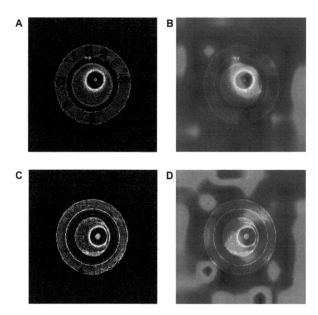

Figure 2.1 Explanations of firearm manufacturer prediction from cartridge case images using a deep neural network. (A, C) depict input images for the method: two cartridge cases fired with firearms of the same manufacturer and model. (B, D) depict explanations of the AI prediction, in the form of a heatmap: red "warmer" regions contributed more to the AI's prediction, blue "cool" regions less. We expect any prediction on firearm manufacturer to be guided by the marks left by the firearm used, not by the image background. The explanation in (B) nicely corresponds with this intuition, showing the network's attention was on the firing pin impression. Surprisingly, exactly the same network and exactly the same explanation method yielded a confusing explanation for a very similar cartridge case image, seemingly indicating the network found parts of the background of most importance (D). Whereas (B) increases our trust in the algorithm, (D) does not. Yet, (B) does not show that the algorithm is fit for purpose, (D) does not show it is not. Although there is merit in using explanations, the decision on whether the algorithm is fit for purpose should be taken based on validation.

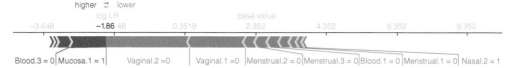

Figure 2.2 Example of a feature importance visualization, explaining a log LR of −1.86 predicted by an AI-based LR method. The LR method looks at presence/absence of 15 mRNA markers for specific body fluids, and returns an LR for H1: vaginal mucosa and/or menstrual secretion is present in the sample, H2: they are not present. For example, the bottom left text "Blood.3 = 0" indicates the third marker for blood is absent. The present sample contained nasal mucosa, leading to only markers for nasal (Nasal.1, Nasal.2) and mucosa (Mucosa.1) to be present. The visualization shows the contribution of features leading to an increase (red) or decrease (blue) of the LR. As expected, the absence of vaginal and menstrual markers leads to a low LR, whereas the mucosa marker (which is also expressed in vaginal mucosa) leads to a higher LR. This explanation increases our trust in the method, as the method uses the features in the way we would expect.

The features of the model are the presence/absence of certain biological markers specific to relevant body fluids. The Shapley value for a feature is interpretable as the amount that the log LR changed due to the measured value for that marker. The sum of the Shapley values is equal to the log LR for the measurement. These methods can be useful for illustrative purposes in court, although we should be aware they do not convey a full understanding of the method (cf. Figure 2.1).

2.3.3 Limitations of Explanations

The main caveat in using explanations is that they can lead to overconfidence, particularly so when they are unsubstantiated, which can be hard for a lay person to determine. If we feel we understand a method, we tend to overestimate the strength of its predictions (Koehler 1991). Historic examples in criminal law are the explanations given for phrenology and lie detectors. In XAI, explanations such as those given by feature importance methods are necessarily approximations – providing all the relevant features would no longer be understandable. This can lead to having too much or too little confidence in the actual method. The different users of a method should understand it well enough for their application, e.g., to decide whether a certain validation is appropriate or sufficient. Yet, we should be wary of relying too much on explanations, and be transparent to ourselves and others that many methods we cannot and need not understand fully.

2.4 Validation (and its Explanation)

This section discusses how empirical validation of new and non-standard forensic methods promotes their acceptance within the forensic community, while their accreditation enables the legal community to assess their value and performance when applied in forensic case work. Validation relies on protocols and experiments to decide on acceptance or rejection, using a set of chosen validation criteria (Meuwly et al. 2017). Together with accreditation, empirical validation can demonstrate compliance with international quality standards (Wilson-Wilde 2018). Note that this differs from theoretical validation, which pertains to proving or disproving mathematical formulae, and is out of the scope of this chapter.

2.4.1 Measure the Method's Performance

In forensic case work the ground truth about the questioned data of the case under examination is unknown for the competing pair of mutually exclusive alternative propositions, P1 and P2, tested. Therefore, before being used in practice, the performance of a method needs to be measured in conditions similar to those of the case. The aim of empirical validation is not to understand the functioning of a method, but to measure its performance in defined conditions.

Protocols, experiments, and validation data for which the ground truth is known define the validation conditions that allow for the demonstration of the acceptance or rejection on chosen validation criteria. This demonstration depends on the relevance of the validation protocol, and in particular of its performance characteristics (*what to measure?*), performance metrics (*how to measure?*) and validation criteria (*what performance is needed to regard a method as valid?*) (Ramos et al. 2020). The demonstration is also largely conditioned by the assumption of representativeness of the validation data: to be able to infer that the performance observed during the validation is comparable to the performance expected in case work, it is not only crucial to have a sufficiently big dataset, but also a sufficiently representative dataset (Vloed et al. 2020).

2.4.2 Approach in Four Steps

The approach proposed hereunder is freely inspired from the methodology for biometric performance testing described in (International Organization for Standardization 2021) and adapted to the empirical validation of forensic evaluation methods. It consists of four steps: technology, forensic application, operational, and case-by-case validation.

The developers of a method (forensic computer scientists, statisticians, and developers) are responsible for the technology and forensic application validation and the users of a method (forensic examiners) are responsible for the operational and case-by-case validation of a method. The phase of empirical validation is necessary to prevent that the method developed exhibits undesirable behavior when applied to forensic case work. The empirical validation needs to be performed on data that has not previously been seen during the phase of method development.

2.4.2.1 Technology Validation

The aim of technology validation is to select the most suitable AI technology to be integrated in an AI-based forensic evaluation method, for example a face or speaker recognition biometric algorithm. In a forensic evaluation method, fundamental errors encompass data capture and extraction errors (failure-to-acquire), metadata transcription and labeling errors (failure-to-label), and algorithmic comparison errors (false negative and false positive). These fundamental errors combine to form forensic evaluation system errors. How these evaluation errors combine depends upon the number of comparisons made possible with the available validation data (International Organization for Standardization 2021).

The technology validation aims to demonstrate whether the algorithm selected for the forensic evaluation method to be developed is fit for its intended use. It consists of testing algorithms using a validation dataset comparable to the data encountered in the applications for which the method is developed. For example, the "Rule of 30" has been proposed by Doddington (Doddington et al. 2000) and has been adopted in ISO 19795–1 (International Organization for Standardization 2021) for helping to determine the size of the dataset: to be 90% confident that the true error rate is within ±30% of the observed error rate, there must be at least 30 errors. This rule comes directly from the binomial distribution assuming independent trials, and may be applied by considering the performance expectations for the validation. Applying the "Rule of 30" would necessitate 3000 positive tests (P1 is true) and 30 000 negative tests (P2 is true), obtained from a set of 3000 positive data and 30 000 negative independent data. The alternative is to compromise on independence by re-using smaller sets, and to be prepared for a loss of statistical significance (Mansfield and Wayman 2002).

The technology validation focuses on the ability of the algorithms to separate between the competing propositions, illustrating their discriminating power. These performance characteristics can be assessed by performance metrics such as the false positive and false negative rates (respectively, FPR and FNR), the equal error rate (EER), and represented graphically by the detection error trade-off (DET) or the receiver operating characteristic (ROC) curve (cf. Figure 2.3).

For example, the ongoing NIST-face verification vendors tests (FVRT) makes extensive use of these metrics and graphical representation to assess and compare state-of-the-art commercial and academic face recognition algorithms ("Face Recognition Vendor Test (FRVT)" n.d.; Grother et al. 2018). When available, the developers of a forensic method can rely on the results of such tests to exclude unsuitable algorithms and select algorithms possibly suited for a defined forensic application.

2.4.2.2 Forensic Application Validation

The aim of forensic application validation is to demonstrate the validity and applicability of AI-based systems designed for applications such as forensic identity verification, identification, intelligence, investigation, and evaluation (Meuwly and Veldhuis 2012). The forensic application validation consists of testing a forensic system, using a validation dataset comparable to the data of forensic cases for which the system is developed. In the field of forensic evaluation, AI-based systems have been developed to compute LRs for source level inference,

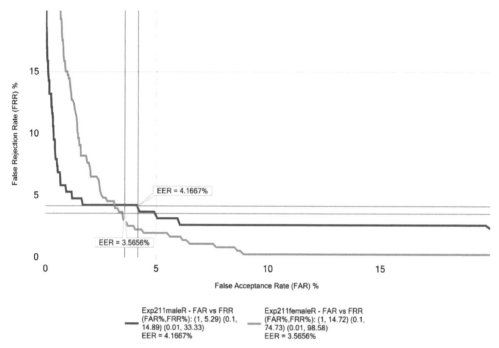

Figure 2.3 Example of comparison of the performance of the software Vocalise 2019 (version 2.7.0.1650) for a dataset of female (pink) and male speakers (blue) (NFI-FRITS Database), using a ROC curve to to visualize the method's false positive and false negative tradeoff. Courtesy of David van der Vloed, Netherlands Forensic Institute.

e.g., speaker recognition (J. Gonzalez-Rodriguez et al. 2007; Kelly et al. 2019; Morrison et al. 2020), face recognition (Jacquet and Champod 2020), fingermark (Stoney et al. 2020), firearms (Riva et al. 2020), or biometric systems (Gonzalez-Rodriguez et al. 2005). Forensic evaluation systems dedicated to the computation of LRs for activity level inference have not yet been developed.

The forensic application validation combines the measurement of primary and secondary performance characteristics to determine the ability of AI-based forensic evaluation systems to compute the best performing LRs. The accuracy, discrimination, and calibration are primary performance characteristics. They relate directly to performance metrics and focus on desired properties of the forensic evaluation systems. The cost log likelihood ratio (C_{llr}) as well as its discrimination (C_{llr}^{min}) and calibration (C_{llr}^{cal}) components (Brümmer and du Preez 2006) and the empirical cost entropy (ECE) as well as its discrimination (ECE^{min}) and calibration (ECE^{cal}) components (Ramos et al. 2013) are metrics designed and applied to measure the accuracy, discrimination, and calibration of forensic evaluation systems, respectively. These primary performance characteristics can be represented graphically by the empirical calibration graph (calibration), the receiver operating characteristics (ROC), and detection error trade-off (DET) curves (discrimination) and the Tippett plot (accuracy) (Meuwly et al. 2017).

The robustness, monotonicity, and generalization are secondary performance characteristics. They describe how the primary performance characteristics behave in various conditions encountered in forensic case work, e.g., when the case work and comparison data are sparse, when their quality differs, or when the conditions of their collection do not correspond to case work conditions (mismatch between the trace material and the control data) (Ramos et al. 2020). The robustness measures the stability of the LRs produced by a forensic evaluation system when the data vary. The monotonicity measures its ability to produce bigger or smaller LRs (in case Proposition P1 or P2 is true) when the quality/quantity of data increases monotonically. The generalization measures the stability of the LRs produced by a system for previously unseen data. The secondary performance characteristics relate to a single primary performance metric or a single graphical representation, e.g., the robustness of the accuracy, the monotonicity of the discrimination, or the generalization of the calibration. As shown by Jacquet et al. (Jacquet and Champod 2020) for face recognition, algorithms selected during the technology validation can exhibit very different performances in a defined forensic application. This result indicates the necessity of the forensic application validation for every new forensic automatic method developed.

2.4.2.3 Operational Validation

The aim of operational validation is to demonstrate the validity of the integration of an AI-based forensic evaluation system in a forensic evaluation case workflow and to demonstrate that forensic examiners are competently using the system. A system can be considered as integrated in the case workflow and ready to be used when the LR computation process and the combination of its results with the results of other automated or human-based interpretation methods has been described and assessed.

Forensic examiners can be considered as competent when they understand the functioning, performance, and limits of the system (knowledge), when they are able to run the system in case work conditions (skill), and when they are able to testify in court about the results of the system and about its validation (behavior). Competence needs to be acquired through a theoretical and practical education program and assessed and monitored on a regular basis.

The developments of early forensic evaluation methods can be considered as a craftsmanship process. When the forensic scientists are engaged in the development of each step: the method, its validation, and its use in case work, the degree of competence of the examiner is already very high at the moment of implementation. The necessity for operational validation is minimal. With the industrialization of the process, the tasks have been divided between the developers and the users of the method. In this situation, the degree of competence of the examiner is very low at the moment of implementation of the method in case work. In such circumstances, the operational validation is essential to ensure the competence of the examiners for this method.

2.4.2.4 Case-by-case Validation

The aim of case-by-case validation is to refine the generic forensic application validation of an AI-based system to a case-specific situation. The approach followed for case-by-case validation is similar to the one described above for forensic application, but with focus on the specific conditions of the forensic case at hand. The forensic application validation is based on the assumption that the validation dataset chosen is comparable to the data of forensic cases for which the system is developed.

The case-by-case validation allows the performance and calibration of the system to be assessed using a dataset closer and more representative of the specific case data, for example the angle, the pose, and the illumination of a face picture, or the recording length, the background noise, or the codec of a speech audio recording. As AI-based methods are statistical by nature, the case-by-case validation also allows the robustness of the system to data scarcity to be studied, a recurring situation in forensic evaluation case work. The aim remains to reduce the risk of error of the method due to an unknown unknown. This tailor-made and last step of the validation is performed by the forensic examiner, as part of the case work process prior to the examination of the trace material.

Note that the case-by-case validation is feasible for automatic forensic evidence evaluation, but not for many other AI applications, e.g., recognizing traffic signs by autonomous vehicles or tagging photos on a personal cell phone. When case-by-case validation is not possible, only generic validation remains, and explainability may well go from "desirable" to "necessary". The medical field is an example outside forensic science where case-by-case validation is feasible, and here arguments very similar to our own are being made in the discussion on explainability (Durán and Jongsma 2021; Ghassemi et al. 2021; McCoy et al. 2022).

2.4.3 Accountability

In forensic science quality is no longer considered as an internal matter for a forensic provider only, but also as an external matter of concern for the requester. Quality assurance (QA) is a mechanism developed and implemented to meet and maintain minimum quality and integrity standards regarding the forensic services and products offered. QA establishes a sense of responsibility, transparency, and accountability at the forensic provider.

Accreditation is an external form of QA. Forensic services and products are evaluated by an external accreditation body that determines the compliance to the applicable standards. Accreditation is both a status and a process. The accreditation status is the provision of a public recognition by the accreditation body that a forensic provider meets the applicable standards. The forensic provider acquires the accreditation status in undergoing a process of external review to demonstrate compliance to the standards and the constant will to improve the quality of its service and products. This includes the accreditation of new and non-standard methods, such as AI-based methods for forensic evaluation. The validation protocols describing the experiments (Ramos et al. 2020), the validation report presenting the technology, forensic application and operational validation results (Meuwly et al. 2017), and the competence of the forensic examiners performing the method are subject to review and acceptance. The documentation (protocol and report) of the case-by-case validation is part of the case report, for example as an annex to the main case work report.

The empirical validation and accreditation of AI-based forensic evaluation methods is a necessary step before their use in case work. This step does not dispense with the preliminary discussion of ethical issues relating to the data used, the purpose of the method, and the proper conduct of its users.

2.5 Conclusion

AI-based methods contribute to a more and more sophisticated automation of professional activities, including forensic evidence evaluation. The contribution of AI methods to forensic evaluation grows at a fast pace as strategies for collecting, digitizing, and structuring data are put in place across forensic fields. Fields we expect to benefit from AI methods first are forensic biometry, for the individualization of human beings, and in fields focusing on the individualization of objects such as firearms and ammunition, toolmarks, or shoemarks.

In this chapter we provide arguments as to why we consider that validation is a necessary stage towards the acceptance of AI-based forensic evaluation, while explainability, although important, remains merely desirable. Where full understanding is beyond our reach, as is the case for most complex AI systems, trust should come from the demonstration of sufficient performance in the circumstances of the forensic case at hand. We have further laid out the four points of view required for this technological, applicative, operational, and case-by-case validation. It is fundamental that the end users of forensic evaluations, the courts, are able to understand how science validates algorithms in order to determine the extent to which the results can be trusted and whether the method is deemed fit for the intended use.

References

Bollé, T., Casey, E., and Jacquet, M. (2020). The role of evaluations in reaching decisions using automated systems supporting forensic analysis. *Forensic Science International: Digital Investigation* 34 (September): 301016.

Bosma, W., Dalm, S., Erwin, V.E. et al. (2020). Establishing phone-pair co-usage by comparing mobility patterns. *Science & Justice: Journal of the Forensic Science Society* 60 (2): 180–190.

Brümmer, N. and du Preez, J. (2006). Application-independent evaluation of speaker detection. *Computer Speech & Language* 20 (2): 230–275.

Campbell, A. (2011). The fingerprint inquiry report. *Edinburgh, Scotland: APS Group Scotland* 790.

Doddington, G.R., Przybocki, M.A., Martin, A.F., and Reynolds, D.A. (2000). The NIST speaker recognition evaluation–overview, methodology, systems, results, perspective. *Speech Communication* 31 (2–3): 225–254.

Doshi-Velez, F. and Kim, B. (2017). Towards a rigorous science of interpretable machine learning. *arXiv [stat.ML]*. arXiv. http://arxiv.org/abs/1702.08608 accessed 17 April 2023.

Durán, J.M. and Jongsma, K.R. (2021). Who is afraid of black box algorithms? On the epistemological and ethical basis of trust in medical AI. *Journal of Medical Ethics* March. https://doi.org/10.1136/medethics-2020-106820.

Egli, N.M., Champod, C., and Margot, P. (2007). Evidence evaluation in fingerprint comparison and automated fingerprint identification systems—modelling within finger variability. *Forensic Science International* 167 (2): 189–195.

Evett, I.W., Jackson, G., and Lambert, J.A. (2000). More on the hierarchy of propositions: exploring the distinction between explanations and propositions. *Science & Justice: Journal of the Forensic Science Society* 40 (1): 3–10.

Face Recognition Vendor Test (FRVT) (n.d.). NIST. https://www.nist.gov/programs-projects/face-recognition-vendor-test-frvt (accessed 11 January 2022).

Ghassemi, M., Oakden-Rayner, L., and Beam, A.L. (2021). The false hope of current approaches to explainable artificial intelligence in health care. *The Lancet. Digital Health* 3 (11): e745–50.

Gonzalez-Rodriguez, J., Rose, P., Ramos, D. et al. (2007). Emulating DNA: rigorous quantification of evidential weight in transparent and testable forensic speaker recognition. *IEEE Transactions on Audio, Speech, and Language Processing* 15 (7): 2104–2115.

Gonzalez-Rodriguez, J., Fierrez-Aguilar, J., Ramos-Castro, D., and Ortega-Garcia, J. (2005). Bayesian analysis of fingerprint, face and signature evidences with automatic biometric systems. *Forensic Science International* 155 (2–3): 126–140.

Goodfellow, I.J., Shlens, J., and Szegedy, C. (2014). Explaining and harnessing adversarial examples. *arXiv [stat.ML]*. arXiv. http://arxiv.org/abs/1412.6572 (accessed 28 March 2023).

Grother, P., Ngan, M., and Hanaoka, K. (2018). Ongoing face recognition vendor test (FRVT) part 2. https://doi.org/10.6028/nist.ir.8238 (accessed 26 December 2021).

Gruber, J.S. and Poza, F.T. (1995). *Voicegram Identification Evidence*. Lawyers Cooperative Pub.

Guidotti, R., Monreale, A., Ruggieri, S. et al. (2018). A survey of methods for explaining black box models. *ACM Computing Surveys* 93, 51 (5): 1–42.

Hall, S.W., Sakzad, A., and Choo, K.-K.R. (2021). Explainable artificial intelligence for digital forensics. *WIREs Forensic Science* June. https://doi.org/10.1002/wfs2.1434.

Haraksim, R., Ramos, D., and Meuwly, D. (2017). Validation of likelihood ratio methods for forensic evidence evaluation handling multimodal score distributions. *IET Biometrics* 6 (2): 61–69.

International Organization for Standardization (2021). Information technology — biometric performance testing and reporting — part 1: principles and framework. 19795-1. https://www.iso.org/standard/73515.html (accessed 22 December 2021).

Jackson, G.C., Aitken, G.G., and Roberts, P. (2013). Case assessment and interpretation of expert evidence: guidance for judges, lawyers, forensic scientists and expert witnesses. In: *Royal Statistical Society*.

Jacquet, M. and Champod, C. (2020). Automated face recognition in forensic science: review and perspectives. *Forensic Science International* 307 (February): 110124.

Phillips, P.J. and Przybocki, M. (2020). Four principles of explainable AI as applied to biometrics and facial forensic algorithms. *arXiv [cs.CV]*. arXiv. http://arxiv.org/abs/2002.01014 (accessed 28 March 2023).

Kelly, F., Alexander, A., Forth, O., and Vloed, D.V.D. (2019). From I-vectors to X-vectors—a generational change in speaker recognition illustrated on the NFI-FRIDA database. In: Proc. 25th Int. Assoc. Forensic Phonetics Acoust. (IAFPA), 1–28.

Kelly, L., Sachan, S., Lei, N. et al. (2020). Explainable artificial intelligence for digital forensics: opportunities, challenges and a drug testing case study. *Digital Forensic Science*. https://doi.org/10.5772/intechopen.93310.

Koehler, D.J. (1991). Explanation, imagination, and confidence in judgment. *Psychological Bulletin* 110 (3): 499–519.

LeCun, Y., Bengio, Y., and Hinton, G. (2015). Deep learning. *Nature* 521 (7553): 436–444.

Leegwater, A.J., Meuwly, D., Sjerps, M. et al. (2017). Performance study of a score-based likelihood ratio system for forensic fingermark comparison. *Journal of Forensic Sciences* 62 (3): 626–640.

Lundberg, S.M. and Lee, S.-I. 2017. A unified approach to interpreting model predictions. In: Proceedings of the 31st International Conference on Neural Information Processing Systems, 4768–4777.

Mansfield, A.J. and Wayman, J.L. (2002). Best practices in testing and reporting performance of biometric devices. http://www.kisa.or.kr/uploadfile/as-is/060405-BestPractices_v2_1-_-1153808236433.pdf.

Matzen, T., Kukurin, C., Judith, V.D.W. et al. (2022). Objectifying evidence evaluation for gunshot residue comparisons using machine learning on criminal case data. *Forensic Science International* 335 (June): 111293.

McCoy, L.G., Connor, T.A., Brenna, S.S. et al. (2022). Believing in black boxes: machine learning for healthcare does not need explainability to be evidence-based. *Journal of Clinical Epidemiology* 142 (February): 252–257.

Meuwly, D. (2022). Reconnaissance de Locuteurs En Sciences Forensiques: L'apport D'une Approche Automatique. http://www.unil.ch/esc/files/live/sites/esc/files/shared/These.Meuwly.pdf.

Meuwly, D., Ramos, D., and Haraksim, R. (2017). A guideline for the validation of likelihood ratio methods used for forensic evidence evaluation. *Forensic Science International* 276 (July): 142–153.

Meuwly, D. and Veldhuis, R. (2012). Forensic biometrics: from two communities to one discipline." In: 2012 BIOSIG - Proceedings of the International Conference of Biometrics Special Interest Group (BIOSIG), 1–12.

Molnar, C. (2020). *Interpretable Machine Learning*. Lulu.com.

Morrison, G.S., Enzinger, E., Ramos, D. et al. (2020). Statistical models in forensic voice comparison. In: *Handbook of Forensic Statistics* (ed. D.L. Banks, K. Kafadar, D.H. Kaye, and M. Tackett), 451–497. CRC Press.

Office of the Inspector General (2006). A review of the FBI's handling of the brandon mayfield case. US Department of Justice, Washington, DC.

Quattrocolo, S., Anglano, C., Canonico, M., and Guazzone, M. (2020). Technical solutions for legal challenges: equality of arms in criminal proceedings. *Global Jurist* 20 (1). https://doi.org/10.1515/gj-2019-0058.

Ramos, D., Gonzalez-Rodriguez, J., Zadora, G., and Aitken, C. (2013). Information-theoretical assessment of the performance of likelihood ratio computation methods. *Journal of Forensic Sciences*. https://doi.org/10.1111/1556-4029.12233.

Ramos, D., Krish, R.P., Fierrez, J., and Meuwly, D. (2017). From biometric scores to forensic likelihood ratios. In: *Handbook of Biometrics for Forensic Science* (ed. M. Tistarelli and C. Champod), 305–327. Cham: Springer International Publishing.

Ramos, D., Maroñas, J., and Almirall, J. (2021). Improving calibration of forensic glass comparisons by considering uncertainty in feature-based elemental data. *Chemometrics and Intelligent Laboratory Systems* 217 (October): 104399.

Ramos, D., Meuwly, D., Haraksim, R., and Berger, C.E.H. (2020). Validation of forensic automatic likelihood ratio methods. In: *Handbook of Forensic Statistics*, (D.L. Banks, K. Kafadar, D.H. Kaye, and M. Tackett)143–162. Chapman and Hall/CRC.

Ribeiro, M.T., Singh, S., and Guestrin, C. (2016). Why should I trust you? In: *Proceedings of the 22nd ACM SIGKDD International Conference on Knowledge Discovery and Data Mining*. New York, NY, USA: ACM. https://doi.org/10.1145/2939672.2939778.

Riva, F., Mattijssen, E.J., Hermsen, R. et al. (2020). Comparison and interpretation of impressed marks left by a firearm on cartridge cases–towards an operational implementation of a likelihood ratio based technique. *Forensic Science International* 313: 110363.

Selvaraju, R.R., Cogswell, M., Das, A. et al. (2017). Grad-cam: visual explanations from deep networks via gradient-based localization. In: *Proceedings of the IEEE International Conference on Computer Vision*, 618–626.

Shapley, L.S. (1951). *Notes on the N-Person Game – II: The Value of an N-Person Game*. RAND Corporation.

Stoney, D.A., Marco, D.D., Champod, C. et al. (2020). Occurrence and associative value of non-identifiable fingermarks. *Forensic Science International* 309 (April): 110219.

Vloed, D.V.D., Kelly, F., and Alexander, A. (2020). Exploring the effects of device variability on forensic speaker comparison using VOCALISE and NFI-FRIDA, a forensically realistic database. In: *Proceedings of the Odyssey Speaker and Lang. Recogn. Workshop*, 402–407.

Wilson-Wilde, L. (2018). The international development of forensic science standards - a review. *Forensic Science International* 288 (July): 1–9.

Ypma, R.J.F., Maaskant-van Wijk, P.A., Gill, R. et al. (2021). Calculating LRs for presence of body fluids from mRNA assay data in mixtures. *Forensic Science International. Genetics* 52 (May): 102455.

CHAPTER 3

Machine Learning for Evidence in Criminal Proceedings: Techno-legal Challenges for Reliability Assurance

Radina Stoykova, Jeanne Mifsud Bonnici, and Katrin Franke
Norwegian University of Science and Technology (NTNU), Gjøvik, Norway

3.1 Introduction: AI in the Intersection of Criminal Procedure and Forensics

This chapter identifies one overarching problem which can significantly impact the successful adoption of artificial intelligence (AI) in general, and machine learning in particular for law enforcement purposes – namely the existing techno-logical, methodological, and legal fragmentation in digital investigations and forensics. This fragmentation problem and the specifics of the new AI technology can lead to notable negative effects on the criminal justice system and distrust in the scientific validity of such methods.

3.1.1 Technical Fragmentation in Digital Investigations

The first major challenges for criminal justice, law enforcement, and forensics are the data volumes and complexities in the investigation stage of the proceedings. Ferguson stated that a normal legal case contains a maximum 100 000 documents, while since 2013 lawyers and police have more often encountered "ridiculously" large cases containing more than 100 million files (Ferguson J. 2016). Data complexities and technical fragmentation lead to situations where the examination of a single user's application requires expertise in multiple domains from file systems to clouds and video forensics. Further, cybercrime is on the rise (Europol 2021), more than 50% of the online content is encrypted,[1] while the potential use of AI by criminals is a serious threat.[2]

---

[1] See statistics by security researcher Scott Helme, "Alexa Top 1 Million Analysis – August 2018" (*Scott Helme*, 24 August 2018). https://scotthelme.co.uk/alexa-top-1-million-analysis-august-2018 accessed 03.12.2022.

[2] See Keynote speech at IFSEC 2018 by Silvino Schlickmann Jr, Assistant-Director Research & Innovation in Interpol. Reported at: Wesley Charnock, "Artificial intelligence: the new cybercrime threat" (*IFSEC Global*, 21 June 2018). https://www.ifsecglobal.com/ifsec/artificial-intelligence-threat accessed 02.12.2022.

This causes a significant disruption to the traditional model of criminal justice (Ashworth and Zedner 2008; Rothschild-Elyassi et al. 2019). Prosecutors are more often unable to deal with all the data collected for evidence which leads to investigations collapsing. For example, it was reported that the US Department of justice stores more than 4 petabytes of information and this is projected to double again by next year (Penn 2022). Prosecutors are criticized by judges for their "disturbing inability" to handle the data or to provide understandable reviews to the defence and judges which causes the trials to collapse. Similarly, in Europe due to limited resources and concerns about efficiency, the investigation process is shortened and minor cases are more often dismissed (Boyne 2016). There is a rise in plea bargaining, negotiated agreements, active judicial case management, and acceptance of pre-trial witness statements (Field 2009). Ultimately, the investigative stage of criminal proceedings becomes more proactive, science-driven, and outcome-determinative (Park et al. 2018; Zawoad and Hasan 2015).

US government officials advocate for a radical reduction of data collection and targeted evidence gathering. However, speedy reviews and selective data collection threaten the quality of digital evidence, the very essence of digital forensics standards, which can cause complete abandonment of scientific data examination in favour of push-button-forensics, and ultimately denial of justice. Rather, more automation and intelligent systems for triage and evidence analysis are needed to support LEA work in a technologically fragmented environment complemented by a suitable reliability validation process.

3.1.2 Legal and Methodological Fragmentation in Digital Investigations

In the absence of a comprehensive legal framework for law enforcement in Europe (Kusak 2017; Mifsud Bonnici, J. P., Tudorica, M. & Cannataci, J. A. 2018; Vermeulen et al. 2010) based on fair trial and criminal justice principles, the legislative regime becomes more fragmented. LEA obligations are scattered across data protection regimes, E-evidence exchange proposals, anti-encryption laws, AI systems regulation in addition to national criminal justice procedures and increasingly unclear status of foreign evidence and cross-jurisdictional cooperation with private or public entities.

In addition, the domain of digital forensics (DF) remains methodologically fragmented and is still shaped by technical capabilities and best practices rather than an international legislative framework. Practitioners who apply their specialities to legal problems, often misrepresent the law (Nijboer and Sprangers 2000), while lawyers and judges tend to trust the science (Edmond and Martire 2016; Edmond and Roberts 2011). This exposes the lack of standards on how to evaluate the reliability and integrity of digital evidence in legal settings (Katilu et al. 2015; Mason and Seng 2017, para. para 6.210 and 6.219; Van Buskirk and Liu 2006). Authors argue that both judges and law enforcement agencies readily accept novel forensics methods and systematically overestimate the weight of expert evidence (Craig Callen 2015; Edmond 2016; Risinger 2018; Smith and Kenneally 2008). In most jurisdictions, judges continue to be provided with no real guidance on how they should determine evidential reliability (Edmond 2012; Horsman 2018a) which also leads to unequal treatment of suspects and defendants (Gross and Mnookin 2003; Risinger 2000).

AI methods, big data analytics, and automated tools to deal with the volumes and complexities of data, require new forensic science standards to ensure the reliability of digital evidence and process quality which currently is underdeveloped. The literature for the past 15 years shows an ongoing reliability and reproducibility crisis in digital forensics (Jakobs and Sprangers 2000; National Research Council 2009; PCAST 2016). Digital forensics specialists do not agree on standard procedures and methods. This leads to proliferation of standards (Kohn et al. 2013; Montasari et al. 2019) or lack of them (Casey 2019; Horsman 2018b; Hughes and Karabiyik 2020; Jones and Vidalis 2019), premature use of novel science and technology, lack of accountability or formal validation in digital forensics (Tully et al. 2020). Exponential backlogs and resource constraints in digital investigations (Montasari and Hill 2019; Scanlon 2016) warn that any effort towards standardization, field governance, entry requirements, and transparency (Doyle 2019; Horsman 2019, 2018a; Vincze 2016), cannot be at the expense of efficiency. As data science and AI are more necessary for investigations, push-button forensics and fast data reviews endangers the very basis of forensic science.

AI techniques can assist law enforcement to overcome data volumes and complexity hurdles. However, the identified legal, technical, and methodological fragmentation in digital forensics for law enforcement is alarming. The premature deployment of AI systems in such a problematic domain might cause significant long-lasting negative effects to the criminal justice system and legal uncertainty as well as distrust in the scientific validity of such methods. Further, in contrast to traditional DF tools, AI-based investigative methods have some specifics which impact their reliability validation and might obstruct effective cross-examination of evidence found using AI.

3.1.3 Specifics of ML-based Investigative Approach

ISO defines machine learning as the process of optimizing model parameters through computational techniques, such that the model's behaviour reflects the data or experience. (ISO/IEC 23053, 2022) ML is a data-driven method as it requires data samples to learn to fulfil a task.

There is a fundamental difference between structural and data driven (statistical) methods for pattern recognition. Structural methods like rule-based classifiers can be very accurate in identifying specific characteristics in datasets if the relevant data features are known and there are not too many of them. For example, if a forensic examiner has clear indicators of compromize, a rule-based classifier can efficiently discover it. However, structural approaches perform poorly when there is too much data and too many features to examine. They also present a problem when the thresholds are too narrow, as slight variation of the traces are aften being overlooked. Therefore, data driven (statistical) methods are preferable when dealing with large investigative corpus, but present challenges of their own.

Firstly, identifying for which investigative tasks ML can be useful, is of vital importance for their successful implementation in the investigative process. ML is best applied to learn characteristics for generalization. For example, ML in marketing is used to find trends or similarities to recommend other products (people who bought this book also bought the following book). Similarly, when applied in criminal investigations one needs to make sure that the ML approach is only applied to generalization tasks. However, too often ML is falsely used to identify outliers, e.g., high-profile criminals, which might lead to false identification of suspects (cross-ref. Chapter Jan Wilhelm). For example, a bank monitoring system can flag suspicious transactions, but without further investigation by experts does not provide proof of fraud.

Secondly, identifying patterns of criminal activity requires that the nature of imbalanced datasets where 95%+ of the data is regular activity of users, while only small percentage is related to anomalous (criminal) patterns in data, is taken into account. Data relevant for investigations is not easily mapped or studied, while also in constant evolution – data features relevant today might not be relevant tomorrow. Consequently, it is not always possible to predict the nature (characteristics) of criminal behaviour at the time of model training. In addition, training datasets often contain only a few training samples of criminal patterns at the time of system design. Ergo, in order to use ML approaches effi-ciently, investigators must study both normal user activity and anomalous (sus-picious) use of systems.

Thirdly, ML methods require a quality criterium regarding how well a new learned model fulfils the learning task. In practice, most of the research in ML for digital forensics is application-based where in-depth study of underlying ML con-cepts or techniques, as well as their limitations, are often replaced with trial-and-error studies. Arguably legal and scientific-regulation efforts are currently focused on technology quality assurance, while how the new ML methods will be integrated in the established forensic science methodology and fair trial investigation standards is often disregarded. Such models require validation procedures to be implemented within the model ensuring continuous testing and optimization, rather than a stand-alone validation.

Finally, there are long-standing issues in traditional forensic sciences (Findley 2011; Nijboer and Sprangers 2000; Saks and Faigman 2008; Wigan and Clarke 2013) which are inherited in data-driven approaches for evidence discovery and have an aggravated impact on human rights. Firstly, data-driven approaches disclose unique characteristics of the behaviour of individuals, confidential, and sensitive data about them which infringes upon the individual's rights. For example, as both normal user activity and criminal patterns in data needs to be studied human rights concerns emerge for larger groups of people rather than only for those linked to a crime. Privacy and fair trial issues emerge in larger scale. For instance, an innocent suspect might be wrongly convicted based on an exaggerated or erroneous forensic report. The danger of such injustice is significantly amplified if a ML model presents flawed evidence analysis, as, for the period in which the error persists, all examined cases with the model might be compromized. Second, ML techniques often look at low level data structures and can disclose and utilize security vulnerabilities in existing software which might infringe upon intellectual properties, trade secrets, and security of systems in general. Finally, there is a tendency for advanced digital forensics methods and techniques to be kept secret for their reuse and to avoid anti-forensics, however, this reduces the possibility for such techniques to be scrutinized in the scientific community and in open court.

> **GAP 1** Criminal evidence systems are not adapted to regulate ML-based evidence discovery not because of a lack of evidence principles and rules, but rather due to the difficulty of transcribing and implementing them in a domain which presents a fundamentally different approach to investigations all together. As law more heavily regulates the design and use of technology, it becomes increasingly difficult for prosecutors and lawyers to understand what the technical implementations corresponding to the formulated legal principles are. This, consequently, deepens the technological and methodological fragmentation in digital investigations.

3.1.4 Scope and Definitions

Ultimately this chapter asks the question: to what extent does the current legislative framework for AI in law enforcement achieve fair trial objectives and do we have sufficient practical solutions and clear standards to ensure reliable validation of AI- evidence?

The focus is not on a concrete AI application for law enforcement and forensics, but on formal criteria for legal compliance and AI reliability validation during investigations. Thus, this work aims to pose the questions: under which conditions can an algorithm be used for forensic purposes, are AI methods reproducible and how can AI-evidence reliability be assessed? It aims to start an open dialog for validation of AI techniques for investigative and pre-trial proceedings in order to bring awareness among different stakeholders, avoid miscarriages of justice due to the use of technology, and prevent an "AI winter in forensics". The provided comparison of legal provisions, technical specifications, and best practices is an initial evaluation of the important elements of a techno-legal policy for AI deployment in law enforcement work as well as a gap analysis of missing solutions.

This chapter uses the term AI systems for law enforcement in the narrow sense of machine learning. Machine learning is selected as an AI domain, which develops rapidly and is broadly tested or adopted for reducing volumes and complexities in law enforcement work. Therefore, it requires more urgent elaboration of legislative challenges. Nevertheless, the legal framework does not distinguish different regimes for AI methods and the findings are applicable to other AI domains by analogy. In contrast to digital forensics which deal only with data born digital, such AI methods can also be applied to physical evidence (like DNA, fingerprint) that has been digitalized. AI methods for digital investigations and evidence should be distinguished also from *AI forensics* which refers to forensic examination of compromized AI systems (Baggili and Behzadan 2019).

Distinction must be made between AI applied in forensic science and applied in criminology. Forensic science is defined as "application of scientific methods to establish factual answers to legal problems" (Årnes 2018, p. 2). Criminology is a social science dealing with *"nature, extent, causes, control, and prevention of the criminal behaviour of both the individual and society"*.[3] Although the use of AI in criminology for crime prediction and crime prevention is out of the scope of this chapter, the findings on what constitutes a scientifically proven method in the digital evidence domain is generalizable to all AI methods.

This chapter is structured as follows: in Section 3.1 the introduction identified the emerging challenges in digital investigations and their regulations, AI forensics specifics, as well as the scope of the chapter. Section 3.2 then identifies the major building blocks of the legislative framework for AI evidence, namely the fair trial principle, the AIA proposal, and the data protection regime, which are examined in their general requirements for AI system design. Section 3.3 introduces the techno-legal challenges in each process of a ML pipeline. Technical challenges and legislative shortcoming are discussed as well as relevant legal compliance and reliability validation techniques. Section 3.4 provides an overview of the identified techno-legal gaps and recommendations for further research.

---

[3] See also Difference between Forensic Science and Criminology (Difference Between | Descriptive Analysis and Comparisons, 2022). http://www.differencebetween.info/difference-between-forensic-science-and-criminology accessed 02.12.2022.

3.2 Legal Framework

New AI legislation has been introduced in the USA,[4] the UK,[5] Canada,[6] Australia (Cox et al. 2022), and China where the AI regulation is already in force.[7] The focus here is only on the European Union (EU) approach. However, the development of AI regulation globally shows a fundamental shift in technology development as for the first time a piece of technology (AI models) has been subject to regulative compliance from its development throughout its entire life cycle, and governance is not only subject to reliability validation from an engineering point of view, but it requires techno-legal assessment of every stage of the processing.

In order to ensure legal compliance and technology robustness in the development of AI systems for forensics, LEAs have to gain the know-how to design accountable information processes where the processing steps in the AI pipeline are conducted according to techno-legal policies. Before examining the techno-legal gaps in the machine learning pipeline, this section provides a brief overview of the legislative framework in the EU. The design and application of AI for law enforcement purposes is subject mainly to the following legislative acts:

- The right to a fair trial principle of criminal procedure
- The draft Artificial Intelligence Act (AIA[8]) – in relation to high-risk AI systems requirements
- The Law Enforcement Directive[9] – data protection regime for the purposes of the prevention, investigation, detection or prosecution of criminal offences or the execution of criminal penalties

---

[4] Report 2022 State of State Legislation on Artificial Intelligence. https://www.inclusivechange.org/ai-governance-solutions and Trends in biometric information regulation in the USA. https://www.adalovelaceinstitute.org/blog/biometrics-regulation-usa; White House Blueprint for an AI Bill of Rights: Making Automated Systems Work for the American People. https://www.whitehouse.gov/ostp/ai-bill-of-rights accessed 02.12.2022.

[5] David Matthews, UK rejects EU approach to artificial intelligence in favour of "pro-innovation" policy (*Science Business*, 19 July 2022). https://sciencebusiness.net/news/uk-rejects-eu-approach-artificial-intelligence-favour-pro-innovation-policy accessed 02.12.2022.

[6] Alex LaCasse, "Canada introduces new federal privacy and AI legislation" (*IAPP*, 16 June 2022). https://iapp.org/news/a/canada-introduces-new-federal-privacy-and-ai-legislation accessed 03.12.2022.

[7] Brian Wm. Higgins, "China's Regulation of Internet Recommender Systems: What US Companies Should Know" (*Blank Rome*, 28 February 2022). https://www.blankrome.com/publications/chinas-regulation-internet-recommender-systems-what-us-companies-should-know accessed 03.12.2022.

[8] Proposal for a Regulation of the European Parliament and of the Council laying down harmonised rules on artificial intelligence (Artificial Intelligence Act) and amending certain union legislative acts COM/2021/206 final [2021]. Disclaimer: The analysis here concerns the draft proposal of AIA which might be changed until its final adoption in 2025.

[9] Directive (EU) 2016/680 of the European Parliament and of the Council of 27 April 2016 on the protection of natural persons with regard to the processing of personal data by competent authorities for the purposes of the prevention, investigation, detection or prosecution of criminal offences or the execution of criminal penalties, and on the free movement of such data, and repealing Council Framework Decision 2008/977/JHA [2016] OJ L119/89.

- The General Data Protection Regulation (GDPR[10]) – data protection regime for any other purpose of processing

This section focuses on the fair trial principle in the context of the AIA proposal and the data protection regime (LED) as the main sources of AI regulation. We provide a brief analysis of the legal requirements related to law enforcement work with AI systems. Further, comparison between the acts illustrates that certain legal challenges remain an area of research and debate. Those steps of the analysis will assist in developing the legal requirements that will be further examined as part of the techno-legal analysis of ML pipelines.

3.2.1 The Fair Trial Principle

The right to a fair trial defines the most important principles in criminal proceedings and evidence law. The principle is universal and provides a common understanding for the design of fair criminal procedures. A detailed analysis of the right to a fair trial is done elsewhere. (Stoykova 2022)

For this chapter, Table 3.1 is a high-level summary of the two main principles of a fair trial: equality of arms and the presumption of innocence. From each principle derived is a specific requirement for evidence procedure (evidence rule) based on European Court of Human Rights (ECtHR) case law. Each evidence rule is interpreted in the context of digital investigations, specifically in relation to AI-evidence

Table 3.1 Fair trial and Evidence requirements.

Principle	Evidence Rules (Requirements)
Equality of Arms	*Fair procedure to evaluate the lawfulness and lawful use of evidence*
	Possibility to challenge evidence: fair disclosure and information about evidence
	(Sufficient) time and facilities to prepare the defence evidence
	Possibility to maintain equality of arms against expert evidence
	Legal assistance in crucial stages of the evidence handling
Presumption of Innocence	*Accurate Fact-finding*
	Protection against prejudicial effects in the evidence procedure
	Protection against reverse burden of proof

---

[10] Regulation (EU) 2016/679 of the European Parliament and of the Council of 27 April 2016 on the protection of natural persons with regard to the processing of personal data and on the free movement of such data, and repealing Directive 95/46/EC (General Data Protection Regulation) (Text with EEA relevance) [2016] OJ L 119/1.

and AI-based investigative methods. This interpretation can provide an initial overview of the legal, technical, and methodological challenges and set the scene for a further gap analysis.

Fair procedure to evaluate the lawfulness and lawful use of evidence means that each party should have the ability to evaluate the **quality** of the evidence (i.e., verify "whether the circumstances in which it was obtained cast doubt on its reliability or accuracy");[11] maintaining **contestability** (including ensuring the "opportunity of challenging the authenticity of the evidence and of opposing its use"); and compensation for reliability shortcomings by introducing **supporting evidence** (i.e., questionable evidence must be evaluated in the light of supporting evidence).[12] Further, the court must be able to assess "whether the proceedings as a whole, *including the way in which evidence was taken*, were fair".[13] To transpose these requirements to the digital domain it is necessary that the datasets for AI training are obtained lawfully, that the origin and integrity of AI evidence can be traced back, and accuracy of each processing step can be validated and contested in a chain of custody. In the case of violation of an individual's rights during the investigation, on the discretion of the judge the evidence might be excluded.

Possibility to challenge evidence refers to the obligation for the prosecution to disclose to the defence all material evidence in their possession for or against the accused;[14] right to the defence to be presented with not only evidence directly relevant to the facts of the case, but also other evidence that might relate to the admissibility, reliability, and completeness of the former.[15] The defence must have the opportunity: *(i)* to be involved in the definition of the criteria for determining what may be relevant[16] and *(ii)* to conduct further searches for exculpatory evidence.[17] It is quite challenging to interpret how these requirements can be transposed to AI-based evidence analysis. What kind of explanation on the AI system or the evidence discovery process will suffice effective challenging of the evidence reliability? Should the defence be involved in certain stages of the AI model development or consequently be provided with opportunity to cross-examine the model and ask the expert relevant questions? Should the defendant have certain access rights to evidence datasets and/or to the AI model itself and under which conditions? In cases when the defence uses their own AI model for exculpatory evidence discovery, who and how should be authorized to validate their findings and compare them to those by the prosecution?

---

[11] Dragojević v. Croatia App no 68955/11 (ECtHR, 15 January 2015) para 129.

[12] Prade v. Germany App no 7215/10 (ECtHR, 3 March 2016) paras 34–35.

[13] Doorson v. the Netherlands App no 20524/92 (ECtHR 26 March 1996) para 67. Emphasis mine.

[14] Rowe and Davis v. the UK ECHR 2000-II 287.

[15] Rowe and Davis v. the UK, cited above, para 66; Mirilashvili v. Russia App no 6293/04 (ECtHR 11 December 2008) para 200; Leas v. Estonia App no 59577/08 (ECtHR 6 March 2012) para 81; Windisch v. Austria App no 12489/86 (ECtHR 27 September 1990) para 28; see also Dowsett v. the UK App no. 39482/98 (ECtHR 24 June 2003) para 41.

[16] Sigurður Einarsson and Others v. Iceland App no 39757/15 (ECtHR 4 June 2019) para 90 and Rook v. Germany App no 1586/15 (ECtHR 25 July 2019) paras 67 and 72.

[17] Sigurður Einarsson and Others v. Iceland, cited above, para 91.

There is a general principle that the defence should have *time and facilities to pre-pare the defence evidence* and to put all relevant defence arguments before the court. In cases where ML models and big data analytics are used for evidence by the prosecution, the relevant rights for the defence should be available. Effective defence against unreliable evidence requires access to datasets and digital forensics expertise and tools in cases where the defence is unable to deal with data volumes and complexities in a case.

ECtHR pays special attention to an expert's competence and credibility. *Possibility to maintain equality of arms against expert evidence* means that the procedural rules must not deprive the defence of challenging expert opinion effectively when this requires specialist knowledge.[18] The defence should be able to contest and comment on the expert's findings,[19] and to be presented with the expert report as well as the expert findings on exculpatory evidence.[20] Note that this requirement refers not only to expert reports on the results of the ML model but also requires explanation and documentation on the concrete dataset, legal basis of processing operations, rights protection and bias mitigation in each case. As argued by Roth "machine conveyances are often in the form of predictive scores and match statistics, which are harder to falsify through validation against a known baseline" (Roth 2017). The accuracy and effect of such predictions in evidence discovery must be clearly stated by the expert. AI systems must allow for the evaluation and interpretation of their processing operations at further stages in the proceedings which might span a period of several years. The question arises, are post hoc challenging of the system and legacy software testing the best solutions or is validation and defence involvement at the time of the evidence discovery a more efficient and fair procedure?

Legal assistance in crucial stages of the evidence handling means that the court has established the essential role of the defence lawyer to test and participate in evidence discovery on pre-trial – namely identification procedures or reconstruction of events and on-site inspections,[21] search and seizure operations,[22] when the accused is taken in custody,[23] and in cross-border witness examination.[24] Similarly, it can be argued that in the crucial stages of AI processing the defence lawyer

---

[18] Stoimenov v. the former Yugoslav Republic of Macedonia App no 17995/02 (ECtHR 5 April 2007) para 38 and Matytsina v. Russia App no 58428/10 (ECtHR 27 March 2014) para 169.

[19] Feldbrugge v. the Netherlands, App no 8562/79 (ECtHR 29 May 1986) and Letinčić v. Croatia App no 7183/11 (ECtHR 3 May 2016) para 50.

[20] Nideröst-Huber v. Switzerland App no 18990/91 (ECtHR 18 February 1997) para 24; Lobo Machado v. Portugal App no 15764/89 (ECtHR 20 February 1996) para 31; Vermeulen v. Belgium App no 19075/91 (ECtHR 20 February 1996) para 33.

[21] İbrahim Öztürk v. Turkey App no 16500/04 (ECtHR 17 February 2009) paras 48–49; Türk v. Turkey App no 51962/12 (ECtHR 31 March 2015) para 47; Mehmet Duman v. Turkey App no 38740/09 (ECtHR 23 October 2018) para 41.

[22] Ayetullah Ay v. Turkey App nos 29084/07 and 1191/08 (ECtHR 27 October 2020) paras 135 and 163.

[23] Simeonovi v. Bulgaria App no 21980/04 (ECtHR 12 May 2017) para 111.

[24] A.M. v Italy 1999-IX 45, paras 26–27.

should be involved, e.g., to define exculpatory hypotheses and search parameters; to understand the application and methodology of AI model predictions; or to evaluate the speech-to-text analysis during interrogation.

Accurate fact-finding is necessary as LEA in criminal investigations must meet the highest burden of proof. However, the law does not require absolute legal certainty but only that the verdict is based on "direct or indirect evidence sufficiently strong in the eyes of the law to establish guilt".[25] *Protection against prejudicial effects in the evidence procedure* means that innocent suspects and defendants must be protected from pre-judgement and claims of guilt early in the investigations. *Protection against reverse burden of proof* means that in certain cases the presumption of innocence is violated when the burden of proof is shifted from the prosecution to the suspect or defendant.[26]

The presumption of innocence must be taken into consideration in the design and use of the AI system to avoid prejudicial effects. AI for recidivism prediction or identification suspect *ab initio* could have embedded bias for inculpatory evidence while assumption of guilt can be set as part of the parameterization of a tool, by the selection of search method and keywords, or can influence the choice of input or interpretation of the output. In the worst case, this could lead to parallel construction of evidence and reverse burden of proof.

In summary, the fair trial principle requires evidence procedures that can validate the origin and accuracy of the evidence, but more importantly whether the process that produced the evidence is fair, accountable, and respects defence rights. In this sense, AI models of evidence discovery and analysis cannot be simply treated as aiding or providing intelligence in investigation. Every use of analytics in evidence procedures has an impact on fundamental rights and freedoms. Fair trial requires rigorous examination of datasets, processing operations, and modelling quality for their impact on legal decision-making.

Legal scholars have identified that an unclear legal basis in combination with lack of standard procedures for novel digital forensics methods can have a tremendous impact on the right to a fair trial (Champod and Vuille 2011; Edmond and Roberts 2011), the presumption of innocence (Campbell 2013; Milaj and Mifsud Bonnici 2014; Sliedregt 2009), the suspects/defendants' rights protection (Wendy De Bondt and Gert Vermeulen 2010), legality of evidence (Gless 2010), and its admissibility (Kusak 2017). This can result in errors and miscarriages of justice. Consequently, AI systems compliance with fair trial principles raises rather fundamental challenges to criminal procedure. It should be further analysed if those challenges are mitigated in the context of the requirements for new investigative measures and within the AI and data protection legislation or gaps persist.

---

[25] Yearbook of the European Convention on Human Rights, 1963, p.740.
[26] Telfner v. Austria App no 33501/96 (ECtHR 20 March 2001) para 15.

3.2.2 Necessity and Proportionality of Investigative Measures

AI-based investigative measures have an impact not only on the fair trial principle but ca also interfere with several other rights such as the right to privacy and data protection, freedom of expression, security, telecommunication secrecy, and the prohibition against discrimination. In order to prevent abuse of investigative power ECtHR developed a necessity and proportionality test, which is further elaborated in the data protection regime. LEA must demonstrate compliance with the test for every new investigative measure.

In order to be justified, according to the ECtHR test, an investigative measure must be provided by law, pursue a legitimate aim, and be necessary in a democratic society. The first two requirements are straightforward. For example, the investigation of child pornography is a legitimate aim, and the penal and procedural code provides for certain powers for LEA to, e.g., search and seize such material. The deciding requirement for the introduction of AI-based technology for search and seizure of child pornography will be the necessity test. According to EDPB[27] it translates to the following checks:

- Pressing social need – although the measure interferes with individuals' rights, the measure is needed to tackle severe, urgent, or imminent danger
- Proportionality – the measure must be proportionate to the legitimate aim being pursued, e.g., evidence led explanation of why the existing measures are no longer sufficient for meeting that need
- Relevant and sufficient reasons – the reasons given to justify the interference are relevant and sufficient, e.g., research, surveys or other information to underpin its reasoning

The requirement for pressing social need means that more serious crimes can justify more intrusive measure, e.g., violent sexual crime is more severe/pressing than burglary and therefore can justify more intrusive measure, such as the use of an AI model for facial recognition to identify the suspect. However, there are many minor crimes of cyberbullying where the data that needs to be analysed is not less than a serious crime and AI can be used to reduce the back log. In this case the seriousness and severity come from the need to avoid denial of justice by dropping all minor cases.

For new AI models to be developed and used in evidence analysis LEA must justify the need of such measures, compare proposed AI models and their intrusiveness to existing measures, and provide reasoning of the efficiency of the measure and all safeguards taken to minimize the interference with individuals' rights. For example, applied research in real live settings is already done in several law enforcement agencies to identify their claimed benefits in comparison to the controversies of surveillance in public spaces. (Yeung 2021)

---

[27] EDPB Opinion 01/2014 on the application of necessity and proportionality concepts and data protection within the law enforcement sector (available at https://ec.europa.eu/justice/article-29/documentation/opinionrecommendation/files/2014/wp211_en.pdf).

Consequently, the fair trial principle requires quality of evidence procedures and procedural rights assurance for the defence in the use of AI models in investigations and trials, while the necessity and proportionality test provide requirements for justification of new AI-based investigative methods.

> **GAP 2** Although the fair trial principle can be interpreted in the context of AI-based investigative measures, there is insufficient legal research as to what are suitable means to satisfy each derived requirement, do we have AI system solutions that can mitigate power imbalance between the parties in the criminal proceedings, and how can effective reliability validation and cross-examination of AI-generated evidence be ensured.

This poses questions like: is it sufficient to have a combination of system design safeguards against prejudicial effects and judicial discretion or are new AI specific defense rights necessary? Similarly, as AI-based evidence discovery methods provide a completely novel approach to investigations are they comparable in their intrusiveness in relation to traditional investigative measures in order to evaluate their proportionality and necessity or is this legal test no longer valid?

Even from the brief analysis here, it becomes clear that AI-investigative systems bring several quite specific challenges to the fair trial doctrine. It should be further examined whether the current EU approach to regulate the design and use of AI systems in law enforcement in combination with the existing data protection regime can sufficiently enforce fair trial compliance as well, or whether domain specific regulation is still necessary to address the gaps.

3.2.3 The AIA Proposal

The draft AIA sets requirements for the design of the AI system and obligations for providers and users of such systems. The definition of AI in the draft AIA is intentionally very broad and is based on the principle of technological neutrality in order to accommodate any future development of AI technology and ensure statue longevity. An AI system is defined as any software developed with machine learning, logic- and knowledge-based, or statistical approaches which are: *(i)* based on human-defined objectives; and *(ii)* can generate outputs such as content, predictions, recommendations, or decisions influencing the environments they interact with. Some have argued that the definition is overbroad as it does not include only machine learning and automated decision-making systems (ADMs) but also simple logic programming which does not have the societal effects that the AIA tries to mitigate. (Ebers et al. 2021; Mökander et al. 2022) The AIA provisions that regulate specifically the use of AI systems for law enforcement purposes are shown in Figure 3.1

LEAs are prohibited from using AI for behavioral manipulation or exploiting vulnerabilities of suspects and defendants. An example is psychological profiling of targeted individuals in order to obtain confessions. Further, AIA sets a ban on the use of AI systems for social scoring such as blacklisting ex-convicts or certain groups of suspects which leads to their unjustified or disproportionate treatment, e.g.,

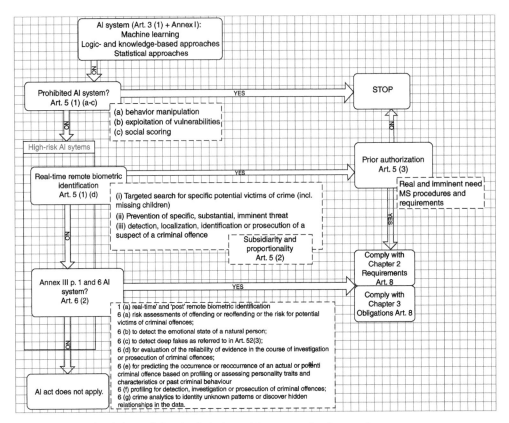

Figure 3.1 Applicability of the draft AIA to AI systems for law enforcement purposes
Credit: Adapted from[28]

increased police searches; extensive data collection and analytics on them. Lastly, Art. 5 AIA prohibits the use of **"real-time" remote biometric identification** systems in publicly spaces for law enforcement purposes. For example, indiscriminate facial recognition of all people in a public area in real time to identify a terrorist is prohibited.[29] Similarly, the use of *Clearview AI* software[30] to identify suspects across billions of images from the internet and social media is also prohibited in Europe. However, this prohibition is subject to exceptions. Such systems can be used only for three purposes – targeted search for potential victims of crime or missing children; for the prevention of threat that is imminent and substantial; and for the detection, identification, and prosecution of a suspect (Art. 5 (1) (d)). In such cases LEA must obtain prior authorization (Ar. 5 (3)) according to MS rules and by proving that (i) there is a real and imminent need and (ii) the investigative

---

[28] Based on: prof. R. Leenes, TILT Digital Legal Lab research initiative, AIA visual map available at: https://www.sectorplandls.nl/wordpress/news/a-visual-guide-to-the-ai-act-by-ronald-leenes. Modified and extended to LEA relevance.

[29] Lucilla Sioli, "A European approach to the regulation of artificial intelligence" (*CEPS Think Tank*, 23 April 2021). https://www.youtube.com/watch?v=X9h8MZIuvKg&ab_channel=CEPSThinkTank accessed 30.11.2022.

[30] See Wikipedia page: https://en.wikipedia.org/wiki/Clearview_AI accessed 30.11.2022.

measure is proportionate and other, less intrusive investigative methods would be unsuccessful or unavailable (Art.5 (2)).

Most of the typical uses of AI for law enforcement purposes are categorized in the draft AIA as high-risk AI systems. High-risk means that they have serious legal implications in relation to fundamental rights and freedoms most notably the right to liberty, privacy and data protection, non-discrimination, and fair trial. Such systems are not prohibited but are subject to restrictions.

High-risk AI systems for law enforcement are specified in Annexure III p.1 and 6 (see Figure 3.1) and must comply with of Chapter 2 (requirements for the AI system) and Chapter 3 (obligations for the providers and users of such systems).

The requirements for the AI system are rather stringent and are summarized in Table 3.2:

Table 3.2 High-risk AI systems requirements.

Risk-management system (Art. 9)	foreseeable risks for the intended purpose
Data and data governance (Art. 10)	high-quality training, validation, and testing data (relevant; representative, accurate) with application-area specific properties; identifying individuals or groups affected
Technical documentation (Art. 11+ Annex IV)	extensive; includes, e.g., general description of the AI system; the elements of the AI system and of the process for its development; the validation and testing procedures used; about the monitoring, functioning and control of the AI system; the risk management system
Record-keeping (Art. 12)	documentation and logs to ensure accountability and transparency
Transparency information (Art. 13)	appropriate degree of transparency to enable users to interpret the system's output and use it
Human oversight (Art. 14)	built-in or user-implemented measures to allow a person to correctly interpret the AI high-risk system's output
Cybersecurity (Art. 15)	including protection against discrimination and adversarial machine learning

Each of the AIA requirements in Table 3.2 as well as challenges in AI for digital forensics will be discussed in Section 3.3 in the relevant sub-section from the ML pipeline. However, the next sub-section examines the AIA act in the context of data protection, which already shows some legislative contradictions in the legal framework.

3.2.4 AI System Development and Legislative Contradictions

The last building block of the legislative framework is data protection compliance for AI systems. When AI is used for the processing of personal data for law enforcement purposes the LED regime needs to be followed, while for any other purpose of processing the GDPR still applies. Here we are comparing some important provisions from AIA, GDPR, and LED in order to identify common principles for AI system development. A closer look at those overall system development requirements already shows discrepancies in the legal regimes which remain currently under legal debate and further research.

AI systems for LEA purposes such as:

- Real-time, remote biometric identification in public spaces
- Biometric categorization (using biometrics to categorize individuals into clusters based on ethnicity, gender, political or sexual orientation, or other grounds on which discrimination is prohibited)
- AI for detecting emotions
- AI for recidivism prediction (prediction of the risk of reoffending)
- Behaviour manipulation and social scoring by the police

will most likely not pass the data protection or necessity and proportionality threshold. Data protection authorities and legal scholars heavily criticized the AIA for not including an absolute ban on such systems (Ebers et al. 2021; EDPB-EDPS 2021; Veale and Borgesius 2021). For example, AIA exceptionally allows the use of real-time, large-scale biometrics for the identification of suspects. However, according to GDPR in such cases LEA must ensure data protection compliance not only in relation to potential suspects but also to all other individuals affected by the measure, which in practice is challenging (Yeung 2021). Moreover, some of those practices cannot prove technological robustness either. For example, AI systems for the detection of emotions are still inaccurate and unreliable (Barrett et al. 2019). A study of an existing recidivism prediction algorithm COMPAS showed that quantifying predictions do not have added value since people without any criminal history can also get high recidivism scores by simply filling in the questionnaire used to feed the algorithm (Dressel and Farid 2018). In addition, historical police data on crime incidence is a notoriously bad source to train prediction algorithms as it contains bias towards minority groups and is not an accurate representation of criminality. Further, identifying variables which correlate to certain legal outcome requires understanding of legal argumentation, which is hard, if not impossible, to quantify and introduces serious concerns in relation to the presumption of innocence and defense rights. Consequently, even though the listed AI systems are still under legal debate, LEA can hardly justify their use under the legal framework in the EU, while national law can still prohibit such use. (Rec. 41 AIA) There is a clear focus on the regulation of biometrics in AIA, but other highly problematic topics in law enforcement work are not addressed, e.g., AI-enabled surveillance such as computer vision or NLP applications. AIA also focuses on system design requirements and accountability, while other aspects like case-based authorization for use or prevention of misuse can complement the regime and consistently regulate such AI-systems instead of generally prohibit them.

GAP 3 Certain AI systems will remain legally problematic in Europe. Even if they can meet the requirements of the draft AIA, they might not comply with the data protection regime and are highly intrusive to fundamental rights. AIA fails to recognize that such systems are not limited to biometrics, while their law enforcement applications require safeguards against misuse beyond system design and monitoring.

3.2.4.1 Lack of Validation Framework + Fragmented Roles and Obligations

The lack of a comprehensive validation framework to avoid tool dependencies and push-button-forensics in law enforcement work is not addressed by the AIA proposal. Rather both AIA and the data protection regime introduce different legal roles with corresponding obligations. This leads to ambiguities between the regimes which runs the risk of LEA using an AI-system without being able to validate it.

The AIA distinguishes between providers and users of AI systems. Providers are those who develop an AI system and place it on the market or into service, while users are those who only purchase the system and use it. The providers of AI systems have considerably more obligations than users to assess the AI system and to ensure compliance with AIA. The data protection regime on the other hand, defines obligations for controllers and processors of personal data. There is no reference in AIA to the data protection classification. The only simplification is that the data protection authority (DPA) will be also be the market surveillance authority (MSA) for law enforcement. There are overlaps in the obligations and they can be easily satisfied if the AI system provider and data controller are the same. An example is when LEAs develop in-house AI systems. This, however, is not a very plausible scenario due to limited resources or expertise in LEA. Rather AI system developers will provide off-the-shelf AI models to be used by LEAs who remain controllers and processors of the data. In such case, compliance with both regimes might be ambiguous for several reasons.

First, the data protection regime does not clarify the status of private companies or research institutions which process data for law enforcement purpose. LED applies only to data processing by competent authorities, which private companies are not, while GDPR does not apply to data processing for law enforcement purpose. It can be argued that LEAs are best suited to identify risks for individual rights. However, they might be in a situation where, as controllers they establish only the data protection risks and measures, while for other risks e.g. in relation to fair trial or non-discrimination it is up to the AI system provider to decide.

Secondly, doubled obligations for compliance and incidents reporting arise. The AI system provider and processor will have to supply the same compliance information, once to the controller (under DP regime) and once to the DPA (under AIA regime). Similarly, LEAs will have to do the same as users of AI system but controllers of datasets for example in the case of data breach. Consequently, the DPA will receive the same information twice.

Commercial or research organizations developing AI models for law enforcement purposes will want to preserve copyrights and profit for the designed models. Even more troubling is that LEA as controllers must establish technical and organizational measures for personal data processing, but they should trust the AI system (commercial) provider on the overall assessment of the AI system accuracy and risks. This provokes high concerns for legitimacy as commercial AI system providers are put in a position to influence not only the evidence processing (as it was up until now with DF tools) but also the criminal justice system as a whole. Moreover, such an arrangement enters contradiction with digital forensics principles for reliability validation. It is already well known, that law enforcement purchasing commercially developed DF tools have multiple drawbacks with validation, multi-purpose tool limitations, and lack of competency by LEA to detect tool errors or interpret results correctly (Marshall and Paige 2018; Nordvik et al. 2021). Those limitations will only be intensified if general-purpose machine learning models are purchased by law enforcement without sufficient understanding of the dependencies the model development has in relation to the characteristics of real investigative data, the specific task and the pre-processing tasks for designing datasets for training and testing machine learning models. Consequently, commercially developed general purpose AI models need to be internally tested by LEA for their specific application and datasets (cross ref chapter explainability/validation Ypma Ramos Meuwly). AI design requirements, as summarized in Table 3.2, are all in relation to the intended purpose of the AI model. Fairness of processing and bias mitigation must be done also in relation to concrete purpose, ergo, if the AI model is used for another purpose a new evaluation is required. For example, a commercial face recognition AI system purchased by LEAs is a repurposing of an AI model which require testing anew by LEA for AIA compliance and application-specific model validation. It is questionable if such complicated testing is economically and technically feasible for each law enforcement agency. An independent validation body might be better suited for this.

Further, as pointed out by data protection authorities, there could be discrepancies between the two regimes in different stages of the modelling or when the model is designed to learn continuously over new datasets (EDPB-EDPS 2021). For example, if an AI system provider is using its own datasets for training and validation of the model, they are controllers and providers in this stage, while LEAs might be providers and controllers for task-specific validation and the production stage. This means that the same actors might have multiple different functions on different stages of the processing. For example, the provider can define some purposes of the AI system during training, but they cannot comply further with the AIA or data protection regime if LEA purchase the AI system for their specific use with their own datasets. If LEA are considered providers they might not have sufficient knowledge about the AI system design or large-enough testing datasets to satisfy AIA requirements (Ebers et al. 2021). In general, the decision to exempt users of AI systems from so many obligations is questionable. The regime of fragmented roles and obligations although an important first step for AI regulation, can hardly replace a domain-specific legislation for law enforcement and undermines legal certainty.

> **GAP 4** Intellectual property rights might require LEA to trust the documentation and self-assessment of the AI system provider rather than test it. This is in a direct contradiction with digital forensic standards and fair trial procedure. A comprehensive reliability validation process must define law enforcement and AI providers obligations for repurposing of commercially developed AI systems.

3.2.4.2 Risk and Privacy Impact Assessment

Art. 9 AIA requires a quality and risk management process for the intended purpose of AI systems. Art.9 AIA expands the scope of privacy risk assessment (Art. 27 LED) to include risks to other fundamental rights. Prior to processing, a description of the envisaged processing operations and assessment of known, foreseeable, and emerging risks should be performed. This could be combined with the assessment of the proportionality of the investigative measure. The UK, published such a practical guide for law enforcement (The UK National Police Chiefs Council 2020). Close cooperation with DPA is required, as they can assist in formulating requirements for the specific AI system.

Risk and privacy impact assessment	
Prior processing	description of the envisaged processing operations; an assessment of the risks to the rights and freedoms of data subjects; known, foreseeable, emerging future risks (Art. 27 LED and Art. 9 AIA)
Dataset construction Pre-processing Feature construction	safeguards, security measures and mechanisms to ensure the protection of personal data and to demonstrate compliance *test* most appropriate risk management measures
System deployment	adequate information to AI system users about the risk (Art 13 AIA)

In Section 3.3 we outline relevant research, practical solutions, and gaps for risk assessment, privacy enhancing strategies, and bias mitigation for AI systems.

3.2.4.3 Transparency Versus Accountability Versus Explainability

As examined in Section 3.2.1 the fair trial principle requires a certain level of transparency and accountability in law enforcement work to enable defence procedural rights and judicial scrutiny. However, there is also a legitimate need to ensure effective prosecution and to protect investigative methods and technology.

Both the data protection and the AIA regime are ambiguous how to balance such opposing interests.

Certain derogations from the principle of transparency are provided for LEA. Art. 4 (1) (a) LED requires only lawful and fair processing, by contrast with GDPR where Art.5 (1) (a) requires transparency as well. Art.13 AIA provides for transparency obligations by the provider of AI system to enable users to interpret the system's output and use it. However, there are no similar obligation towards the individuals affected by this system. Similarly, under Art. 52 LEA are not obliged to inform individuals that they are interacting with an AI system such as chatbot, deep fake, or emotional recognition model. This exemption was criticized by data protection authority as too broad. Data protection authorities emphasized that safeguards for prevention and detection have to be stronger because of the presumption of innocence (EDPB-EDPS 2021). Moreover, the use of such systems by LEA must be evaluated in respect to defence rights or the prohibitions of entrapment and indictment. The provision is a clear example that fair trial considerations are not addressed, and it is up to the providers of such systems to assess those risks which undermine legal certainty.

Surprisingly, Art.13 avoids the well-known concept of explainable AI and only refers that AI systems should be *sufficiently* transparent to enable users to *interpret* the system's output and use it appropriately. However, the use of AI systems for evidence analysis, requires AI system tuning and reliability testing which far exceeds the modest interpretation of output. The AIA does not give further guidance on what measures can satisfy interpretability requirements and what kind of explanations are suitable for criminal proceedings. This question is left to standardization bodies with the help of the increased academic research to develop domain specific guidelines.

The principle of accountability is much stronger in LEA context where data protection rules (Art. 5 (2) GDPR and Art. 4 (4) LED) are extended with AI system specific requirements for record-keeping, logging features, and extensive technical documentation requirements including general description of the AI system; the elements of the AI system and of the process for its development; the validation and testing procedures used; about the monitoring, functioning and control of the AI system; the risk management system (Art. 11–12 AIA). However, Art. 12 is vaguely formulated referring to a level of traceability appropriate to the intendent purpose and apart from some specific requirements for biometric systems leaves matters of compliance and implementation to recognized standards and specifications. The additional accountability requirement for human oversight of the system is also rather ambiguous. Art. 14 requires the provider or user of AI system to implement measure for a person to fully understand the capacities and limitations of the high-risk AI system, to duly monitor its operation, and mitigate automation bias (automatically relying or over-relying on the output produced by a high-risk AI system). In addition to the repeated vague requirement for interpretable output, the provision demands a possibility for a human to disregard, override or reverse the output of the high-risk AI system and to intervene or interrupt the system through a "stop" button or a similar procedure.

The last two requirements go against the very purpose of AI systems to automate tasks. As no specific criteria is provided what might justify such intervention, it is questionable if the human intervention will mitigate risks in the system or to the contrary – introduce bias and limit understanding of it. In fact, risks, errors, and bias in AI systems are usually systematic in nature and need continuous testing and re-evaluation of the system by experts with diverse datasets and scenarios. Pulling the plug of an AI system should be the result of validation testing and specific standards rather than selective decisions. In addition, evaluation of fundamental rights risks imposed by AI systems requires a multi-stakeholder debate where the technology (AI system) is decoupled from its social purpose. This will result in: *(i)* tasks suitable for full automation, *(ii)* task requiring continuous human-machine interaction (where expert knowledge should be represented as subjective measurements affecting the system performance) and *(iii)* tasks that should remain the primary concern of human evaluation. For example, policymakers might decide that ML model for evidence detection can be fully automated, its reliability assessment requires machine-human assistance, while its evaluation for a legal decision (e.g., if the suspect should be taken into custody) should be reserved to human discretion. Similarly, for some tasks like bullet trajectory calculation AI systems can outperform humans. In such case the need for human intervention, apart from reliability validation, is quite limited. Therefore, if the human oversight provision is not supported by clear validation standards and policy decisions it could turn into an arbitrary and even automation hampering decision with limited benefits for consistent decision making and treatment of individuals.

> **GAP 5** Full transparency in law enforcement work is undesirable and might clash with obligations for efficient prosecution. However, the imprecise formulation of the derogations from the principle of transparency in AIA undermines legal certainty. Arguably, new accountability or interpretability requirements for AI systems in law enforcement work cannot be introduced without clarifying their meaning in the criminal procedure. Consequently, specific questions such as defense rights to cross-examine and challenge AI-generated evidence, forensic interpretation and reporting of AI system output, chain of custody requirements, authorization, or procedural safeguards against AI system misuse by law enforcement etc. – will remain jurisdiction-specific and therefore deepening the identified technological, methodological, and legal fragmentation in digital investigations.

3.2.4.4 Individual Rights

Notably, AIA is based on product safety regulations and focuses on AI system design requirements and obligations but does not encompass any specific rights for individuals subject to the AI model prediction. By contrast, in the data protection regime, the accountability and fairness obligations are strengthened with data subject rights. However, to ensure effective prosecution those rights are curtailed in the LED, in comparison to GDPR. As AI systems produce automated or semi-automated decisions the related data subject rights are of particular interest. This sub-section also examines the data rights regime in the context of fair trial in order to provide a first incentive on the adequacy of the legal regime.

Art. 13(2) (f) and 14(2) (g) GDPR defines the right to information about the source of data, modalities and conditions of data processing, including information about *the logic involved* and *the consequences* related to automated decision-making and profiling. The EDPB clarified that in order to understand the automated decision the individual affected should receive information about the categories of data used (as input), testing data that the process is fair, as well as the criteria relied on (features, classes) and differences between classes and scenarios in which the individual can fall under more beneficial category (EDPB 2018). The same right in Art. 13 LED is significantly curtailed and does not refer to automated decision making or source of data. It is up to the member states to decide on appropriate level of information, while EDPB guidelines for law enforcement are missing. Art .15 GDPR requires further data subjects to have access to the personal data used as input and to information to verify the lawfulness of the processing. In relation to profiling, EDPB emphasized that important is to specify *"envisaged consequences* of the processing, rather than an explanation of a *particular* decision". Once again, no equivalent obligation exists for law enforcement in Art. 14 LED.

Both Art.16 GDPR and Art. 16 LED codify a right to rectification of personal data. However, under LED law enforcement are permitted to restrict or refuse erasure. Similarly, while under Art. 21 GDPR the data subject has a right to object the data processing, no similar provision exists in LED.

Finally, there is a general prohibition of decisions based solely on automated processing that produce legal effect or significantly impact individuals (Art. 22 GDPR) although the provision is subject to exceptions. There are inconsistencies in the data protection regime as to the regulation of inferred data, which is interpreted only in GDPR context. In relation to data portability EDPB gave an opinion that inferences from the analysis of data provided by the data subject does not fall under the scope of the data portability right (EDPB 2016). However, in relation to profiling, decisions based on profiling or fully automated decisions the EDPB emphasized that the individuals should enjoy their rights to information, access, and erasure in respect to the input data *as well as the data about observed behaviour or inferred data* (EDPB 2018). The same guideline gives best practice guidelines on information to be provided about the functioning of machine learning systems and how they impact the individual, however, simultaneously emphasize Rec. 63 provision that data subject rights should not interfere with intellectual property rights. The data subject at minimum has the right to obtain human intervention on the part of the controller, to express his or her point of view and to contest the decision. Those provisions already create a complex balancing rights situation which however is not interpreted in the context of the LED regime.

Art. 11 LED addresses automated decisions and profiling but it is not formulated as data subject right. The scope of the LED provision is limited to only *fully* automated decisions, which *adversely* or significantly affect the individual. Such decisions are not completely prohibited but instead the member states can decide when and under which safeguards they are necessary. Further, no right to contest or object automated decisions is explicitly codified, but only suggested in Recital 38. There are no specific requirements for semi-automated decisions – they are subject only to the general data protection principles. Consequently, the LED regime significantly limits the data subject rights and is very vague in terms of automated decisions and profiling, while AIA does not refer to any individual rights. In different contexts, legal scholars question the existence of a right to explanation of automated decision making, its scope or its utility. Some argued that a right to explanation cannot be derived from the GDPR regime (Goodman and Flaxman 2017; Wachter et al. 2017), while other refer to the limited practical utility of Art. 22 GDPR due to its numerous conditions and exceptions (Mendoza and Bygrave 2017). This legal uncertainty leads to at least two significant gaps in the regime.

GAP 6 The data subject rights regime in LED does not really contribute to fair trial objectives.

By contrast to the limited rights of information, access, and erasure in the LED regime, the principle of fair trial requires extensive procedural safeguards for suspects and defendants to receive information relevant to the lawfulness and reliability of the AI-based investigative measure and to be sufficiently informed about the model in order to actively cross-examine and challenge the processing operations on valid grounds. In automated or semi – automated decision making, including profiling, the expert evidence doctrine, requires not only explanation of the scientific validity of the AI model, but arguably active defence rights to request or participate in certain processing stages in order for the model to identify exculpatory evidence. While source code disclosure or extensive examination of the system functionality might not be necessary if sufficient validation data is provided, certain stages of the processing such as pre-processing, feature and algorithm selection or output interpretation are determinative to the reliability of the evidence and to the effective exercising of the defence rights. Contrary to the data protection regime, explanation is necessary not only in respect to the envisaged consequences of the decision, but also on all subjective and objective measurements that influenced the model. Presumably, the AIA requirements for high-risk AI systems will support forensic examiners and investigators in evaluating the output of such systems. However, they do not resolve the legal uncertainty around explanation rights in relation to defence rights transposition to AI-based investigative outcomes.

GAP 7 There is a lack of feasibility studies on (i) transposition of defense rights to AI systems and (ii) interpretation of data subject rights in the context of fair trial.

Complex questions arise with respect to the protection of data subject rights and defence rights in the context of AI-based investigative measures. From fair trial point of view, the risk from (semi-) automated evidence processing and decision making far exceeds the concept of personal data and its protection. In order to avoid contradictions between data subject rights and defence rights they must be interpreted simultaneously and consistently in order to design a specific regime for AI-supported investigative procedures. This again supports the argument that rethinking of the legal framework and the criminal justice principles is required to reflect the impact of new technology on individual rights.

So far, we have clarified the main legal requirements and challenges for AI systems development in law enforcement. Furthermore, these high-level requirements must be further elaborated within the processes that apply at each step of the AI modelling. The next section discusses the techno-legal challenges in each process of the AI system for digital forensics and law enforcement purposes, which use machine learning. The analysis follows the ISO/IEC 23053:2022 *machine learning pipeline* and identifies relevant research in reliability validation, best practices, and legal compliance techniques. The created roadmap can be used and extended as a template for LEAs in each investigative task to begin with designing an accountable and legally compliant ML process. The broader goal of the gap analysis is to avoid and "AI winter in forensics" or fear of the legislation, while simultaneously expose shortcoming of the AI legal regime from practitioner point of view. The identified techno-legal challenges can serve as a roadmap for further research.

3.3 Machine Learning Pipelines: Techno-legal Challenges

The determinative stages of the ML pipeline according to ISO/IEC 23053:2022 are: tasking, data acquisition, pre-processing, and modelling (feature extraction and selection and algorithm selection). Each of those stages is connected to the legislative requirements to identify practical solutions and gaps for compliance.

The purpose of the techno-legal gap analysis in this section is threefold. It aims firstly to identify LEA needs in each stage of the ML pipeline. Secondly, it examines best practices, existing implementation solutions, and standards for ML processes which can facilitate the efficient deployment of AI in law enforcement work, technical robustness, and legal compliance. Finally, the identified gaps in each processing stage aim to outline broader techno-legal perspective on AI for further research.

3.3.1 Task + Purpose Limitation and Data Minimization

It is crucial for law enforcement to identify for which investigative tasks machine learning models are useful and for which they are not. ML methods can be used in several stages of the digital investigation process, e.g., hypothesis generation, examination (filtering, pre-processing), or analysis, but they are suitable only for specific, generalization-related investigative tasks. ISO/IEC 23053:2022 defines three main ML tasks: classification, clustering, and regression.

Classification tasks are defined as the prediction of the assignment of an instance of input data to a defined category or class. (ISO/IEC 23053, 2022) The most common classification tasks in investigations are related to file system metadata analysis (Hargreaves and Patterson 2012; Mohammad and Alqahtani 2019; Serhal and Le-Khac 2021), malware and network analysis (Du et al. 2020), detection of relevant digital traces such as child abuse image and predatory chats detection (Borj et al. 2021; Ngejane et al. 2021). However, there are significant differences in the progress made in different domains. For example, malware and intrusion detection classification tasks are advancing faster as global shared and labelled datasets are available, and extensive research and sharing is enabled by the IT security community. In other domains, like file systems which are more specific to digital forensics, rather than the security field, the advancements are slow, few papers exist, mapping single experiments rather than systematic work. Classification tasks are strongly dependant on correct representation of the expert forensic knowledge and interpretation of crime related data properties. Recent use of classification for recidivism prediction stumbled upon racial bias and skewed data outputs mostly due to biased historical arrest data (Larson et al. 2016) and difficulties to quantify variables that reliably correlate to prediction of recidivism.

Clustering tasks are still insufficiently researched in digital forensics. There are some examples of clustering for pre-processing and link mining (Flaglien 2018), data recovery (Du et al. 2020; Nassif and Hruschka 2013), topic modelling (Porter 2018) or improving search output (Beebe and Liu 2014).

Regression is not so often used for law enforcement purposes. Skimming through research databases showed one example where a regression model was used to predict future crime patterns and development of criminal activity (Awal et al. 2016), which is a rather criminology related task.

The purpose limitation principle in Art. 8 LED states two requirements: (i) data should be collected for specified, legitimate, and explicit purposes and (ii) not processed in a way incompatible with those purposes. Note that Art. 6 GDPR gives six different legal grounds to justify processing and specific requirements for further processing, while LEA Art. 8 LED provides only one: if necessary for the performance of a task carried out by a competent authority for the purposes of the Directive and based on Union or Member State law. Consent is not a valid ground for law enforcement processing. Art. 4 (b) does not state any specific requirements for further processing except compatible use (Table 3.3).

LEA purposes are (Art. 4 in conj. Art. 1(1)): prevention, investigation, detection, or prosecution of criminal offences, execution of criminal penalties, including prevention of threats to public security. If LEA process data for any other purpose GDPR apply. For example, if data was collected to investigate drug trafficking it can be processed for a new law enforcement purpose, e.g., the

Table 3.3 Task purpose limitation/Repurposing of datasets and models.

	Purpose limitation	**Compatible use: Repurposing of datasets**
Art. 4 LED	– specified, legitimate and explicit – provided by law – necessary and proportionate – prevention, investigation, detection, or prosecution of criminal offences	– in scope of LED – provided by law – necessary and proportionate – scientific, statistical, or historical research + appropriate safeguards
Chapter 2 AIA	AI system design compliance according to the intended purpose self-assessment by the provider	Repurposing of models – new AIA compliance validation – application-specific model validation – no exception for research

detection of organized criminal groups as long as this is authorized by law, necessary, and proportionate (Art. 4 (2)). Consequently, the purpose of the limitation principle in LED is defined flexibly and can accommodate big data forensics and the creation of datasets for ML models for law enforcement, as well as data reuse between different competent authorities. It has been argued that the purpose limitation principle is often a matter of skilful legal drafting and there are no clear mechanisms to verify or enforce the principle in different stages of processing (Biega and Finck 2021). Further, from a theoretical point of view, scholars emphasize that the principle is at odds with knowledge discovery in databases where "they lose the social norms associated with intra-context processing of data" (Koops 2013). The assessment of the design of high-risk AI system and its compliance with Chapter 2 of AIA should be done by the provider also in relation to the intended purpose. However, AI modelling includes several processing stages and sub-processes which follow the same investigative purpose but might be associated with very different social risks. For example, algorithms which perform pre-processing tasks are at risk of evidence loss during outlier removal or expert bias in labelling, although they might be compliant with a legitimate purpose of processing.

It can be beneficial to abandon the unfruitful discussion on if and to what extent the purpose limitation principle applies to AI models. In order to preserve meaning, the principle should be rather interpreted within the technical term tasking (as investitive or forensic hypothesis) and its crucial importance for reliability validation. *Tasking* is a determinative stage in the ML pipeline because it defines the scope and boundaries of the processing, i.e., it allows assessment of why a data source was acquired, examined, or analysed. As part of the reliability validation process the *task* influences the selection of the methods and tools, the pre-processing, and the selection of relevant data features. Disclosure of the digital forensics task is of importance for the defence to understand hypothesis and assumptions, their potential impact on the processing operations, and if alternative hypotheses, e.g., for exculpatory evidence, were tested by the examiner. In exercise of its right to participate in determinative stages of the processing, in particular cases, the defence may request under the judge's, discretion testing of other hypotheses that might acquit the defendant or reduce the charges. In a broader context, explicitly formulated tasks can serve for proportionality assessment of the investigative measure, purpose limitation, and legal authorization. The AI model and the dataset should be built for a specific purpose, defined in the task, and any repurposing of the model or the datasets must be compatible with this purpose.

In addition, there are some practical hurdles in relation to repurposing of datasets and AI models to be outlined. LEAs and DF examiners work with partial information, uncertainties, and incomplete representation of past events. In the initial stages of the investigation LEAs might not be able to define a specified and explicit purpose for processing. Even if they define such a purpose *ab initio*, evidence discovery requires low level data retrieval and examination, which might lead to the discovery of personal data which is not intended to be processed but is a by-product of the examination. Even if such data is not related to the investigation and not of any relevance to the investigative purpose, its processing might still be necessary for testing the reliability of the evidence discovery process or the tool retrieval results. Further the data minimization principle requires the collection only of relevant and not excessive data for the purpose of the investigation (Art. 4 (1) (c) LED) and Art. 10 AIA have similar requirements for ML training and validation datasets. Simultaneously, a principle in digital forensics is to acquire all the data on a device in order to preserve its integrity. Applying data minimization in the initial collection of data might jeopardize the reliability of the evidence and risks exculpatory evidence to be missed. Moreover, before training an AI model it is not possible to know which data is excessive.

Art. 4 (3) LED provides that the processing of personal data for scientific, statistical, or historical research purposes is allowed if it is subject to appropriate safeguards for the rights and freedoms of data subjects. However, there is no similar exception in AIA which makes unclear the legal status of AI models developed by researchers for law enforcement purposes (Ebers et al. 2021).

Art. 9 LED defines that further processing of private companies' data to law enforcement is governed by GDPR, and once LEA receive the data it falls under the LED regime. However, the provision does not clarify which data protection regime applies to private entities such as digital forensics companies or AI models' and tools developers who process personal data specifically for law enforcement purposes.

GAP 8 It remains unclear how to interpret the purpose limitation principle for AI systems. Reliable digital evidence discovery requires checks and balances to resolve the tension between data protection and reliability validation of evidence processing for each forensic task separately, which cannot be known *ab initio*. Rather than insisting on purpose limitation *ab initio*, a more suitable approach is to define guidelines for legally compliant tasks and safeguards for each processing stage in AI modelling.

3.3.2 Dataset Engineering and Data Governance

Digital forensics experts and data scientists still consider dataset design as an engineering task. *Hutchinson* describes datasets as "technical infrastructure and their development as an important engineering output to view and structure knowledge in defined infrastructures and standardized interfaces, creating value by enabling rapid iteration and new forms of processes" (Hutchinson et al. 2021, pp. 560–561). Data for machine learning models can be structured, semi- or unstructured, user- or machine-generated, user- or machine labelled. From a legal point of view however, datasets are heterogenous digital assets with specific rights and obligations. User-generated data falls under personal data protection, intellectual property, confidentiality, and trade secrets protection. Machine-generated data once acquired could fall under the *sui generis* database right. Similarly, labelled training datasets for ML models can be subject to intellectual property rights.

The dataset must be acquired specifically for the purpose of the AI model and the threshold for data governance in law is set quite high. Art. 10 AIA requires high-quality training, validation, and testing datasets. Datasets must be relevant, representative, accurate, and to have application-area specific properties. AI providers must also ensure that datasets are error-free. GDPR and the LED similarly codify the principles of accuracy and data minimization. Note that, Article 5(1)(c) GDPR requires adequate, relevant and *limited to what is necessary* data, while the working in Article 4(1)(c) LED is different: data must be adequate, relevant and *not excessive*. This gives more leeway for LEA to collect and analyse data, unlike companies who are obliged to check periodically if data is still necessary and if not to delete it (De Hert and Sajfert 2021).

Nevertheless, practitioners know that real datasets are messy and rarely error free. The requirement was described as technically not feasible and hampering innovation (Ebers et al. 2021). However, Art. 10 AIA needs to be met only sufficiently in relation to the purpose of AI system (Veale and Borgesius 2021). Ebers et al. argue that some privacy by design techniques like differential privacy intentionally introduce noise in the datasets in order to protect personal data, which might degrade the accuracy of the data. Further, privacy by default and by design might collide with requirements for dataset quality, fairness, and model performance. Similarly, in order to mitigate bias and affected groups by the ML model, it is often required that more data is collected, which shows again tension between the principles of accuracy and data minimization or fairness (Finck and Biega 2021). Another example are the algorithms which might require more data to improve performance accuracy, which again introduces a trade-off between accuracy and data minimization. However, there are examples of techniques for enlarging datasets by preserving their statistical properties such as data augmentation and perturbation that do not necessarily impact accuracy and also do not require more personal data collection (Borj et al. 2021).

The identified legal requirements for datasets show that the design, description, and attributes of reusable datasets for the training and validation of machine learning models is an area of ongoing techno-legal research and standardization. An EU study reported that currently there are no universally agreed standards for data quality assessments for machine learning datasets (de Miguel Beriain et al. 2022, p. 27).

From a fair trial perspective, the selection of the datasets to be acquired, examined, or analysed is determinative, as it allows verification of the origin and integrity of the digital evidence discovered. The description of the data source and its unique identification, the acquisition space, and its integrity verification, as well as the storage path to one or more datasets used in the digital forensic investigation are requirements of the validation process. The defence must have knowledge of the raw data material in order to challenge the lawfulness and lawful use of the datasets, their quality, and the potential impact of the data processing in the investigation on its integrity and reliability. In cases where the prosecution is in possession of the only forensically preserved datasets of interest to the defence, the judge is in a position to evaluate the conditions under which the defence can be granted access to the forensic copies.

3.3.2.1 Problems with DF Datasets

In digital forensics, dataset is defined as a set of related, discrete elements that have varying meanings based on the context and are used in some type of experiment or analysis (Grajeda et al. 2017).

> **GAP 9** The main problems with datasets for AI modelling in law enforcement are the lack of training, validation, and testing datasets for research as well as data protection and intellectual property rights which limit further the availability and reuse of datasets. In addition, certain trade-offs between real and synthetic datasets are identified.

3.3.2.1.1 Lack of Training, Validation, and Testing Datasets

The lack of real, high-quality, publicly available datasets for research and development of ML techniques in law enforcement is identified as one of the major problems in the field (Baggili and Breitinger 2015). Moreover, criminal (anomalous) data patterns change over time, which requires ML models to be retrained and re-evaluated continuously on several, diverse datasets.

A common problem, described by Solanke, is the overuse of the limited available datasets for testing digital forensics methods and tools which leads to "solutions gradually adapting to a dataset over time" (Solanke and Biasiotti 2022). This leads to generalizability questions when methods are tested only on one dataset as well as relevance issues as these datasets become outdated. For example, the DARPA dataset, largely used for intrusion detection development, was criticized as being out of date as it does not include many actual attacks and also in terms of the quality of the dataset development (Torrano-Gimenez et al. 2015). Others argue that most of the public datasets for digital forensics research are suffering from "insufficient diversity, poor timeliness, unrealistic or missing background noise [...and] unknown ground truth" (Göbel et al. 2022).

The quality of the dataset impacts the performance of the ML model and whether it is going to generalize well. Investigative data is usually heterogenous, with a large amount of noise as it is extracted from users' activity on different devices, while criminals might take anti-forensics actions to damage or destroy the data. Acquired data is often imbalanced, incomplete, and sparse. For example, a study of ML techniques for detecting suspicious files in file system metadata concluded that the influence of imbalanced classes for the model's performance is insufficiently studied (Du and Scanlon 2019). High dimensionality and class over-laps, if not addressed correctly, might lead to poor generalization, unreliable parameter estimation, and reproducibility problems. Often ML methods for evidence analysis are applied on DF tool outputs (Serhal and Le-Khac 2021; and Du Scanlon 2019). This means that there is an assumption that the tool acquired and interpreted the dataset correctly, which is an inherent limitation of statistical models. Current all-in-one DF tools do not allow parameters to be tuned during data acquisition for the purpose of ML which shifts the focus on pre-processing techniques.

> **GAP 10** Before developing the ML model where pre-processing and relevant feature engineering are performed there is no possibility to know if the training, validation, and testing datasets have statistical features and are of sufficient quality for the specific task at hand.

For example, it might be that the dataset has statistical features to solve a particular problem, but the examiner did not discover them. It also might be that the dataset simply does not have the characteristics required by the forensic task. Initial estimation of the dataset characteristics can be done based on previous models, but this requires systematic research and development in the ML models for each specific task.

3.3.2.1.2 Data Protection and Intellectual Property Limitations

In addition, legal requirements for data protection and intellectual property are often seen as a major barrier for access and research of real datasets and ever-increasing demands for synthetic ones (Grajeda et al. 2017; Horsman and Lyle 2021; Solanke and Biasiotti 2022). To the contrary, as examined in Section 3.2.4 many of the principles of data governance and data protection can be met in big datasets for law enforcement purposes. In addition, the legislation is in favour of creating free flow of information and altruistic data sharing in the public domain provided that the legal requirements are met. However, from our personal experience enabling access to investigative data and compliance with data protection requirements (which soon will also include AIA compliance) is a complex, bureaucratic, and time-consuming process. A study in mobile forensics, also reported the hurdles to get access to real investigative data and that much of the ML research in this sub-domain is done on a "dataset made available to the researchers by an Italian LEA" (Serhal and Le-Khac 2021). In addition, the current *sui generis* database right in the EU might render many high-quality, labelled datasets proprietary, which is criticized in the literature as hampering AI innovation (Kop 2021).

Another legal and technical problem is repurposing of datasets, e.g., which were not created for the purpose of digital forensics but end up being used in this way such as the Enron dataset (Horsman and Lyle 2021). Repurposing will always require a new legal evaluation and a validation of the dataset for its suitability to be used (1) in the domain of digital forensics; (2) for the purpose of training ML models; (3) and for the specific forensic task.

Training datasets are dependent on, and might become rapidly obsolete with, new versions of underlying technologies. For example, Hargreaves et al. trained neural network for timeline reconstruction in file systems and reported that a new training dataset is required for newer versions of the applications running on the file system (Hargreaves and Patterson 2012).

3.3.2.1.3 Real and Synthetic Datasets

The digital investigations are dependent on access to real, up-to-date datasets, while the utility of synthetic datasets is limited. Nevertheless, currently most available datasets for academic DF research are synthetic and only around 1/3 originated from real data (Grajeda et al. 2017).

Real datasets refer to data generated by a user(s) during usual activity and interaction with the system. A synthetic dataset is a dataset generated under controlled testing conditions, for instance, computer-generated, simulation or experiment (Grajeda et al. 2017).

Nevertheless, both real and synthetic datasets have advantages and disadvantages to be considered. Real datasets represent the behaviour of computer-users and allow ML models to learn patterns encountered in investigative data. However, as examined by NIST, in such datasets the ground truth is hard to determine, there is large amount of noise, effort is required to obtain sufficient datasets so that there is coverage of all features, and creating the dataset takes significant effort including access authorization and legal compliance (US National Institute of Standards and Technology 2022). In synthetic datasets the ground truth is usually known. They can be kept small, allow noise control and selecting attributes that can reduce dimensionality, class imbalance, and mislabelled classes problems. Synthetic datasets can be designed to fit different investigative or testing scenarios, they can easily adapt to changes in the underlying software and support sharing, reuse, and reproducibility studies as well as public disclosure of results without legal restrictions. However, it is questionable whether synthetic data can be designed well enough to resemble real-world criminal activity and whether a ML model trained on synthetic dataset will perform well on real data. For example, researchers wrote a simulator to detect money laundering which used "aggregated anonymized data from a real financial dataset to generate synthetic data that closely resembles the transactions dynamics, statistical properties and causal dynamics observed in the original dataset, while incorporating any malicious behaviour of interest" (Lopez-Rojas and Barneaud 2019). They reported, that the false negatives (undetected fraud) were considerably less under strict controls. Other identified drawbacks were that it is difficult to build a realistic model due to the complexity of variables and parameters, biased information and class overlap remains an issue (Lopez-Rojas and Axelsson 2012).

The comparison shows that synthetic datasets can be used for cross-comparison of algorithms and to test their accuracy according to data attributes and a concrete investigative problem. For example, they can be used to analyse the statistical properties of the given dataset in order to choose the appropriate feature selection algorithm. In order to understand if the learned patterns on a synthetic data are transferable to real-world data the examiner must be able to clearly describe the differences between synthetic and real data. This might be quite challenging in practice.

GAP 11 Apart from research and model development activities or method validation testing – synthetic datasets can hardly replace knowledge that can be extracted from real-world situations.

As a recommendation for dataset engineering reliability and validation a three-step schema can be used:

  i. Initial development and modelling on public dataset – for comparison of algorithms performance
 ii. Experiment on a synthetic dataset designed as close to a real one as possible (in cooperation with law enforcement)
iii. Application of the AI model to real law enforcement dataset (internally)

3.3.2.2 Dataset Sustainability

There is an argument for dataset sustainability which might require a legislative initiative to differentiate between explorative and operational data analysis. Explorative data analysis (EDA) is a typical data engineering task as it requires that the data is looked at from as many angles as possible to identify interesting features, facts about the dataset, or new phenomenon (Morgenthaler 2009). EDA is independent of the ML model or specific tasks. Therefore, EDA can be performed by an independent dataset engineering centre which is concerned only with dataset quality validation. It also ensures sustainability and legal compliance as it provides for reuse of datasets rather than collection of datasets for each task.

Operational data analysis (ODA) comes into play once the dataset is needed for a specific task. Therefore, ODA is part of the ML modelling, and in particular feature engineering, and is based on the preliminary EDA. If legal authorization is different for EDA and ODA bodies this will allow better validation of the datasets once in dataset design and once in dataset modelling, while at the same time will ensure continuous reuse of datasets for domain-specific tasks.

GAP 12 Even if the production of high-quality datasets for AI models is emerging as a new techno-legal niche, legislative efforts are simultaneously abstract and demanding. Arguably most LEA have neither the resources nor the know-how for dataset engineering. More centralized efforts for rapid generation and reuse of high-quality datasets for AI in law enforcement, including differentiation between explorative and operational data analysis – are required.

3.3.3 Pre-processing for Input: Trade-offs between Accuracy and Computational Costs

Art. 10 (2) (c) AIA requires quality procedures and documentation on annotation, labelling, cleaning, enrichment, and aggregation of training, validation, and testing datasets.

The raw dataset can contain structured or unstructured data in different formats or an aggregation of heterogenous datasets. In a broad sense, pre-processing is conducted during dataset engineering encompassing tasks like indexing and data recovery (e.g., decryption; decompression), aggregation of datasets, format unification, fixing incomplete or removing redundant data, sorting or filtering based on data reduction and triage methods (e.g., hash analysis; data deduplication) (see Section 3.2.2). Data protection measures like the removal of identifying attributes, anonymization, or pseudonymization are usually done during pre-processing in dataset engineering according to the privacy impact assessment. (ISO/IEC 23053, 2022)

By contrast, *pre-processing for input (in narrow sense)* means that the data is prepared and transformed for the specific forensic task. It refers to tasks that improve the quality of the data, e.g., by normalization, labelling, data cleaning, or augmentation.

The pre-processing is part of the validation process because data transformation impacts the accuracy and reliability of the data in the range relevant for the investigation. Pre-processing may introduce alteration and information-loss to be accounted for and thereby impacts the accuracy of the feature selection and results.

Statistics show that it is the most time-consuming and expertise-demanding task, requiring 60% of the time to build a model (CrowdFlower 2016). Pre-processing has two distinct phases: data preparation and data sampling are examined here. However, feature extraction and selection, although classified as data reduction pre-processing tasks, are part of the modelling (processing) and are examined in the next section.

GAP 13 The impact of pre-processing techniques on the ML model performance is insufficiently researched. As pre-processing techniques are task and dataset specific, their full documentation for validation purposes should be mandated. Regrettably, in current practices such information is largely omitted.

A study in topic modelling for network link analysis in dark web chats demonstrated that LDA algorithms are sensitive to pre-processing and following a strict and iterative pre-processing and hyperparameters tuning can improve the performance of the algorithm. (Johnsen and Franke 2019) The authors emphasized that information on pre-processing techniques in topic modelling is missing, while such techniques vary widely. The impact of pre-processing in data mining is well-explored in other domains such as marketing (Crone et al. 2006) and medicine. (Benhar et al. 2020) The studies show that the impact of pre-processing techniques varies by ML model, indicating that for each ML algorithm and setup only a specific set of pre-processing techniques will achieve accuracy improvement, while others may have no impact.

A common mistake in ML is the violation of the strict separation between training, validation, and testing datasets during pre-processing. Although the whole dataset is split in three, often features or parameters are calculated for the whole. This leads to overestimation of the ML model accuracy and undetected biases and is described as data snooping. (Arp et al. 2021)

Pre-processing for input creates a working dataset which can be constructed according to purpose limitation and data minimization principles to ensure that LEAs select for processing only data relevant for the evidence discovery task. Pre-processing is a determinative stage also because exculpatory evidence can be missed during pre-processing. Since sometimes the detection of outliers might be crucial for the investigation, cutting them at a very early stage might be undesirable. The decision of which pre-processing methods are to be employed is crucial in order to evaluate if the data is of sufficient quality and nature to support or refute the investigative hypothesis. As this decision depends on the sufficient understanding of the dataset and includes subjective evaluation it has to be assessed for prejudicial effects arising from assumptions of guilt or early "tunnel vision". Disclosure of the pre-processing methods and their justification can assist the judge to assess if the defence should be given an opportunity to be involved in the selection of the pre-processing methods or to comment and challenge on the data range for further processing.

Pre-processing techniques are very task and domain specific and insufficiently studied for digital forensics. Improving reliability and robustness of acquisition and pre-processing techniques is crucial for data protection and AIA compliance. For example, outlier removal, data normalization, labelling, feature extraction and selection, are all forms of data minimization and data governance. De-identification is also a pre-processing technique for removing the association between a set of identifying attributes and the data principal. (ISO/IEC 23053, 2022)

GAP 14 There is a need for a taxonomy of pre-processing techniques and their advantages and disadvantages in the context of data protection, data governance, and bias mitigation requirements.

3.3.3.1 Data Cleaning

Common data cleaning methods include outlier removal and missing values imputation. There are statistical methods for outlier removal which are suitable for numeric data and clustering methods. In DF outliers might degrade the learning process as irrelevant or redundant data impact both speed and accuracy. To the contrary, outliers can be also of great importance for the investigation as they can represent evidence for abnormalities associated with suspicious activities. Therefore, methods where the outliers can be studied and visualized might be of greater utility than completely removing them *ab initio*. However, studying outliers in large, complex datasets from different sources manually is very resource and time consuming. Therefore, clustering techniques can be used as an initial data cleaning approach. For example, Flaglien et al. observed that classification of files for detection of malware involved in online banking fraud is inefficient, because of the lack of details about specific malware characteristics or signatures (Flaglien 2018). As a pre-processing step the authors used clustering to derive structured representation and visualization of common linked patterns from all involved sources. This allowed the investigators with domain specific knowledge to further classify files of interest. Consequently, clustering methods for data cleaning have advantages over statistical outlier removal.

3.3.3.2 Normalization

Normalization is used to tackle big differences in the range of numerical features and to ensure that the features are comparable when training an ML model. There are data-range, distribution, and structure-based approaches. Many real datasets in digital forensics exhibit non-uniform, skewed distributions. (Nagy 1983) data-range methods such as quantile function[31] are better suited to handle normalization problems in such datasets as they allow probability distribution to be studied. Normalization tasks can be also studied according to the digital forensics domain. For example, for IoT ML models Kebande et al. also recommended domain specific based on a uniform random variable, based on ranks or based on some scaling approaches (Kebande et al. 2020).

3.3.3.3 Labelling

Labelling is defined as a process to assign a target variable to a sample. In the classical case, digital forensic expert knowledge is used for labelling a training dataset. Labelling is mostly done manually and is very time consuming. For

---

[31] See Wikipedia page. https://en.wikipedia.org/wiki/Quantile accessed 30.11.2022.

example, Serhal et al. examined machine learning based solutions with features extracted from file metadata to identify possible smart phone files of interest regarding terrorism. Only 6% of the files were marked of interest to the investigation. Files of interest depend on the type of the investigation task. However, terrorism is a very broad term and does not limit the investigative task. As the labelling is highly subjective validation information should include the reasoning behind the selection and possible disagreements between experts in order to mitigate bias and to prove that the labelling was relevant to the task.

As the amount of data increases, manual labelling of data based on expert knowledge although important, might no longer be feasible. In addition to expert knowledge labelling, automated approaches can be tested such as semi-supervized or machine-labelling. Sub-samples can be labelled by the expert and a classifier can further machine label the whole dataset. Other techniques like deep learning for image captioning (Hossain et al. 2019) or word masking based on BERT (Devlin et al. 2019) where models have to predict words missing from a sentence, can be used for automation of the labelling process. However, those approaches depend on good pre-processing to ensure that samples are representative and relevant. Previous studies in defining useful features for a concrete investigative problem can be useful.

3.3.3.4 Data Augmentation

The performance evaluation is not reliable if the testing set is too small (Kononenko and Kukar 2007, p. 81). Data augmentation can be used to enlarge the dataset to improve performance by generating synthetic data that have similar data distributions to the real data (Fan et al. 2021).

Data perturbation and augmentation to enlarge and improve the utility of a real dataset was demonstrated by researchers of predatory chat detection (Borj et al. 2021). These pre-processing techniques can be also used to ensure compliance with data protection as the added synthetic data can prevent re-identification of individuals. However, the reliability of the synthetic data depends on expert knowledge and correct identification of relevant data attributes.

3.3.4 Modelling

ISO defines as part of the modelling feature extraction and selection, algorithm selection, and hyperparameter tuning. From a legal point of view, the modelling processes are related also to ensuring fairness of processing, accountability, and explainability.

3.3.4.1 Feature Extraction and Selection

In many cases the data points of interest are significantly outnumbered by the available features. High dimensionality problems, class variances, and small disjuncts can cause overfitting, poor generalization, unreliable parameter prediction, and high computational costs. Dimensionality reduction algorithms have a significant impact on what is considered relevant data for evidence.

Feature extraction and selection is one of the most important processes to tackle those issues. It requires combined knowledge and reasoning about statistical properties of data as well as their forensic properties. From a technical point of view, choosing sufficiently representative features for the dataset is crucial for improvement of data quality and classification algorithm performance as well as for reliability validation. From a legal standpoint, this task is relevant to comply with purpose limitation and data minimization principles and to prove data governance, bias mitigation, and fairness of processing. Nevertheless (Qadir and Noor 2021), report that researchers often neglect the feature selection process.

> **GAP 15** Studies of feature selection algorithms and their dependences on dataset characteristics are scarce.

Feature extraction aims to construct relevant features from the original dataset. Feature selection is used to decide which is the smallest number of features relevant to the classification problem that does not affect classifier accuracy. (Nguyen, thesis) Usually, feature selection is used to handle redundant and irrelevant data, while feature extraction methods are proposed to handle class noise problems. It is suggested, that feature selection methods that handle redundant and irrelevant features at once are more robust compared to methods that discretely handle feature redundancy and/or irrelevant features (Khalid).

All feature construction methods have limitations. Further, the *ugly duckling* rule (Duda et al. 2001, p. 461) states that in the absence of assumptions there is no best feature representation, ergo, there is always subjectivity and, therefore, bias concerns in feature selection. Further, adding more features to the model does not improve statistical significance. For example, in recidivism prediction researchers showed that a simple linear predictor with only two features performs nearly equivalent to COMPAS with its 137 features (Dressel and Farid 2018). Therefore, DF experts should not restrict themselves to any one feature selection method but use multiple robust feature selection methods instead and compare the results (Fan et al. 2021; Khalid et al. 2014; Nguyen et al. 2010). For example, Qadir and Noor, 2021 report that "decision Tree give best results for features like PE and n-grams while Neural Networks give overall good results with various features". Further, Nguyen et al. showed that feature selection algorithms perform differently depending on whether the dataset has features that are linearly or non-linearly correlated to the class label and to each other. For example, one of the most popular, feature extraction methods is principal component analysis (PCA) as it covers standard deviation, covariance, and eigenvectors and is largely recommended in ML for file systems analysis (Du and Scanlon 2019; Mohammad and Alqahtani 2019), in biometrics (Karamizadeh et al. 2013), and in image forgery detection. Those studies discuss that PCA requires feature normalization to a certain range as forensic data is heterogenous. In addition, PCA works on linearly correlated features. In order to avoid information loss and optimize accuracy, nonlinear feature extraction methods should be explored (Fan et al. 2021). For feature selection, it is also known that Pearson's correlation coefficient works only on linearly correlated features. Further, feature selection and extraction depend on sufficient understanding of the data structure and contextual knowledge or special expertise about the forensic task. Combining expert knowledge and automatic feature selection methods is considered more reliable than focusing on single approach (Torrano-Gimenez et al. 2015).

The requirement for diversifying feature selection and extraction methods is related also to the sensitivity of the classifier to the feature selection method and the data. For example, a study in forensic document author identification compared different feature selection methods and their impact on different classifiers (Chitrakar 2013). Importantly, the research showed that *(i)* some feature selection method perform well on small datasets but do not scale well; *(ii)* some classifiers performed better with specific feature selection methods. Classification accuracy achieved with different feature construction strategies is highly sensitive to the type of data (Khalid 2014) and therefore domain specific.

The process of feature selection must be fully documented and traceable. Issues with *feature selection* are related to inappropriate selection method, e.g., insufficient detection of statistical properties representative for the dataset and heuristic feature search strategies. The defence should be given knowledge of the feature selection and extraction method in order to be able to challenge on valid grounds the digital evidence relevance and probative value. Forensic feature extraction should be done in a deterministic way to ensure that no data is omitted or transformed at random, to allow recomputing of results under different hypotheses, and to enable exculpatory evidence search when the defence has a well-founded request.

> **GAP 16** The limitations of feature selection and extraction methods must be studied with respect to the dataset characteristics. Appropriate feature construction requires combining expert knowledge and automatic feature selection methods. Research in digital forensics expert knowledge that can be used for different machine learning tasks is still scarce.

3.3.4.2 Algorithm Selection and Evaluation Metrics

According to the *no free lunch theorem* there is no superior algorithm for solving a problem (Duda et al. 2001). However, testing algorithm performance shows that some algorithms can outperform others because they match a particular problem better. Consequently, there are no problem-independent reasons to choose one algorithm over another. Ergo, the algorithms for pre-processing, feature extraction, and classifiers must be tested and documented for reliability validation in a way that allows evaluation of their suitability and limitations in relation to the different law enforcement tasks and dataset characteristics.

In criminology, intelligence, or security investigation there is no burden or standard of proof and all algorithms can be used if suitable to the dataset and the task. In contrast, in order to comply with fair trial requirements and the high burden of proof in criminal investigations, only deterministic algorithms should be used. Algorithms that do not depend on heuristics give reproducible results and allow validation of audit trail, and explainability in further proceedings. However, some deterministic algorithms, like deep learning might be not explainable.

As digital forensics actions comprise automated processing and human-machine interactions, the reliability of *algorithm selection* for each processing operation has two elements: algorithmic accountability (objective measurements); and human interaction (subjective measurements). Objective measurements are related to the algorithm type, hyperparameters tuning, limitations, and software implementation. Subjective measurements are related to the assumptions and constraints imposed on the method by the examiner during parameterization. For example, the most routine task of a forensic examiner is the search for relevant data. The logic of the processing consists of three elements: the search space (working dataset); the search method (e.g., Boolean, string) and the search target (e.g., keywords). The first two elements can be objectively-measured while the third is subjective. The search space (dataset) might be challenged on lawfulness grounds if LEA lacked or exceeded authorization or otherwise violated the legal basis for acquiring the data. The judge can also decide on the expert's competency and on the need to validate the adequacy of the search method and algorithm according to the forensic task in case this is challenged. The search target can be re-examined for cognitive bias and rerun with different control parameters (keywords). In addition, documenting subjective and objective measurements in processing benefits LEAs by allowing them to trace back processing operations to systematically correct errors and verify inferences from different data sources. The law requires clear separation of facts from inferences, which is translated for digital evidence and system design as strict separation of the objective and subjective measurements in the processing operation, but accounting for both.

Appropriate performance evaluation metrics is another important validation issue that needs to be examined in the context of criminal investigations. Solanke gives a general overview of evaluation metrics for classification, clustering, and regression tasks in ML (Solanke and Biasiotti 2022) but specifics of the dataset or the context always impact this decision. For example, in highly imbalanced datasets F1 score is preferred, as accuracy measures are strongly influenced by the majority class for all predictions and, therefore, generally unsuitable (Du and Scanlon 2019). IoT forensics require context-based evaluation metrics due to the lack of initial information about such devices (Kebande et al. 2020). Misclassification, misinterpretation or missing features might result in false negatives. This can be detrimental for the outcome of the investigation (and potentially trial) in cases where important or exculpatory evidence is missed. The general recommendation in digital investigations is to prioritize high recall scores.

In commercial digital forensics tools the algorithm and its implementation are fixed. This means that reliability validation requires disclosure of the general characteristics and limitations of the known algorithms and on demand disclosure of the algorithm's implementation. Implementation errors in the underlying software can have a legal impact as well. For example, a vulnerability in the encryption implementation for Android mobile phones which leads to data leakage and can be exploited by LEAs for data acquisition was discovered (Alendal et al. 2021). This requires legal safeguards in respect to the authorization of offensive evidence acquisition methods which undermine security, responsible disclosure of security vulnerabilities discovered by LEAs (Fukami et al. 2021), and awareness of such errors that can potentially destroy evidence if criminals discover them first. Errors related to the implementation of algorithms in software are systematic in nature. Therefore, NIST recommends error mitigation analysis rather than statistical error rate which is only useful for random errors (US National Institute of Standards and Technology 2022).

> **GAP 17** Heuristics in algorithm selection and parameterization are not sufficiently accounted for in investigation. Subjective measurements in algorithm selection and algorithm implementation errors can degrade its performance and lead to data leakages.

3.3.4.3 Fairness of Processing and Bias Mitigation

Mitigation of bias and discrimination in AI systems is a central legislative concern. Art. 10 (5) AIA states that for the purpose of bias mitigation providers may process special categories of personal data defined in Art. 9 GDPR and Art. 10 LED such as race, ethnicity, political opinions, religious or philosophical beliefs, genetic, biometric or health data. GDPR and LED, in contrast, restrict the processing of sensitive data, especially in the context of automated decisions and profiling (Art. 22 GDPR and Art. 11 LED). EDPS and EDPB criticized this provision as not sufficiently clear to create a legal basis for the processing of sensitive data, and especially in the context of LED additional protective measures need to be designed and assessed for compliance with data protection (EDPB-EDPS 2021). AIA does not provide a definition of bias or what forms of biases are prohibited (Ebers et al. 2021). In addition, the legal concept of bias is very complex. It refers to both direct discrimination (where individuals or groups are suffering harm based on their protected attributes) and indirect discrimination (apparently neutral provision, criterion or practice would put persons of a racial or ethnic origin at a particular disadvantage compared with other persons).[32] Assessment of bias requires evaluation of how the processing impacts concrete individuals as well as specific groups and it refers to more complex social problems embedded in data. Scholars have shown the need to process protected attributes in order to achieve equal treatment

---

[32] See Art. 2 (a) and (b) of Council Directive 2000/43/EC of 29 June 2000 implementing the principle of equal treatment between persons irrespective of racial or ethnic origin [2000] OJ L180/22.

and fairness of processing (Hardt et al. 2016), but an open question is still who and how should they conduct such processing (Veale and Binns 2017). Further, ML models can find correlations in data which can disadvantage certain groups in society or reinforce stereotypes in a contra-intuitive way which requires further discussion on the correct legal response (Wachter 2022). Research shows that data-driven approaches amplify confirmation bias (Schwartz et al. 2022) and subsequently amplify biases in humans (Glickman and Sharot 2022).

Fairness of processing and bias mitigation require an overall assessment of the ML model and depending on the model different techniques can be used during pre-processing, processing, or post-processing. A recent study discusses statistical bias and discrimination and explores the techniques proposed to develop more fair processing in different ML models (de Miguel Beriain et al. 2022). NIST also published a guideline to bias mitigation for AI systems (Schwartz et al. 2022). The guidelines summarize current state of the art techniques to mitigate bias in ML models which can be applied in different stages of processing. They are highly model, task, and data specific and not specifically designed for law enforcement purposes.

> **GAP 18** An emerging techno-legal problem is that the draft AIA leaves bias mitigation to providers of AI systems, but recent studies show extreme socio-technical complexity which makes questionable the ability of AI developers to act as governors. Overlaps or differences between statistical bias and the legal concept of discriminatory bias must be studied in greater depth as to how they can be mitigated effectively in AI modelling. Considering that bias mitigation is highly specific to the data, model, and the domain, while law enforcement is a domain of high-sensitivity – rather specific guidelines are needed.

3.3.4.4 Explainability in AI Forensics

The question whether individuals should have a right to explanation is under legal debate and the AIA refers to interpretability but does not clarify any requirements for desired level of transparency and accountability. In fact, based on a classification of the level of explainable AI for digital forensics (Hall et al. 2022), the AIA requires merely output interpretation which could be interpreted as comprehensible AI models showing relevant features and confidence scores. However, we refer to the concept of *truly explainable* models where the line of reasoning for the decision-making process, human-understandable features of the input data and individual decision can be deconstructed to provide justification. There are several techno-legal incentives that fully explainable and interactive AI systems are the way forward in digital investigations.

Explainability in AI (XAI) enables compliance with fair trial procedural guarantees. Legal and AI scholars criticize the need for a right to explanation from data protection point of view as a vague concept, legally unclear as to when explanation is to be sought, what an explanation entails, to what extent ML experts can provide the information actually needed for legal decision making, and multiple practical limitations of explanations which may lead to a false sense of transparency (Ananny and Crawford 2018; Edwards and Veale 2017). However, in criminal proceedings fair trial obligations clearly require explanations with respect to AI systems used in evidence discovery. XAI is crucial for the preparation and cross-examination of expert report, to map expert findings on exculpatory evidence, and to facilitate defence queries on later stages of the proceedings. AI systems introduce information asymmetries between the parties in criminal proceedings which need to be mitigated in the light of the equality of arms principle.

Further XAI is helpful for identifying bias and prejudicial effects embedded in the model which can significantly impact innocent suspects. Arp et al. examined research in advantages and limitations for explainable deep learning and argued that explainability is a crucial element for identifying spurious correlations in datasets. Such correlations occur when artifacts unrelated to the problem create shortcut patterns for separating the classes and lead to the adaptation of the model to those patterns, rather than task-related patterns (Arp et al. 2021).

The type of explanation is domain specific and depends on the AI model. Some models like small decision trees are readily explainable, while others like neural network might not be fully susceptible to human understanding. From a legal point of view, Edwards and Veale provide a taxonomy for "*subject-centric* explanations focussing on particular regions of a model around a query […] for interactive exploration, as do explanation systems based on learning a model from outside rather than taking it apart (*pedagogical* versus decompositional explanations) in dodging developers' worries of intellectual property or trade secrets disclosure". Further, Atkinson provides a theoretical overview of techniques used in AI and law for explainability (Atkinson et al. 2020). The study supports the view that it is not so much required to examine the design and all components of AI systems but rather explanation is sought as to "why a particular classification is appropriate" or "the key data items which gave rise to the inference", where "the explanation is presented not in probabilistic terms but as scenarios or arguments" or case comparison to similar cases. For example, Lau and Biedermann propose the use of nearest neighbour data to explain to individuals why they are classified in a certain group (e.g., as suspects) (Lau and Biedermann 2019). There are also tools which assist the forensic examiner to understand the impact of the selected features on the output (Bollé et al. 2020) Bollé also emphasize that current machine learning approaches are not designed to measure the performance of the system for a given purpose, to assist forensic practitioners in understanding the criteria for reaching given output, or how such output can be evaluated in the context of the forensic hypotheses.

A comprehensive overview of XAI for digital forensics referred to many specific challenges such as a large number of features (e.g., pieces of evidence), missing data, multiple conflicting decision criteria, and the need for interactive learning (Kelly et al. 2020). Nevertheless, the authors emphasize the importance not only of XAI but of interactive machine-expert learning such as fuzzy rule-based models combined with knowledge base and rules provided by experts for optimizing results.

It is a common misconception among data scientists that if the AI system is used only to provide intelligence for the investigation, but not for the evaluation of evidence, LEAs are exempt from transparency and accountability obligations (Hall et al. 2022). In fact, the use of AI systems early in the investigation stage may have significant impact on the presumption of innocence and on the evaluation of the lawfulness of the investigative measures and evidence based on AI intelligence.

It should be noted that process level accountability does not require full transparency such as source code disclosure *per se*. Reviewing source code abstractly is a complex and time-consuming task, which in addition is ineffective to reliably detect errors in complex machine operations. As argued by Taylor et. al. "more crucial than a review of source code, is the ability to have access to outputs that demonstrate each step of a calculation" (Taylor et al. 2017). Only in certain specified cases should source code be made available for scrutiny, for example where similar errors occur across various tools, indicating the use of a common library is a root cause. Nevertheless, in most cases process-level documentation of the parameters of the processing according to validation criteria is the minimum that can enable sufficient legal and scientific scrutiny to satisfy fair trial and demonstrate coherence in the digital evidence discovery without degrading efficiency. Further, there is a need for accountability information to be automatically generated in parallel with the processing operations so that certain reliability validation tasks can be automated for more complex methods. Lastly, as argued there are different techniques for validation of digital forensics methods and tools which might be adapted to different levels of accountability and explainability.

> **GAP 19** It is unclear to what extend explainability of AI models have benefits for the criminal proceedings beyond validation. Different levels and types of explainability might be required according to the recipient, e.g., AI user or other parties in the proceedings or the specific use of AI system, e.g., identifying suspect, assessment of reliability of inculpatory evidence, or identifying a vehicle. Explainability is currently not interpreted in the context of defence rights.

3.4 AI Use in Investigations: AI System Design + Data Protection = Fair Trial?

It is questionable if data protection principles (LED) in combination with AI systems design requirements (AIA) ensures sufficient protection of individuals in relation to the use of AI systems in criminal investigations.

As argued, the purpose limitation principle is often a matter of skilful legal drafting and there are no clear mechanisms to verify or enforce the principle in different stages of processing. Data minimization, individual and group bias mitigation, and data quality principles can often contradict each other and lead to trade-offs in practice.

The accountability regime created by GDPR and LED for personal data, is extended by AIA to the whole AI supply chain (EDPB-EDPS 2021). However, those rules are high-level and in the absence of concrete guidelines of how to evaluate which AI model is permissible for which purpose or which safeguards are sufficient to mitigate bias and error, the high standard of legal certainty in criminal procedure cannot be met. Moreover, the AIA and LED accountability process is insufficiently interpreted in the context of other fundamental principles in criminal procedure, in relation to fair trial requirements, and in respect to existing digital forensics standards. Such considerations are even more important to address potential misuses of AI systems in criminal proceedings and power imbalances AI can introduce in the criminal procedure.

It is questionable, whether providers of AI systems are best suited to perform evaluation of systems impact on the presumption of innocence or its compliance with fundamental criminal justice values. For example, is there a need for new defence rights in relation to AI technology or how the existing ones are interpreted as a matter of public policy? Further complex intellectual property and security issues arise from the examination of proprietary software by law enforcement, which are currently not regulated sufficiently. Moreover, some fundamental principles in digital forensics such as data integrity preservation collide with data protection and AIA design regime.

In the absence of a legal regime to align fair trial objectives in AI-assisted criminal procedures, important questions of legitimacy and legal certainty arise both in terms of suitable transposition of defence rights to AI models, as well as suitable validation and standardization in AI forensics. For example, algorithmic prevention and detection of crime interfere seriously with the presumption of innocence. In the current legislative framework, such a risk to the presumption of innocence presumably will be evaluated only by the AI system provider under Art. 9 AIA risk assessment. Public-private partnerships and providers of AI-evidence systems should not be responsible for risk assessments that can have effects on the criminal proceedings as this not only introduces power imbalances between prosecution and defence or between the LEA and the AI system providers but also makes the rights and guarantees for defendants very uncertain. As identified a reliability validation framework and independent validation bodies are a necessity for datasets, algorithms, and AI models testing. However, the legislator's focus on accountability and validation is insufficient to replace the missing procedural rights framework in criminal proceedings.

Digital investigations require increased EU-wide and international cooperation and evidence exchange. Current and proposed legislation in the EU aims to provide legal instruments to enable and facilitate cooperation between law enforcement agencies. However, the legislative framework does little to harmonize evidence law, establish principles for digital forensics, or enable defence rights in relation to the increased use of technology in criminal procedure (Gless 2013; Kusak 2019; Wendy De Bondt and Gert Vermeulen 2010). For example, the EU commission developed the E-evidence proposals, which aim to facilitate European Production and Preservation orders[33] and in addition entered into negotiations with the USA for an agreement on cross-border access to electronic evidence.[34] Analysis of these developments is out of scope here, but it should be noted that these legislative initiatives do not address defence procedural rights, digital forensics questions or evidence reliability standards. As argued by Tosza, the EIO regime does not "attempt to unify or harmonise the law of evidence", while the proposed European production order lacks "any safeguards for ensuring the accuracy and reliability of digital data for criminal proceedings" (Tosza 2020). Art. 2(4) AIA also excludes the use of AI systems for law enforcement international cooperation from its scope. Apart from the data protection concerns this exclusion once again confirms that international criminal procedure issues in relation to technology-facilitated investigations are largely overlooked in the current legal framework. This raises questions on evidence forum shopping and parallel construction of evidence, as well as procedures to examine and challenge AI-generated evidence from international investigations.

Finally, LEA use of AI has specifics which require foreseeable, domain-specific, and precise regulatory approach rooted in criminal justice values and their transposition to AI technology. Moreover, an international agreement or standards on cross-border procedures and evidence exchange is an important guarantee for fair trials but currently underdeveloped in the legislative reforms. The complex interaction between GDPR, LED, AIA, and fair trial principle leads to fragmentation and legal uncertainty and might cause inconsistent interpretation, implementation, and enforcement of diverse techno-legal rules among different law enforcement agencies, which might lead to a different level of competence and evidence quality, different treatment of defendants, and poor integration of AI systems in LEA work.

Active participation of the defence or audit trails for determinative stages in evidence processing may face practical concerns. The need to produce accountability information could reduce efficiency due to increased algorithmic complexity, increased data volume, and the multitude of machine-human operations to be logged in a short period of time. Additionally, there may be confidentiality concerns around certain novel digital forensics methods and tools, which means that access to process-level documentation might be undesirable. Finally, the processing operations, even when documented, might display a level of complexity that is hard to comprehend for a human without deployment of further, likely unavailable, technical means for analysing the documentation. These

---

[33] Proposal for a Regulation of the European Parliament and of the Council on European Production and Preservation Orders for electronic evidence in criminal matters.COM/2018/225 final and additional Directive of the European Parliament and of the Council laying down harmonised rules on the appointment of legal representatives for the purpose of gathering evidence in criminal proceedings. COM (2018) 226 final.
[34] Information note 7295/21 from the European Commission services following the stock-taking meeting with the US on an EU-US Agreement on cross-border access to electronic evidence, 26 March 2021 (LIMITE).

hurdles, require rethinking of the question what kind of procedural rights and safeguards in the AI evidence discovery process will suffice effective challenging of the evidence reliability?

3.5 Conclusion

This chapter started with the questions is the current legislative framework for AI in law enforcement clear and sufficient to ensure fair trial and whether we have sufficient implementation solutions and standards to ensure compliance and reliability validation of AI evidence. It was argued that the adoption of AI-based investigative solutions can face significant hurdles due to the current technical, methodological, and legal fragmentation in digital investigations. The study identified multiple gaps in the legislation and its transposition to AI systems which can be summarized as three common issues: *(i)* how to translate high-level, legal principles into practical implementation solutions; *(ii)* the inevitable trade-offs between some principles in practice *(iii)* the technical feasibility of legal compliance.

The current EU approach to regulate the design and use of AI systems in combination with the existing data protection regime cannot sufficiently enforce fair trial compliance. A domain specific regulation for law enforcement is necessary to address:
- the technological, methodological, and legal fragmentation in digital investigations (Gap 1)
- the need for fair trial compliance of AI-based investigative measures (Gap 2)
- LEA specific risks/ harms and mitigation mechanisms (e.g., AI systems beyond biometrics), which intrusiveness is amplified due to their use specifically in the law enforcement domain such as computer vision, NLP, transfer learning (Gap 3)
- repurposing of commercially developed AI systems and training datasets (Gap 4)
- misuse of AI systems by law enforcement (Gap 5)
- transposition of defence rights to AI systems (Gaps 6 and 7)
- legally compliant AI-based investigative tasks and safeguards on each processing stage (Gap 8)
- the need for dataset engineering for law enforcement purposes and the limitations of both real and synthetic datasets with respect to data quality (Gaps 9–12)
- testing of the legal implications of different processes in the pipeline and their impact on the overall model performance in specific AI applications (Gaps 13–17)
- the techno-legal complexities with bias mitigation in criminal procedure which can be hardly addressed by the current AIA regime (Gap 18)
- explainability of AI systems in different stages of the criminal proceedings and in the context of defence rights. (Gap 19)

The identified gaps need to be addressed in order to prevent their negative effects on the criminal justice system and potential distrust in the scientific validity of AI-driven investigative methods. Designing of techno-legal policies, best practices, and guidelines for every stage of the ML pipeline becomes a crucial component for

LEAs to enable AI systems in investigations, but also to deliver a practical process design which can be gradually improved in the long term. The gap analysis here is a first step towards such policies as it maps legal requirements and best practices for compliance against the ML pipeline by also discussing the emerging challenges. Further research is needed to analyse in-depth each processing step and within concrete LEA applications. From both technical and legal points of view reliable pre-processing and feature construction is identified as the most pressing need.

References

Alendal, G., Axelsson, S., and Dyrkolbotn, G.O. (2021). Chip chop — smashing the mobile phone secure chip for fun and digital forensics. *Forensic Science International: Digital Investigation* 37: 301191. https://doi.org/10.1016/j.fsidi.2021.301191.

Ananny, M. and Crawford, K. (2018). Seeing without knowing: limitations of the transparency ideal and its application to algorithmic accountability. *New Media & Society* 20: 973–989. https://doi.org/10.1177/1461444816676645.

Årnes, A. (ed.) (2018). *Digital Forensics: An Academic Introduction*. Hoboken, NJ: John Wiley & Sons Inc.

Arp, D., Quiring, E., Pendlebury, F. et al. (2021). Dos and don'ts of machine learning in computer security. https://doi.org/10.48550/arXiv.2010.09470.

Ashworth, A. and Zedner, L. (2008). Defending the criminal law: reflections on the changing character of crime, procedure, and sanctions. *Criminal Law, Philosophy* 2: 21–51. https://doi.org/10.1007/s11572-007-9033-2.

Atkinson, K., Bench-Capon, T., and Bollegala, D. (2020). Explanation in AI and law: past, present and future. *Artificial Intelligence* 289.

Awal, M.A., Rabbi, J., Hossain, S.I., and Hashem, M.M.A. (2016). Using linear regression to forecast future trends in crime of Bangladesh. 2016 5th International Conference on Informatics, Electronics and Vision (ICIEV). Presented at the 2016 5th International Conference on Informatics, Electronics and Vision (ICIEV), 333–338. https://doi.org/10.1109/ICIEV.2016.7760021.

Baggili, I. and Behzadan, V. (2019). Founding the domain of AI Forensics. https://doi.org/10.48550/arXiv.1912.06497.

Baggili, I. and Breitinger, F. (2015). Data sources for advancing cyber forensics: what the social world has to offer. Electrical & Computer Engineering and Computer Science Faculty Publications.

Barrett, L.F., Adolphs, R., Marsella, S. et al. (2019). Emotional expressions reconsidered: challenges to inferring emotion from human facial movements. *Psychological Science in the Public Interest* 20: 1–68. https://doi.org/10.1177/1529100619832930.

Beebe, N.L. and Liu, L. (2014). Ranking algorithms for digital forensic string search hits. *Digital Investigation* 11: S124–S132. https://doi.org/10.1016/j.diin.2014.05.007.

Benhar, H., Idri, A., and Fernández-Alemán, J.L. (2020). Data preprocessing for heart disease classification: a systematic literature review. *Computer Methods and Programs in Biomedicine* 195: 105635. https://doi.org/10.1016/j.cmpb.2020.105635.

Biega, A.J. and Finck, M. (2021). Reviving purpose limitation and data minimisation in data-driven systems. *Technology and Regulation* 44–61. https://doi.org/10.26116/techreg.2021.004.

Bollé, T., Casey, E., and Jacquet, M. (2020). The role of evaluations in reaching decisions using automated systems supporting forensic analysis. *Forensic Science International: Digital Investigation* 34: 301016. https://doi.org/10.1016/j.fsidi.2020.301016.

Borj, P.R., Raja, K., and Bours, P. (2021). Detecting sexual predatory chats by perturbed data and balanced ensembles. 2021 International Conference of the Biometrics Special Interest Group (BIOSIG). Presented at the 2021 International Conference of the Biometrics Special Interest Group (BIOSIG), 1–5. https://doi.org/10.1109/BIOSIG52210.2021.9548303.

Boyne, S.M. (2016). Procedural economy in pre-trial procedure: developments in Germany and the United States. Comparative Criminal Procedure.

Callen, C. (2015). Human deliberation in fact-finding and human rights in the law of evidence. https://lawexplores.com/human-deliberation-in-fact-finding-and-human-rights-in-the-law-of-evidence (accessed 20 July 2020).

Campbell, L. (2013). Criminal labels, the European convention on human rights and the presumption of innocence. *The Modern Law Review* 76: 681–707. https://doi.org/10.1111/1468-2230.12030.

Casey, E. (2019). The chequered past and risky future of digital forensics. *Australian Journal of Forensic Sciences* 51: 649–664. https://doi.org/10.1080/00450618.2018.1554090.

Champod, C. and Vuille, J. (2011). Scientific evidence in Europe – admissibility, evaluation and equality of arms. *International Commentary on Evidence* 9: https://doi.org/10.2202/1554-4567.1123.

Chitrakar, A.S. (2013). Author identification from text-based communications: identifying generalized features and computational methods.

Cox, J., Lewih, A., and Rahman, R. (2022). AI, machine learning & big data laws and regulations | Australia | GLI [WWW Document]. GLI - Global Legal Insights - International legal business solutions. https://www.globallegalinsights.com/practice-areas/ai-machine-learning-and-big-data-laws-and-regulations/australia (accessed 18 August 2022).

Crone, S.F., Lessmann, S., and Stahlbock, R. (2006). The impact of preprocessing on data mining: an evaluation of classifier sensitivity in direct marketing. *European Journal of Operational Research* 173: 781–800. https://doi.org/10.1016/j.ejor.2005.07.023.

CrowdFlower (2016). Data science report.

De Bondt, W. and Vermeulen, G. (2010). The procedural rights debate: a bridge too far or still not far enough? *EUCRIM (Freiburg)* 4: 163–167.

De Hert, P. and Sajfert, J. (2021). The fundamental right to personal data protection in criminal investigations and proceedings: framing big data policing through the purpose limitation and data minimisation principles of the Directive (EU) 2016/680. https://doi.org/10.2139/ssrn.4016491.

de Miguel Beriain, I., Jiménez, P.N., and José Rementería, M. (2022). Auditing the quality of datasets used in algorithmic decision-making systems. European Parliament/ Directorate General for Parliamentary Research Services (EPRS), LU.

Devlin, J., Chang, M.-W., Lee, K., and Toutanova, K. (2019). BERT: pre-training of deep bidirectional transformers for language understanding. https://doi.org/10.48550/arXiv.1810.04805.

Doyle, S. (2019). *Quality Management in Forensic Science*. London and San Diego: Elsevier/ Academic Press.

Dressel, J. and Farid, H. (2018). The accuracy, fairness, and limits of predicting recidivism. *Science Advances* 4: eaao5580. https://doi.org/10.1126/sciadv.aao5580.

Du, X., Hargreaves, C., Sheppard, J. et al. (2020). SoK: exploring the state of the art and the future potential of artificial intelligence in digital forensic investigation. Proceedings of the 15th International Conference on Availability, Reliability and Security. Presented at the ARES 2020: The 15th International Conference on Availability, Reliability and Security, ACM, Virtual Event Ireland, 1–10. https://doi.org/10.1145/3407023.3407068.

Du, X. and Scanlon, M. (2019). Methodology for the automated metadata-based classification of incriminating digital forensic artefacts. Proceedings of the 14th International Conference on Availability, Reliability and Security, 1–8. https://doi.org/10.1145/3339252.3340517.

Duda, R.O., Hart, P.E., and Stork, D.G. (2001). *Pattern Classification*, 2e. New York: Wiley.

Ebers, M., Hoch, V.R.S., Rosenkranz, F. et al. (2021). The European commission's proposal for an artificial intelligence act—a critical assessment by members of the Robotics and AI Law Society (RAILS). *Multidisciplinary Scientific Journal* 4: 589–603. https://doi.org/10.3390/j4040043.

Edmond, G. (2012). Is reliability sufficient? the law commission and expert evidence in international and interdisciplinary perspective (part 1). *The International Journal of Evidence & Proof* 16: 30–65. https://doi.org/10.1350/ijep.2012.16.1.391.

Edmond, G. (2016). Legal versus non-legal approaches to forensic science evidence. *The International Journal of Evidence & Proof* 20: 3–28. https://doi.org/10.1177/1365712715613470.

Edmond, G. and Martire, K. (2016). Forensic science in criminal courts. Australian Bar Review. 367–384.

Edmond, G. and Roberts, A. (2011). Procedural fairness, the criminal trial and forensic science and medicine. *Sydney Law Review* 33: 36.

EDPB (2016). Guidelines on the right to data portability.

EDPB (2018). Guidelines on automated individual decision-making and profiling for the purposes of regulation 2016/679.

EDPB-EDPS (2021). Joint opinion 5/2021 on the proposal for a regulation of the European Parliament and of the Council laying down harmonised rules on artificial intelligence (Artificial Intelligence Act) | European Data Protection Board.

Edwards, L. and Veale, M. (2017). Slave to the algorithm? Why a "right to an explanation" is probably not the remedy you are looking for. *Duke Law & Technology Review* 16: 18–84.

Europol (2021). Internet Organised Crime Threat Assessment (IOCTA) 2021 [WWW Document]. Europol. https://www.europol.europa.eu/publications-events/main-reports/internet-organised-crime-threat-assessment-iocta-2021 (accessed 26 August 2022).

Fan, C., Chen, M., Wang, X. et al. (2021). A review on data preprocessing techniques toward efficient and reliable knowledge discovery from building operational data. *Frontiers in Energy Research* 9: 652801. https://doi.org/10.3389/fenrg.2021.652801.

Ferguson, J. (2016). Defining big data in the e-Discovery World [WWW Document]. LawJournalNewsletters.com. http://www.lawjournalnewsletters.com/sites/lawjournalnewsletters/2015/12/31/defining-big-data-in-the-e-discovery-world (accessed 26 March 2020).

Field, S. (2009). Fair trials and procedural tradition in Europe. *Oxford Journal of Legal Studies* 29: 365–387. https://doi.org/10.1093/ojls/gqp004.

Finck, M. and Biega, A. (2021). Reviving purpose limitation and data minimisation in personalisation, profiling and decision-making systems. https://doi.org/10.2139/ssrn.3749078.

Findley, K. (2011). Innocents at risk: adversary imbalance, forensic science, and the search for truth. *Seton Hall Law Review* 38.

Flaglien, A. (2018). Cross-computer malware detection in digital forensics.

Fukami, A., Stoykova, R., and Geradts, Z. (2021). A new model for forensic data extraction from encrypted mobile devices. *Forensic Science International: Digital Investigation* 38: 301169. https://doi.org/10.1016/j.fsidi.2021.301169.

Gless, S. (2010). Truth or due process? the use of illegally gathered evidence in criminal trials – Germany. *SSRN Journal*. https://doi.org/10.2139/ssrn.1743530.

Gless, S. (2013). Transnational cooperation in criminal matters and the guarantee of a fair trial: approaches to a general principle. *ULR* 9: 90. https://doi.org/10.18352/ulr.244.

Glickman, M. and Sharot, T. (2022). Biased AI systems produce biased humans. https://doi.org/10.31219/osf.io/c4e7r.

Göbel, T., Maltan, S., Türr, J. et al. (2022). ForTrace – A holistic forensic data set synthesis framework. *Forensic Science International: Digital Investigation*, Selected Papers of the Ninth Annual DFRWS Europe Conference 40: 301344. https://doi.org/10.1016/j.fsidi.2022.301344.

Goodman, B. and Flaxman, S. (2017). European Union regulations on algorithmic decision-making and a "right to explanation". *AIMag* 38: 50–57. https://doi.org/10.1609/aimag.v38i3.2741.

Grajeda, C., Breitinger, F., and Baggili, I. (2017). Availability of datasets for digital forensics – and what is missing. *Digital Investigation* 22: S94–S105. https://doi.org/10.1016/j.diin.2017.06.004.

Gross, S. and Mnookin, J. (2003). Expert information and expert evidence: a preliminary taxonomy. Articles.

Hall, S.W., Sakzad, A., and Choo, K.R. (2022). Explainable artificial intelligence for digital forensics. *WIREs Forensic Science* 4. https://doi.org/10.1002/wfs2.1434.

Hardt, M., Price, E., and Srebro, N. (2016). Equality of opportunity in supervised learning. https://doi.org/10.48550/arXiv.1610.02413.

Hargreaves, C. and Patterson, J. (2012). An automated timeline reconstruction approach for digital forensic investigations. *Digital Investigation*, The Proceedings of the Twelfth Annual DFRWS Conference 9: S69–S79. https://doi.org/10/gcx6dn.

Horsman, G. (2018a). Framework for Reliable Experimental Design (FRED): a research framework to ensure the dependable interpretation of digital data for digital forensics. *Computers & Security* 73: 294–306. https://doi.org/10/gcx6dd.

Horsman, G. (2018b). Framework for Reliable Experimental Design (FRED): a research framework to ensure the dependable interpretation of digital data for digital forensics. *Computers & Security* 73: 294–306. https://doi.org/10.1016/j.cose.2017.11.009.

Horsman, G. (2019). Formalising investigative decision making in digital forensics: proposing the Digital Evidence Reporting and Decision Support (DERDS) framework. *Digital Investigation* 28: 146–151. https://doi.org/10.1016/j.diin.2019.01.007.

Horsman, G. and Lyle, J.R. (2021). Dataset construction challenges for digital forensics. *Forensic Science International: Digital Investigation* 38: 301264. https://doi.org/10.1016/j.fsidi.2021.301264.

Hossain, M.D.Z., Sohel, F., Shiratuddin, M.F., and Laga, H. (2019). A comprehensive survey of deep learning for image captioning. *ACM Computing Surveys* 51, 118: 1–36. https://doi.org/10.1145/3295748.

Hughes, N. and Karabiyik, U. (2020). Towards reliable digital forensics investigations through measurement science. *WIREs Forensic Science N/a* e1367. https://doi.org/10.1002/wfs2.1367.

Hutchinson, B., Smart, A., Hanna, A. et al. (2021). Towards accountability for machine learning datasets: practices from software engineering and infrastructure. Proceedings of the 2021 ACM Conference on Fairness, Accountability, and Transparency, FAccT '21, 560–575. Association for Computing Machinery, New York, NY, USA. https://doi.org/10.1145/3442188.3445918.

ISO/IEC 23053 (2022). Framework for Artificial Intelligence (AI) systems using Machine Learning (ML).

Jakobs, L.E.M.P. and Sprangers, W.J.J.M. (2000). A European view on forensic expertise and counter-expertise. *Criminal Law Forum* 11: 375–392. https://doi.org/10.1023/A:1009481107061.

Johnsen, J.W. and Franke, K. (2019). The impact of preprocessing in natural language for open source intelligence and criminal investigation. 2019 IEEE International Conference on Big Data (Big Data). Presented at the 2019 IEEE International Conference on Big Data (Big Data), 4248–4254. IEEE, Los Angeles, CA, USA. https://doi.org/10.1109/BigData47090.2019.9006006.

Jones, A. and Vidalis, S. (2019). Rethinking digital forensics. *Annals of Emerging Technologies in Computing* 3: 41–53. https://doi.org/10.33166/AETiC.2019.02.005.

Karamizadeh, S., Abdullah, S.M., Manaf, A.A. et al. (2013). An overview of principal component analysis. *JSIP* 04: 173–175. https://doi.org/10.4236/jsip.2013.43B031.

Katilu, V.M., Franqueira, V.N.L., and Angelopoulou, O. (2015). Challenges of data provenance for cloud forensic investigations. 2015 10th International Conference on Availability, Reliability and Security. Presented at the 2015 10th International Conference on Availability, Reliability and Security. 312–317. https://doi.org/10.1109/ARES.2015.54.

Kebande, V.R., Ikuesan, R.A., Karie, N.M. et al. (2020). Quantifying the need for supervised machine learning in conducting live forensic analysis of emergent configurations (ECO) in IoT environments. *Forensic Science International: Reports* 2: 100122. https://doi.org/10.1016/j.fsir.2020.100122.

Kelly, L., Sachan, S., Ni, L. et al. (2020). Explainable artificial intelligence for digital forensics: opportunities, challenges and a drug testing case study, digital forensic science. *IntechOpen*. https://doi.org/10.5772/intechopen.93310.

Khalid, S., Khalil, T., and Nasreen, S. (2014). A survey of feature selection and feature extraction techniques in machine learning. 2014 Science and Information Conference. Presented at the 2014 Science and Information Conference. 372–378. https://doi.org/10.1109/SAI.2014.6918213.

Kloosterman, A., Mapes, A., Geradts, Z. et al. (2015). The interface between forensic science and technology: how technology could cause a paradigm shift in the role of forensic institutes in the criminal justice system. *Philosophical Transactions of the Royal Society of London. Series B, Biological Sciences* 370. https://doi.org/10.1098/rstb.2014.0264.

Kohn, M.D., Eloff, M.M., and Eloff, J.H.P. (2013). Integrated digital forensic process model. *Computers & Security* 38: 103–115. https://doi.org/10.1016/j.cose.2013.05.001.

Kononenko, I. and Kukar, M. (2007). *Machine Learning and Data Mining: Introduction to Principles and Algorithms*. Chichester, UK: Horwood Publishing.

Koops, B.-J. (2013). On decision transparency, or how to enhance data protection after the computational turn.

Kop, M. (2021). The right to process data for machine learning purposes in the EU. *Harvard Journal of Law & Technology* 34.

Kusak, M. (2017). Common EU minimum standards for enhancing mutual admissibility of evidence gathered in criminal matters. *European Journal on Criminal Policy and Research* 23: 337–352. https://doi.org/10.1007/s10610-017-9339-0.

Kusak, M. (2019). Mutual admissibility of evidence and the European investigation order: aspirations lost in reality. *ERA Forum* 19: 391–400. https://doi.org/10.1007/s12027-018-0537-0.

Larson, J., Mattu, S., Kirchner, L., and Angwin, J. (2016). How we analyzed the COMPAS Recidivism Algorithm [WWW Document]. ProPublica. https://www.propublica.org/article/how-we-analyzed-the-compas-recidivism-algorithm?token=Tu5C70R2pCBv8Yj33AkMh2E-mHz3d6iu (accessed 20 August 2022).

Lau, T. and Biedermann, A. (2019). Assessing AI output in legal decision-making with nearest neighbors.

Lopez-Rojas, E.A. and Axelsson, S. (2012). Money laundering detection using synthetic data. The 27th Annual workshop of the Swedish Artificial Intelligence Society (SAIS) 9.

Lopez-Rojas, E.A. and Barneaud, C. (2019). Advantages of the PaySim simulator for improving financial fraud controls. In: *Intelligent Computing, Advances in Intelligent Systems and Computing* (ed. K. Arai, R. Bhatia, and S. Kapoor), 727–736. Cham: Springer International Publishing. https://doi.org/10.1007/978-3-030-22868-2_51.

Marshall, A. and Paige, R. (2018). Requirements in digital forensics method definition: observations from a UK study.

Mason, S. and Seng, D. (2017). *Electronic Evidence*, 4e, University of London: Institute of Advanced Legal Studies. https://doi.org/10.14296/517.9781911507079.

Mendoza, I. and Bygrave, L.A. (2017). The right not to be subject to automated decisions based on profiling. In: *EU Internet Law: Regulation and Enforcement* (ed. T.-E. Synodinou, P. Jougleux, C. Markou, and T. Prastitou), 77–98. Cham: Springer International Publishing. https://doi.org/10.1007/978-3-319-64955-9_4.

Mifsud Bonnici, J.P., Tudorica, M., and Cannataci, J.A. (2018). The European legal framework on electronic evidence: complex and in need of reform. In: *Handling and Exchanging Electronic Evidence across Europe, Law, Governance and Technology Series* (ed. M.A. Biasiotti, J. Cannataci, J.P. Mifsud Bonnici, and F. Turchi). Cham: Springer International Publishing. Imprint: Springer. https://doi.org/10.1007/978-3-319-74872-6.

Milaj, J. and Mifsud Bonnici, J.P. (2014). Unwitting subjects of surveillance and the presumption of innocence. *Computer Law & Security Review* 30: 419–428. https://doi.org/10.1016/j.clsr.2014.05.009.

Mohammad, R.M.A. and Alqahtani, M. (2019). A comparison of machine learning techniques for file system forensics analysis. *Journal of Information Security and Applications* 46: 53–61. https://doi.org/10.1016/j.jisa.2019.02.009.

Mökander, J., Juneja, P., Watson, D.S., and Floridi, L. (2022). The US Algorithmic Accountability Act of 2022 vs. The EU Artificial Intelligence Act: what can they learn from each other? *Minds & Machines* 32: 751–758. https://doi.org/10.1007/s11023-022-09612-y.

Montasari, R. and Hill, R. (2019). Next-generation digital forensics: challenges and future paradigms. 2019 IEEE 12th International Conference on Global Security, Safety and Sustainability (ICGS3). Presented at the 2019 IEEE 12th International Conference on Global Security, Safety and Sustainability (ICGS3), 205–212. https://doi.org/10.1109/ICGS3.2019.8688020.

Montasari, R., Hill, R., Carpenter, V., and Hosseinian-Far, A. (2019). The Standardised Digital Forensic Investigation Process Model (SDFIPM). In: *Blockchain and Clinical Trial: Securing Patient Data, Advanced Sciences and Technologies for Security Applications* (ed. H. Jahankhani, S. Kendzierskyj, A. Jamal, et al.), 169–209. Cham: Springer International Publishing. https://doi.org/10.1007/978-3-030-11289-9_8.

Morgenthaler, S. (2009). Exploratory data analysis. *WIREs Computational Statistics* 1: 33–44. https://doi.org/10.1002/wics.2.

Nagy, G. (1983). Candide's practical principles of experimental pattern recognition. *CSE Journal Article* 3.

Nassif, L.F.D.C. and Hruschka, E.R. (2013). Document clustering for forensic analysis: an approach for improving computer inspection. *IEEE Transactions on Information Forensics and Security* 8: 46–54. https://doi.org/10.1109/TIFS.2012.2223679.

National Research Council (2009). Strengthening forensic science in the United States: a path forward. https://doi.org/10.17226/12589.

Ngejane, C.H., Eloff, J.H.P., Sefara, T.J., and Marivate, V.N. (2021). Digital forensics supported by machine learning for the detection of online sexual predatory chats. *Forensic Science International: Digital Investigation* 36: 301109. https://doi.org/10.1016/j.fsidi.2021.301109.

Nguyen, H.T., Franke, K., and Petrovic, S. (2010). Towards a generic feature-selection measure for intrusion detection. 2010 20th International Conference on Pattern Recognition 1529–1532. https://doi.org/10.1109/ICPR.2010.378.

Nijboer, J.F. and Sprangers, W.J.J.M. (eds.) (2000). Harmonisation in forensic expertise: an inquiry into the desirability of and opportunities for international standards. Criminal sciences. Thela Thesis, Amsterdam.

Nordvik, R., Stoykova, R., Franke, K. et al. (2021). Reliability validation for file system interpretation. *Forensic Science International: Digital Investigation* 37: 301174. https://doi.org/10.1016/j.fsidi.2021.301174.

Park, S., Akatyev, N., Jang, Y. et al. (2018). A comparative study on data protection legislations and government standards to implement Digital Forensic Readiness as mandatory requirement. *Digital Investigation* 24: S93–S100. https://doi.org/10.1016/j.diin.2018.01.012.

Penn, B. (2022). Prosecutors drowning in data urged to collect less evidence [WWW Document]. Bloomberg Law. https://news.bloomberglaw.com/us-law-week/evidence-avalanche-prompts-less-is-more-pivot-by-us-prosecutors (accessed 26 August 2022).

Porter, K. (2018). Analyzing the DarkNetMarkets subreddit for evolutions of tools and trends using LDA topic modeling. *Digital Investigation* 26: S87–S97. https://doi.org/10.1016/j.diin.2018.04.023.

Risinger, D. (2018). The five functions of forensic science and the validation issues they raise: a piece to incite discussion on validation. *Seton Hall Law Review* 48.

Risinger, D.M. (2000). Navigating expert reliability: are criminal standards of certainty being left on the dock? (SSRN Scholarly Paper No. ID 251033). Social Science Research Network, Rochester, NY.

Roth, A. (2017). Machine testimony. *The Yale Law Journal* 126: 1972–2259.

Rothschild-Elyassi, G., Koehler, J., and Simon, J. (2019). Actuarial justice. In: *The Handbook of Social Control* (ed. M. Deflem), 194–206. Chichester, UK: John Wiley & Sons, Ltd. https://doi.org/10.1002/9781119372394.ch14.

Saks, M. and Faigman, D.L. (2008). Failed forensics: how forensic science lost its way and how it might yet find it. *Annual Review of Law and Social Science* 4: 149–171. https://doi.org/10.1146/annurev.lawsocsci.4.110707.172303.

Saks, M.J. and Koehler, J.J. (2005). The coming paradigm shift in forensic identification science. *Science* 309: 892–895. https://doi.org/10.1126/science.1111565.

Scanlon, M. (2016). Battling the digital forensic backlog through data deduplication. https://doi.org/10.1109/INTECH.2016.7845139.

Schwartz, R., Vassilev, A., Greene, K.K. et al. (2022). Towards a standard for identifying and managing bias in artificial intelligence (Special Publication 1270). NIST.

Serhal, C. and Le-Khac, N.-A. (2021). Machine learning based approach to analyze file meta data for smart phone file triage. *Forensic Science International: Digital Investigation* 37: 301194. https://doi.org/10.1016/j.fsidi.2021.301194.

Sliedregt, E.V. (2009). A contemporary reflection on the presumption of innocence. *Revue Internationale de Droit Penal* 80: 247–267.

Smith, F.C. and Kenneally, E.E. (2008). Electronic evidence and digital forensics testimony in court. In: *Handbook of Digital and Multimedia Forensic Evidence* (ed. J.J. Barbara), 103–132. Totowa, NJ: Humana Press. https://doi.org/10.1007/978-1-59745-577-0_8.

Solanke, A.A. and Biasiotti, M.A. (2022). Digital forensics AI: evaluating, standardizing and optimizing digital evidence mining techniques. *Künstliche Intelligenz*. https://doi.org/10.1007/s13218-022-00763-9.

Stoykova, A. (2022). Standards for Digital Evidence: an inquiry into the opportunities for fair trial safeguards through digital forensics standards in criminal investigations (Thesis fully internal (DIV)). University of Groningen, [Groningen]. https://doi.org/10.33612/diss.222646186.

Taylor, D.A., Bright, J.-A., and Buckleton, J. (2017). Commentary: a "source" of error: computer code, criminal defendants, and the constitution. *Frontiers in Genetics* 8. https://doi.org/10.3389/fgene.2017.00033.

Torrano-Gimenez, C., Nguyen, H.T., Alvarez, G., and Franke, K. (2015). Combining expert knowledge with automatic feature extraction for reliable web attack detection. *Security and Communication Networks* 8: 2750–2767. https://doi.org/10.1002/sec.603.

Tosza, S. (2020). All evidence is equal, but electronic evidence is more equal than any other: the relationship between the European Investigation Order and the European Production Order. *New Journal of European Criminal Law* 11: 161–183. https://doi.org/10.1177/2032284420919802.

Tully, G., Cohen, N., Compton, D. et al. (2020). Quality standards for digital forensics: learning from experience in England & Wales. *Forensic Science International: Digital Investigation* 32: 200905. https://doi.org/10.1016/j.fsidi.2020.200905.

The UK National Police Chiefs Council (2020). law enforcement data service: data protection impact assessment (DPIA) 67.

US National Institute of Standards and Technology (2022). Digital investigation techniques: a NIST scientific foundation review. NIST.

The US President's Council of Advisors on Science and Technology (PCAST) (2016). Forensic science in criminal courts: ensuring scientific validity of feature-comparison methods [WWW Document]. https://obamawhitehouse.archives.gov/blog/2016/09/20/pcast-releases-report-forensic-science-criminal-courts (accessed 6 March 2020).

Van Buskirk, E. and Liu, V.T. (2006). Digital evidence: challenging the presumption of reliability. *Journal of Digital Forensic Practice* 1: 19–26. https://doi.org/10/bh459r.

Veale, M. and Binns, R. (2017). Fairer machine learning in the real world: mitigating discrimination without collecting sensitive data [WWW Document]. https://journals.sagepub.com/doi/full/10.1177/2053951717743530 (accessed 21 August 2022).

Veale, M. and Borgesius, F.Z. (2021). Demystifying the draft EU Artificial Intelligence Act. *Computer Law Review International* 22: 97–112. https://doi.org/10.9785/cri-2021-220402.

Vermeulen, G., De Bondt, W., and van Damme, Y. (2010). *EU Cross-border Gathering and Use of Evidence in Criminal Matters: Towards Mutual Recognition of Investigative Measures and Free Movement of Evidence?* Maklu, Antwerpen; Portland: IRCP-series.

Vincze, E.A. (2016). Challenges in digital forensics. *Police Practice and Research* 17: 183–194. https://doi.org/10.1080/15614263.2015.1128163.

Wachter, S. (2022). The theory of artificial immutability: protecting algorithmic groups under anti-discrimination law. https://doi.org/10.2139/ssrn.4099100.

Wachter, S., Mittelstadt, B., and Floridi, L. (2017). Why a right to explanation of automated decision-making does not exist in the general data protection regulation. *International Data Privacy Law* 7: 76–99. https://doi.org/10.1093/idpl/ipx005.

Wigan, M.R. and Clarke, R. (2013). Big data's big unintended consequences. *Computer* 46: 46–53. https://doi.org/10.1109/MC.2013.195.

Yeung, K. (2021). Data for policy 2021 keynote lecture: "the production of 'regulatory science' through in-the-wild technology testing: live facial recognition technology as the Thalidomide of AI?".

Zawoad, S. and Hasan, R. (2015). Digital Forensics in the Age of Big Data: Challenges Approaches and Opportunities, IEEE 17th International Conference on High-Performance Computing and Communications 2015 IEEE 7th International Symposium on Cyberspace Safety and Security and 2015 IEEE 12th International Conference on Embedded Software and Systems, pp. 1320–1325.

CHAPTER 4

Formalising Representation and Interpretation of Digital Evidence to Reinforce Reasoning and Automated Analysis

Eoghan Casey and Timothy Bollé

Ecole des Sciences Criminelles, Police Scientifique, UNIL Lausanne, Switzerland

4.1 Introduction

Cybercrime is growing so rapidly throughout the world, that it is difficult to measure and establish a baseline (Caneppele and Aebi 2019). Cyber-investigations have grown in quantity and complexity as reported in the Europol EC3 Internet Organised Crime Threat Assessment (Europol 2021). The massive amount of information being generated in cyberjustice and cybersecurity contexts are rapidly increasing in variety and complexity. Massive amounts of data, make it more difficult to find useful evidence, like looking for a needle in a digital haystack. Automation and artificial intelligence (AI) are being applied to accelerate forensic analysis of digital evidence, but little attention is given to representing results in a manner that supports robust reasoning. As a result, decisions are being made without sufficient support mechanisms, leading to misinterpretation and wrong decisions. Mistakes and missed opportunities in cybersecurity and cyberjustice contexts can have severe consequences, ranging from financial loss, privacy exposure, wrongful convictions, and unapprehended offenders.

The problem is made worse when forensic practitioners are taught to report digital evidence simply as observations, which often results in the false logic of presenting hypotheses as facts. Such false facts misrepresent digital evidence and raise the risk of incorrect decisions. Observed traces could have an alternative explanation from the seemingly obvious one. To provide factfinders with an appropriate level of trust in digital forensic findings it is necessary to formally represent inferences made from observed traces.

Artificial Intelligence (AI) in Forensic Sciences, First Edition. Edited by Zeno Geradts and Katrin Franke.
© 2024 John Wiley & Sons Ltd. Published 2024 by John Wiley & Sons Ltd.

To deal with these trends, there is a growing need for formalized representation and interpretation of digital traces, clearly differentiating between observations and inferences, to strengthen automation and reasoning in forensic investigations.

When analysing digital traces, it is essential to comprehend observed traces as the results of activity, not the activity itself. Establishing a link between a person's actions in the physical world and the digital traces on a device involves inference which has inherent uncertainty (Pollitt et al. 2018). This process typically involves inference, i.e., evaluating observed traces in light of alternative hypotheses to determine the most likely causal action (*inferred action*) as shown in Figure 4.1. Examples of physical actions on a device include facial authentication, inserting a SIM card into a device, movement of a device (e.g., shaking, rotating, exercise), and fingers operating a device via the screen/keyboard. A physical action typically executes virtual actions in the context of a user account, such as unlocking a device, opening a web page, sending a message, and initiating a call. In many forensic investigations, it is necessary both to establish a retrodictive link from the digital traces to a virtual action and to an action that someone performed in the physical world. For instance, on an Android device, it can be inferred that the user accessed a specific webpage based on the combined observations of the Chrome History database being modified, the addition of a URL entry, and the creation of cached content.

In some situations, inferences based on observable objects result in classification and identification, as well as activities. Forensic analysis of child sexual abuse materials (CSAM) cases use artificial intelligence to estimate the victim's age and to classify sexual acts (Sanchez et al. 2019). In addition, image and video data are analysed to make inferences about entities, including people (identification) and vehicles (classification). The inherent uncertainty in any inference is exacerbated by real world complications. For example, stickers or graffiti on traffic signs can cause a neural network to misclassify stop signs as "speed limit 45" signs (Eykholt et al. 2018).

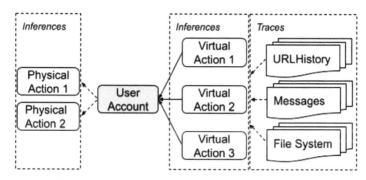

Figure 4.1 Inferring physical actions and virtual actions from observed digital evidence.

This chapter presents illustrative examples of computed similarity, ML classification of digital traces, including making inferences based on computed similarity, object recognition, and application activity logs. This chapter describes the use of ontologies to establish a common conceptualization of digital traces and to formalize evidence-based inferences to support the codification of scientific practices. This work supports human reasoning to make the final determination of how probable or uncertain the link is between the detected traces and user actions.

4.2 Background and Related Work

Existing tools used for analysing digital traces store large quantities of data in non-standard proprietary formats, often without a coherent conceptual model. For example, presenting locations extracted from a mobile device as locations of the device itself is false logic that can lead to misinterpretations (FSR 2021). In Figure 4.2, presentation of location-related information as device locations can cause confusion about their actual meaning. The geolocation information labelled with Device as the origin in Figure 4.2 are actually locations from a map app that are attached to a WhatsApp message, and are not necessarily the location of the device at that time.

The risk of misinterpretation increases when digital forensic tools present digital traces in a manner that does not clearly differentiate between concepts. Figure 4.3 depicts communication between devices but uses an icon of a person, which assumes that only one person used the device at all times. Such assumptions are dangerous in an investigation, potentially implicating the wrong individual. Therefore, it is important to consider alternative hypotheses, and assess the strength/probability of the digital evidence in light of each possibility (Casey 2020).

Existing digital forensic analysis methods focus on unstructured data rather than ontology-based understanding. Natural language processing (NLP) is used on unstructured data to extract entities such as names of people, organisations,

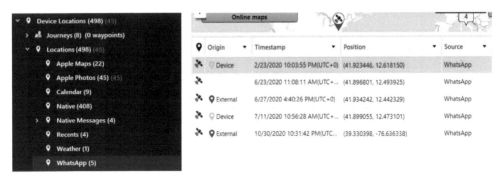

Figure 4.2 Longitude and latitude information being presented as device locations.

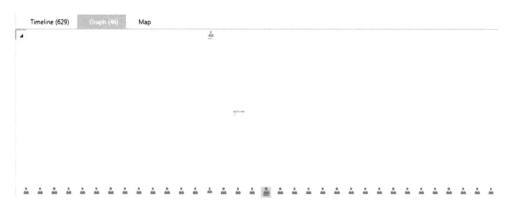

Figure 4.3 Information relating to a mobile device being represented using a person icon.

and places (Ukwen and Karabatak 2021). Machine learning is used on multi-media to classify objects and recognize faces (Du et al. 2020). Machine learning is also used to classify potential grooming behaviour in chat logs (Ebrahimi et al. 2016). Representation of these analysis methods and results is not standardized, and the way they are presented can create confusion and misinterpretation. To support computer-assisted analysis, including automated inferencing, it is necessary to first extract and structure the (meta)data from the unstructured data based on an ontology, and then analyse the structured (meta)data and produce results in a standard structure for further processing or reporting.

Automated systems for detecting criminal acts and identifying perpetrators can have unexpected results, such as the situation involving business woman Dong Mingzhu. Mingzhu's face was used in an advertisement for her company. Facial recognition systems identified her face in the advertisement on the side of a bus, which was located in the middle of the road, and concluded that Mingzhu was jaywalking. As a result, Mingzhu's face and name were displayed on a billboard used to publicly expose people who break traffic laws (BBC 2018).

In 2019, the forensic software developers of Axiom used an early version of the CASE ontology to form graphs and timelines of events with the goal of exploring the use of graph neural networks with Cypher6, a human readable graph query language (Henseler and Hyde 2019).

This work addresses the need for ontology-structured representation of data, analysis results, and evidence-based inferences to strengthen reasoning and automated analysis.

4.3 Method

A path to robust reasoning involves formally representing automated analysis and evidence-based inferences. In order to represent automated processing of digital traces, including computed similarity and machine learning classification, it is necessary to represent the method/tool used (AnalyticTool), the execution of the method/tool (AnalysisAction), and the result of the analysis (AnalyticResult). An inference is defined as an opinion that is formed on the basis of observed objects, including tangible traces and analytic results, in light of a given hypothesis. An inference can, therefore, be represented as the AnalyticResult of a hypothesis test AnalysisAction as depicted in Figure 4.4.

When making an inference, the first step is to clearly articulate the question to address in the form of a hypothesis or proposition.

Illustrative examples in this chapter include the following questions:

1. Are there non-obvious links between devices/cases? Automated analysis computes similarity between email addresses found in different devices/cases to automatically produce a link when the similarity score exceeds a given threshold.
2. What object(s) does the photograph contain?
3. What physical action was performed on the device?
4. Where was the device located when the photograph was taken?
5. Was the photograph a selfie or taken on a different device?

The next step is to treat available data sources, exposing the information they contain in a manner that enables analysis. Formalizing the structured representation of extracted information supports automated normalization, combination, correlation, and validation (Casey et al. 2017). Then it is necessary to take into account the limitations of the digital evidence, including inaccurate or incorrect information (Bollé et al. 2020). Finally, express a degree of uncertainty in the inference, considering alternatives (Casey 2020).

The simplest example is a computed similarity or ML classification. Figure 4.5 depicts such a scenario, with a similarity comparison meeting a preset threshold. Performing an AnalysisAction using an AnalyticTool to process input data and produce an AnalyticResult such as a similarity score that meets the threshold, establishing a relationship between the inputs.

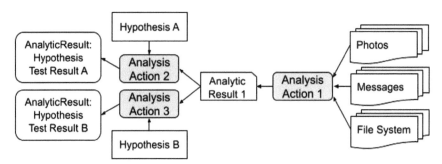

Figure 4.4 Representing inferences as results from hypothesis testing of observed digital evidence and associated analytic results.

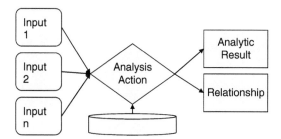

Figure 4.5 Simple example of an AnalysisAction operating on input data using an AnalyticTool to produce an AnalyticResult (e.g., similarity score or classification confidence). When a threshold is set and met by the AnalyticResult, a Relationship can be drawn between the inputs (e.g., similar emails).

4.4 Representing Digital Traces

A lack of formalization in representation of digital traces increases the risks of misinterpretation. To support robust reasoning and automated analysis, it is necessary to organize digital traces in a way that codifies their characteristics, context, and meaning in a way that makes sense. Such sense making is more than creating a data model. Ontologies are being developed to capture the core concepts of cyber-investigation and create a culture of common comprehension. The result of these community-driven activities is a common language for expressing digital traces and related cyber-investigation information such as evidence provenance and forensic processing. In addition to interoperability, semantic structure speeds up recognition of important concepts/entities in data, and the links/patterns.

The ontology-based open source cyber-investigation analysis standard expression (CASE) supports standardized representation, interoperability, and automation in cyber-investigations (https://caseontology.org). This standard provides a machine-understandable representation of cyber-information and its context, including links between items and how data were handled, transferred, processed, analysed, and interpreted. CASE combines multiple forms of knowledge representation to maximize expressivity and extensibility, increasing opportunities for applying artificial intelligence. The properties and classifications of a thing are represented using facets, context of and links between things are represented using relationships and references, the semantic structure is underpinned by ontology. The increased organization of data, metadata, and their context that is encouraged through CASE provides an enriched lattice of information, opening new opportunities for contextual analysis, pattern recognition, machine learning, semantic reasoning, and visualization.

The scope of the CASE ontology covers investigations in any context, including in criminal, cybersecurity, and intelligence. Digital traces include data sources (mobile devices, storage media, memory) and well-known digital objects such as files and folders, messages (email, chat), documents (PDF, Word), multimedia (pictures, video, audio) and logs (browser history, events).

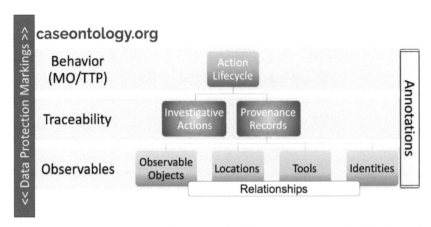

Figure 4.6 CASE encompasses essential concepts for the representation of cyber-investigations.

CASE ensures that analysis results can be traced back to their source(s), keeping track of when, where, and who used which tools to perform investigative actions on data sources. These details are generally referred to as provenance (e.g., chain of custody) and lineage (e.g., chain of evidence). CASE provides a formal representation of analytic results, including inferences, based on evaluation of digital evidence given alternative hypotheses. Furthermore, data markings are baked into CASE to support protection of information in order to prevent privacy violations, exposure of secrets, and other mishandling of sensitive information. The concepts represented in CASE are summarized in Figure 4.6.

An example of CASE is provided here representing an email message and associated email address (badquinn3@gmail.com) that establishes a link between two seemingly independent investigations (see Listings 4.1a and 4.1b). Full details of this illustrative example are available here: https://caseontology.org/examples/crossover

```
{
    "@id": "kb:Investigation1-85c7b8d1-54e0-4023-847a-20e0f55dd48e",
    "@type": "case-investigation:Investigation",
    "uco-core:name": "CROSSOVER_2018_11191001",
    "case-investigation:focus": "Bank Robbery (UBS Lausanne)",
    "uco-core:description": "Forensic treatment of storage media recovered from
getaway car and suspects apartment during investigation of bank robbery.",
            "uco-core:object": "list of uuids in investigation1"
    },
```

Listing 4.1a In Investigation 1, CASE representation of email configured in WhatsApp on a mobile device.

```
{
    "@id": "kb:EmailMessage-c5efd42c-d771-43aa-afe5-6b30740348e3",
    "@type": "uco-observable:EmailMessage",
    "uco-core:hasFacet": [
        {
            "@type": "uco-observable:EmailMessageFacet",
            "uco-observable:body": "",
            "uco-observable:from": {
                "@id": "kb:EmailAddress-d2bc0936-e1c5-4b55-8a1b-af2b3a2b145c"
            },
            "uco-observable:isRead": true,
            "uco-observable:messageID": "2320dc68-65a3-4f05-8884-945992231a1e",
            "uco-observable:sender": {
                "@id": "kb:EmailAddress-d2bc0936-e1c5-4b55-8a1b-af2b3a2b145c"
            },
            "uco-observable:sentTime": {
                "@type": "xsd:dateTime",
                "@value": "2018-11-20T00:00:30+00:00"
            },
            "uco-observable:subject": "Bank transfer ?",
            "uco-observable:to": {
                "@id": "kb:EmailAccount-ca4bc5e3-33a7-4457-b106-d0213e248979"
            }
        }
    ]
},
{
    "@id": "kb:EmailAccount-ca4bc5e3-33a7-4457-b106-d0213e248979",
    "uco-core:hasFacet": {
        "@type": "uco-observable:EmailAddressFacet",
        "uco-observable:emailAddress": {
            "@id": "kb:EmailAddress-5f63c12b-115a-474f-b1b2-15ebdb2fce31"
        }
    }
},
{
    "@id": "kb:EmailAddress-5f63c12b-115a-474f-b1b2-15ebdb2fce31",
    "@type": "uco-observable:EmailAddress",
    "uco-core:hasFacet": {
        "@type": "uco-observable:EmailAddressFacet",
        "uco-observable:addressValue": "badquinn3@gmail.com"
    }
},
```

Listing 4.1a (Cont'd)

```
    {
        "@id": "kb:investigation2-2ca2b7dd-da07-4ad4-9deb-0a0c4c6ff4f6",
        "@type": "case-investigation:Investigation",
        "uco-core:name": "CROSSOVER_2018_12111001",
        "case-investigation:focus": "Weapon of Mass Destruction (Deathly Hallows)",
        "uco-core:description": "The subject Ares Lupin was arrested on suspicion of
acquiring a weapon of mass destruction. The Samsung smartphone he was carrying was
preserved as evidence.",
        "uco-core:object": [
            "list of uuids in investigation2"
        ]
    },
    {
        "@id": "kb:emailmessage-2c032220-8c21-11e9-9c99-0c4de9c21b53",
        "@type": "uco-observable:EmailMessage",
        "uco-core:hasFacet": [
            {
                "@type": "uco-observable:EmailMessageFacet",
                "uco-observable:application": {
                    "@id": "kb:gmail-a1ce9965-ba9c-4fa1-9bfe-58c68ecaadc5"
                },
                "uco-observable:sender": {
                    "@id": "kb:emailaccount-99d72bac-8c21-11e9-8902-0c4de9c21b53"
                },
                "uco-observable:sentTime": {
                    "@type": "xsd:dateTime",
                    "@value": "2018-11-20T21:28:07.00Z"
                },
                "uco-observable:subject": "Re: Bank transfer ?",
                "uco-observable:bodyRaw": {
                    "@id": "kb:contentdata-f3b4a8da-d3ba-46b7-a7a0-3c17ec13648d"
                },
                "uco-observable:fromRef": null,
                "uco-observable:toRef": null,
                "uco-observable:ccRefs": null,
                "uco-observable:bccRefs": null,
                "uco-observable:messageID":
"CAKBqNfyKo+pvHkJy6kwO82jTbkNA@mail.gmail.com"
            }
        ]
    },
    {
        "@id": "kb:emailaccount-99d72bac-8c21-11e9-8902-0c4de9c21b53",
        "@type": "uco-observable:EmailAccount",
        "uco-core:hasFacet": [
            {
                "@type": "uco-observable:DigitalAccountFacet",
```

Listing 4.1b In Investigation 2, CASE representation of email configured in Outlook on computer.

```
                    "uco-observable:displayName": "Harley Quinn"
             },
             {
                 "@type": "uco-observable:EmailAccountFacet",
                 "uco-observable:emailAddress": {
                     "@id": "kb:emailaddress-456a2bac-8c21-11e9-8902-0c4de9c24de5"
                 }
             }
         ]
     },
     {
         "@id": "kb:emailaddress-456a2bac-8c21-11e9-8902-0c4de9c24de5",
         "@type": "uco-observable:EmailAddress",
         "uco-core:hasFacet": [
             {
                 "@type": "uco-observable:EmailAddressFacet",
                 "uco-observable:addressValue": "badquinn3@gmail.com"
             }
         ]
     }
}
```

Listing 4.1b (Cont'd)

Figure 4.7 provides a conceptualization of the information in Figures 4.2 and 4.3. A simplistic representation of this information using CASE is Listing 4.2, using relationships with an expression of confidence. These relationships are the result of evidence-based inferences as discussed later in the chapter.

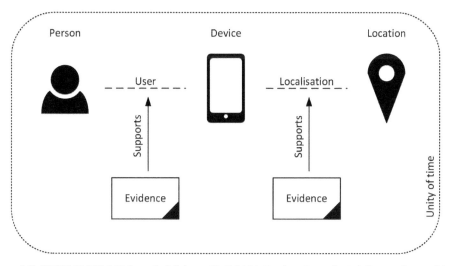

Figure 4.7 DFRWS EU 2022 or Spichiger, H (2022) Evaluation of Mobile Device Evidence under Person-Level, Location-Focused Propositions.

```
{
    "@id": "kb:location-b3c631d4-d1d8-4613-b2b6-f9be6b534a87",
    "@type": "uco-location:Location",
    "uco-core:hasFacet": {
        "@type": "uco-location:LatLongCoordinatesFacet",
        "uco-location:latitude": {
            "@type": "xsd:decimal",
            "@value": "46.53722222222222"
        },
        "uco-location:longitude": {
            "@type": "xsd:decimal",
            "@value": "6.579166666666667"
        },
        "uco-location:altitude": null
    }
},
{
    "@id": "kb:relationship-62290f53-aadd-4f09-8739-8fb51d9901bd",
    "@type": "uco-core:Relationship",
    "uco-core:source": {
        "@id": "kb:device-689a0a0f-ec1d-4dac-83a8-1e0ad31f1a3b"
    },
    "uco-core:target": {
        "@id": "kb:location-b3c631d4-d1d8-4613-b2b6-f9be6b534a87"
    },
    "uco-core:kindOfRelationship": "Located_At",
    "uco-core:isDirectional": true,
    "uco-core:hasFacet": [
        {
            "@type": "uco-core:ConfidenceFacet",
            "uco-core:confidence": {
                "@type": "xsd:nonNegativeInteger",
                "@value": "95"
            }
        }
    ]
},
{
    "@id": "kb:device-689a0a0f-ec1d-4dac-83a8-1e0ad31f1a3b",
    "@type": "uco-observable:MobileDevice",
    "uco-core:hasFacet": [
        {
            "@type": "uco-observable:DeviceFacet",
            "uco-observable:manufacturer": {
                "@id": "kb:Org-052d6e3b-545a-46e3-a2f2-ffaaebf5e498"
            },
```

Listing 4.2 CASE representation of location-related information from a mobile device and linked to a person.

```
                 "uco-observable:model": "SM-G925F",
                 "uco-observable:serialNumber": "RF8H31GS5SF"
           },
           {
                 "@type": "uco-observable:MobileDeviceFacet",
                 "uco-observable:bluetoothDeviceName": "Galaxy S6 edge",
                 "uco-observable:IMEI": "356420075722843"
           },
           {
                 "@type": "uco-observable:OperatingSystemFacet",
                 "uco-core:name": "Android",
                 "uco-observable:manufacturer": {
                       "@id": "kb:org-052d6e3b-545a-46e3-a2f2-ffaaebf5e498"
                 }
           }
     ]
   },
   {
       "@id": "kb:relationship-52d77034-b990-458f-817f-b32aefe87b73",
       "@type": "uco-core:Relationship",
       "uco-core:source": {
             "@id": "kb:person-109289b8-be65-4b7c-b1f4-b2a8e0d7e0a8"
       },
       "uco-core:target": {
             "@id": "kb:device-689a0a0f-ec1d-4dac-83a8-1e0ad31f1a3b"
       },
       "uco-core:kindOfRelationship": "Has_Device",
       "uco-core:isDirectional": true,
       "uco-core:hasFacet": [
             {
                   "@type": "uco-core:ConfidenceFacet",
                   "uco-core:confidence": {
                         "@type": "xsd:nonNegativeInteger",
                         "@value": "90"
                   }
             }
       ]
   },
   {
       "@id": "kb:person-109289b8-be65-4b7c-b1f4-b2a8e0d7e0a8",
       "@type": "uco-identity:Identity",
       "uco-core:hasFacet": [
             {
                   "@type": "uco-identity:SimpleNameFacet",
                   "uco-identity:givenName": "Eoghan",
                   "uco-identity:familyName": "Casey"
             }
       ]
   }
```

Listing 4.2 (Cont'd)

4.5 Representing Computed Similarity

Many tools are required to process digital traces, in particular to correlate and draw links between them. Such methods can be used across data coming from multiple devices in a single case, or across multiple cases. This could help develop new investigative leads or generate new forensic intelligence, in a crime analysis context.

For example, in a forensic intelligence context, the similarity between two email addresses used in online fraud can be computed using the Levenshtein distance (Bollé et al. 2018). The links drawn from such analysis will help create or expand a series of crimes where a same group of authors is responsible for multiple offences. These computer-assisted insights can enhance understanding of the crime ecosystem and help regroup related investigations. The representation of a tool for computing Levenshtein distance of email addresses is shown in Listing 4.3.

```
{
  "@id": "configuredtool-6e80cd16-59b7-4d86-9183-85286ff7337d",
  "@type": "uco-tool:ConfiguredTool"
  "uco-core:name": "string/metric/levenshtein",
  "uco-tool:toolType": "string metric",
  "uco-tool:creator": {
      "@id": "kb:organization-126cf13d-e9ca-490a-8097-71b4cf31e255"
      },
  "uco-tool:version": "esc-levenshtein-1.0",
  "uco-configuration:usesConfiguration": {
      "@id": "kb:configuration-031e8ecb-54be-44a3-b3f0-d9f1f17f54e6",
        "@type": "uco-configuration:Configuration",
        "uco-configuration:configurationEntry": [
            {
                "@type": "uco-configuration:ConfigurationEntry",
                "uco-configuration:itemName": "Algorithm used",
                "uco-configuration:itemValue": "Levenshtein"
            },
            {
                "@type": "uco-configuration:ConfigurationEntry",
                "uco-configuration:itemName": "DecisionThreshold",
                "uco-configuration:itemValue": "0.80"
            },
            {
                "@type": "uco-configuration:ConfigurationEntry",
                "uco-configuration:itemName": "TrainingSet",
            "uco-configuration:itemDescription": "Police dataset v.01.2022",
                "uco-configuration:itemObject": {
          "@id": "trainingdataset-5c17d706-65e7-4aba-8f2d-d2b5eb4a5871"
                }
            }
        ]
      }
}
```

Listing 4.3 AnalyticTool represented using CASE.

An AnalysisAction uses the tool represented in Listing 4.3 on the inputs (two email addresses being compared) to produce an AnalyticResult and, if the threshold is met, a relationship between the inputs is also produced, as represented in Listing 4.4.

```
{
    "@id": "kb:analysisaction-b55c0247-0a47-4325-86d7-a53d89c7f5a5",
    "@type": "uco-action:AnalysisAction",
    "uco-core:name": "computed string similarity",
    "uco-core:startTime": {
        "@type": "xsd:dateTime",
        "@value": "2022-05-10T08:49:00.00Z"
    },
    "uco-core:endTime": {
        "@type": "xsd:dateTime",
        "@value": "2022-05-10T09:54:00.00Z"
    },
    "uco-action:location": {
        "@id": "kb:lab-0561586e-a5cf-451a-b7af-8198c2ac45ab"
    },
    "uco-action:performer": {
        "@id": "kb:analyst-6e8202bc-140b-4b0e-b60b-4ea740c6980d"
    },
    "uco-action:instrument": {
        "@id": "kb:configuredtool-6e80cd16-59b7-4d86-9183-85286ff7337d"
    },
    "uco-action:environment": {
        "@id": "kb:forensiccomputer-d93c0c7d-3976-4b15-9bc6-97e1589aede1"
    },
    "uco-action:object": [
        {
            "@id": "kb:emailaddress1-ab45e7d0-921d-49a9-9ec3-2ab669101dc4"
        },
        {
            "@id": "kb:emailaddress2-f6643823-c690-48b8-91a5-c2c392212e0f"
        }
    ],
    "uco-action:result": [
        {
            "@id": "kb:analyticresult-f9854b19-4aa3-43d4-9891-73e2995cd596"
        },
        {
            "@id": "kb:relationship-776c0739-18b0-48ae-a33a-63eb0d66b196"
        }
    ]
},
```

Listing 4.4 AnalysisAction represented using CASE.

Listing 4.5 provides the representation of the AnalyticResult and Relationship between "timbolle" and "timbole" (imagine we found two email addresses – timbolle@ … and timbole@ … – in two different investigations).

```
{
    "@id": "analyticresult-f9854b19-4aa3-43d4-9891-73e2995cd596",
    "@type": "uco-analysis:AnalyticResult",
"uco-analysis:originatingAction": "analysisaction-b55c0247-0a47-4325-86d7-a53d89c7f5a5",
        "hasFacet": [
        {
            "@type": "analysis:ComputedDistanceResultFacet",
            "drafting:algorithm": "levenshtein",
            "drafting:value": 0.875
        },
        {
            "@type": "analysis:ClassificationResultFacet",
            "drafting:class": "similar emails",
            "drafting:confidence": "exceeds 0.8 decision threshold"
        },
        ]
    },
    {
        "@id": "kb:relationship-776c0739-18b0-48ae-a33a-63eb0d66b196",
        "@type": "uco-core:Relationship",
        "uco-core:source": {
            "@id": "kb:emailaddress1-ab45e7d0-921d-49a9-9ec3-2ab669101dc4"
        },
        "uco-core:target": {
            "@id": "kb:emailaddress2-f6643823-c690-48b8-91a5-c2c392212e0f"
        },
        "uco-core:kindOfRelationship": "Similar_To",
        "uco-core:isDirectional": true,
    },
```

Listing 4.5 AnalyticResult represented using CASE.

A visual depiction of the links produced by this computer-assisted process are shown in Figure 4.8.

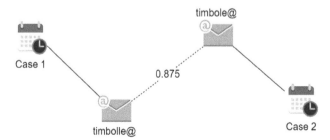

Figure 4.8 Result provided by the tool. The dotted line indicates a possible link between the two email addresses and their Levenshtein similarity score.

4.6 Representing ML Classification

As the volume and variety of data available in investigations is becoming more and more important, there is a need to use automated tools and in particular tools for automated classification, using machine learning techniques. The results of such automated tools need to be integrated in a much larger decision making process, usually involving a human analyst. For example, Figure 4.9 shows ML

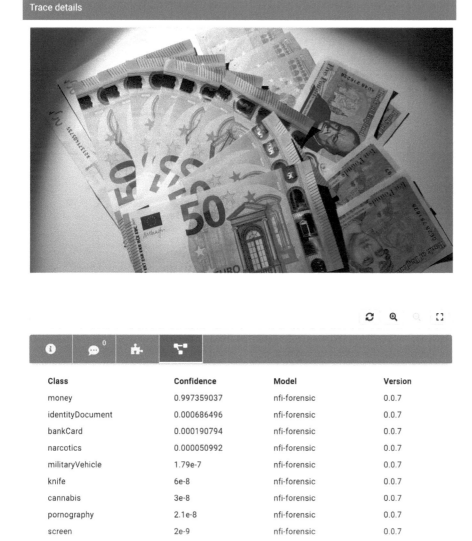

Class	Confidence	Model	Version
money	0.997359037	nfi-forensic	0.0.7
identityDocument	0.000686496	nfi-forensic	0.0.7
bankCard	0.000190794	nfi-forensic	0.0.7
narcotics	0.000050992	nfi-forensic	0.0.7
militaryVehicle	1.79e-7	nfi-forensic	0.0.7
knife	6e-8	nfi-forensic	0.0.7
cannabis	3e-8	nfi-forensic	0.0.7
pornography	2.1e-8	nfi-forensic	0.0.7
screen	2e-9	nfi-forensic	0.0.7
shippingContainer	1e-9	nfi-forensic	0.0.7
envelope	0.298	bvlc_googlenet	v1

Figure 4.9 High confidence classification of digital photograph as depicting money (Hansken presentation of traces in crossover case).

classification of a photograph containing money using the Netherland Forensic Institute's Digital Forensics as a Service (DFaaS) platform called Hansken, which is covered in Chapter 5 (van Beek and Henseler).

To support such automated analysis, it is necessary to represent results of machine learning classification. Other benefits are to help with transparency and auditability of the actions performed in the investigation.

Machine learning systems are tools that can be represented as such in the CASE ontology. The name, the version, and the type of tools should be represented. An important aspect of machine learning concerns the data on which the model was trained and tested. This information can also be documented within the ontology alongside other configuration parameters. The representation of the Hansken tool and result in Figure 4.9 using CASE is presented in Listing 4.6. AnalysisAction is not represented here, but follows the same pattern as Listing 4.5.

```
{
    "@id": "analyticresult-3b715c0f-e80c-4643-b43f-3776e7857ce1",
    "@type": "uco-analysis:AnalyticResult",
    "uco-analysis:originatingAction": "analysisaction-195b443c-124b-41cb-9902-33d44367b43e",
    "hasFacet": [
        {
            "@type": "analysis:ClassificationResultFacet",
            "drafting:className": "money",
            "drafting:confidence": 0.997359037
        }
    ]
},
{
    "@id": "configuredtool-ecc27934-80ea-408d-a106-f827c35fcf80",
    "@type": "uco-tool:ConfiguredTool"
    "uco-core:name": "Hansken",
    "uco-tool:toolType": "DFaaS",
    "uco-tool:creator": "NFI",
    "uco-tool:version": "1.0",
    "uco-configuration:usesConfiguration": {
        "@id": "kb:configuration-031e8ecb-54be-44a3-b3f0-d9f1f17f54e6",
        "@type": "uco-configuration:Configuration",
        "uco-configuration:configurationEntry": [
            {
                "@type": "uco-configuration:ConfigurationEntry",
                "uco-configuration:itemName": "Algorithm used",
                "uco-configuration:itemValue": "Levenshtein"
            },
```

Listing 4.6 Analytic results of ML classification represented using CASE.

```
                   {
                       "@type": "uco-configuration:ConfigurationEntry",
                       "uco-configuration:itemName": "Classifier",
                       "uco-configuration:itemValue": "nfi-forensic"
                   },
                   {
                       "@type": "uco-configuration:ConfigurationEntry",
                       "uco-configuration:itemName": "TrainingSet",
                       "uco-configuration:itemValue": "0.0.7",
                   }
               ]
           }
       }
```

Listing 4.6 (Cont'd)

Another application of artificial intelligence to digital traces is the analysis of application usage logs to automatically detect actions of interest on computing devices, particularly actions that require the physical presence of the user (Moutiez 2020).

A challenge may reside in classification tools that were not specifically designed for forensic purposes but could still find useful applications.

4.7 Representing Hypothesis Test Results (a.k.a. Inferences)

As described in the method section above, inferences can be represented as an hypothesis test AnalyticResult, which is shown in Listing 4.7 using CASE:

```
    {
        "@id": "kb:hypothesisA-f9c1cb5f-6356-40ef-8049-740a0478bc6a",
        "@type": "uco-drafting:Hypothesis",
        "drafting:statement": "money"
    },
    {
        "@id": "kb:hypothesisB-b52eb0ae-e220-470d-a5fd-f72a851a83c5",
        "@type": "uco-drafting:Hypothesis",
        "drafting:statement": "not money"
    },
    {
        "@id": "kb:analysisaction-ff46b490-4cb1-4d04-99ff-b49d84757248",
        "@type": "uco-action:AnalysisAction",
        "uco-core:name": "image classification",
        "uco-core:startTime": {
            "@type": "xsd:dateTime",
            "@value": "2022-08-10T09:33:00.00Z"
        },
```

Listing 4.7 Based on Hypothesis Test Result proposal at https://github.com/casework/
CASE-Examples/tree/ONT-434/examples/illustrations/inference accessed 5 April 2023.

```
            "uco-core:endTime": {
                "@type": "xsd:dateTime",
                "@value": "2022-08-10T09:54:00.00Z"
            },
            "uco-action:location": {
                "@id": "kb:nfilab-7dca9a20-d07c-464f-bdd4-41604c1132e9"
            },
            "uco-action:performer": {
                "@id": "kb:analyst-5b3621af-1827-4a3b-bfd1-8d6187d6bfca"
            },
            "uco-action:instrument": {
                "@id": "kb:configuredtool-ecc27934-80ea-408d-a106-f827c35fcf80"
            },
            "uco-action:environment": {
                "@id": "kb:forensicserver-b4e583ab-a923-484c-a472-78dbeb69a41e"
            },
            "uco-action:object": [
                {
                    "@id": "kb:photo-figure9-0816f57c-b857-41a9-93dd-1390daf48ff5"
                },
                {
                    "@id": "kb:analyticresult-2d260b45-13be-4a55-9f40-02844cf1b55c"
                },
                {
                    "@id": "kb:hypothesisA-f9c1cb5f-6356-40ef-8049-740a0478bc6a"
                }
            ],
            "uco-action:result": [
                {
                    "@id": "kb:analyticresult-f2fbad16-4763-4dbd-95fd-0128ff33c8e3"
                }
            ]
        },
    {
        "@id": "kb:analyticresult-f2fbad16-4763-4dbd-95fd-0128ff33c8e3",
        "@type": [
            "uco-analysis:AnalyticResult",
            "uco-analysis:HypothesisTestResult"
        ],
        "uco-action:originatingAnalysisAction": "kb:analysisaction-ff46b490-4cb1-4d04-
99ff-b49d84757248",
        "uco-core:hasFacet": [
            {
                "@type": "uco-analysis:HypothesisTestResultFacet",
                "drafting:evidenceEvaluation": {
                    "@type": "xsd:decimal",
                    "@value": "0.95"
                },
                "drafting:evaluationType": "Probability",
```

Listing 4.7 (Cont'd)

```
            "drafting:conclusion": "true",
            "drafting:evaluationRationale": "Image appears to con-
tain Euro and British money"
          }
      ]
    },
<ANALYSIS ACTION ON HYPOTHESIS B EXCLUDED FOR BREVITY>
    {
        "@id": "kb:analysisresult-4FFBA459-1D80-491D-BF1B-575EE800D21E",
        "@type": [
            "uco-analysis:AnalyticResult",
            "uco-analysis:HypothesisTestResult"
        ],
    "uco-analysis:originatingAnalysisAction": "kb:analysisaction-d15ef795-baff-4d7c-a9d0-
0c4bdec70f71",
        "uco-core:hasFacet": [
          {
            "@type": "uco-analysis:HypothesisTestResultFacet",
            "drafting:evidenceEvaluation": {
                "@type": "xsd:decimal",
                "@value": "0.05"
            },
            "drafting:evaluationType": "Probability",
            "drafting:conclusion": "true",
            "drafting:evaluationRationale": "Image con-
tains what appears to be money but not confirmed to be real bank-
notes based on serial numbers or watermarks"
          }
      ]
    },
```

Listing 4.7 (Cont'd)

This approach applies a logical method for evidence-based evaluation, with consideration of alternatives and expression of uncertainty. The representation is designed to provide transparency into rationale and facilitate comparison of competing opinions.

Applying the principles of scientific interpretation, it is necessary to consider alternative hypotheses (Biedermann and Kotsoglou 2020).

4.7.1 Location Example

Figure 4.10 shows a photograph extracted from a forensic copy of the Samsung Galaxy device in the Crossover dataset, and processed using the Hansken DFaaS system. The content of the photograph contains a boarding gate B8 in an airport, with the text "FR 9435" and "DUBLIN" extracted using optical character recognition (OCR).

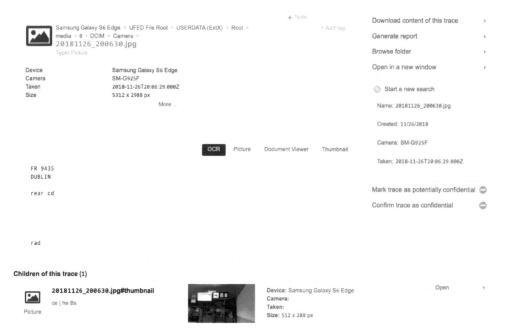

Figure 4.10 Photograph extracted from mobile device and processed using the Hansken DFaaS platform.

Given the above photograph taken in an airport, the following hypotheses tests are considered.

An AnalysisAction could be performed, taking both hypothesis test results as input, resulting in a "Located_At" relationship between the Samsung device and its likely location at Ciampino airport similar to Listing 4.2.

```
{                                          {
"@id": "kb:hypothesisA-83C7F9A7-8644-4CA1-  "@id": "kb:hypothesisB-9A38C54E-2C6D-4663-
A4C1-639A585EDE5C",                        B4B5-7CBBC3FE8974",
 "@type": "drafting:Hypothesis",           "@type": "drafting:Hypothesis",
 "drafting:statement":"Device used to take  "drafting:statement":"Device used to take
photo_20181126_200630.jpg was located at   photo_20181126_200630.jpg was located
Ciampino Airport"                          elsewhere"
        },                                         },
{                                          {
"@id":  "AnalyticResult-B6F21575-B9C1-4721-  "@id": "AnalyticResult-BB9EA3E1-562B-4DF4-
8AD8-508E3CED1CB6",                        8103-659B4447F694",
 "@type": "AnalyticResult",                 "@type": "AnalyticResult",
"uco-analysis:originatingAnalysisAction":  "uco-analysis:originatingAnalysisAction":
"kb:AnalysisAction-071A4373-6CDD-4E73-BBFB-  "kb:AnalysisAction-6EFC15B8-BF46-42FC-
B2BFCB176C75",                             9B33-CE5DCC3D2415",
        "uco-core:hasFacet": [                     "uco-core:hasFacet": [
```

Listing 4.8 Hypothesis test results (inferences) on the device location represented using CASE.

```
{                                              {
        "@type": "uco-                                "@type": "uco-
analysis:HypothesisTestResultFacet",           analysis:HypothesisTestResultFacet",
        "drafting:evidenceEvaluation":                 "drafting:evidenceEvaluation":
        {                                              {
                "@type": "xsd:decimal",                        "@type": "xsd:decimal",
                "@value": "0.95"                               "@value": "0.01"
        },                                             },
                "drafting:evaluationType":                     "drafting:evaluationType":
"Probability",                                 "Probability",
                "drafting:evaluationRationale":        "drafting:evaluationRationale": "Path of
"Path of the picture, Exif metadata, flight    the picture, Exif metadata, flight number
number (OCR), destination (OCR), and date"     (OCR), destination (OCR), and date"
        }                                              }
    ]                                              ]
    },                                             },
```

Listing 4.8 (Cont'd)

4.7.2 Identification Example

Figure 4.11 shows a photograph extracted from the Samsung Galaxy device in the Crossover dataset. The forensic question could be phrased: was the photo a selfie of Eoghan Casey taken using the Samsung device? This question must be evaluated as two pairs of hypothesis:

H1.1) the photo was taken using the Samsung device
H1.2) the photo was taken on some other Samsung device
H2.1) the person depicted in the photo is Eoghan Casey
H2.2) the person depicted in the photo is some other person

The hypothesis test results for H1.1 and H1.2 can be represented based on forensic examination of the Samsung device and evaluation of the observed traces:

```
{                                              {
"@id": "kb:hypothesisA-54A0288F-0E20-4C97-      "@id": "kb:hypothesisB-2C8344A3-90CD-419B-
819D-8C4436C00911",                            AB1E-91F2581B3CFC",
  "@type": "drafting:Hypothesis",               "@type": "drafting:Hypothesis",
  "drafting:statement":"Photo taken using the   "drafting:statement":"Photo taken using
Samsung device"                                another Samsung device"
        },                                             },
{                                              {
  "@id": "AnalyticResult-72C17E2D-AFC5-4BB4-    "@id": "AnalyticResult-70C7B893-
A7BE-CFDCEBB5CE2B",                            90DC-45F5-B915-075039854C0C",
  "@type": "AnalyticResult",                     "@type": "AnalyticResult",
```

Listing 4.9 Hypothesis test results on the photo source represented using CASE.

```
"uco-analysis:originatingAnalysisAction":          "uco-analysis:originatingAnalysisAction":
"kb:AnalysisAction-4F5B3925-874C-467A-8612-        "kb:AnalysisAction-017D4792-2B80-4552-
8F6A0E0D44B5",                                     BCF0-7687BEE2FCE3",
        "uco-core:hasFacet": [                             "uco-core:hasFacet": [
        {                                                  {
                        "@type": "uco-                                     "@type": "uco-
analysis:HypothesisTestResultFacet",               analysis:HypothesisTestResultFacet",
            "drafting:evidenceEvaluation":                     "drafting:evidenceEvaluation":
            {                                                  {
                "@type": "xsd:decimal",                            "@type": "xsd:decimal",
                "@value": "0.99"                                   "@value": "0.01"
            },                                                 },
                "drafting:evaluationType":                         "drafting:evaluationType":
"Probability",                                     "Probability",
                "drafting:evaluationRationale":                    "drafting:evaluationRationale":
"Path of the picture, Exif metadata, flight        Path of the picture, Exif metadata, flight
number, destination and date."                     number, destination and date."
            }                                                  }
        ]                                                  ]
    },                                                 },
```

Listing 4.9 (Cont'd)

An AnalysisAction can be performed, taking the hypothesis test results for H1.1 and H1.2 as input, resulting in a "Depicted_In" relationship between the person and photo, assigning a confidence of 99 (see Listing 4.10). Another AnalysisAction can be performed, taking the hypothesis test results for H2.1 and H2.2 as input, resulting in a "Taken_Using" relationship between the photo and device, assigning a confidence of 99 (see Listing 4.10). Another analysis action can be performed, taking these relationships as input, resulting in a "Has_Device" relationship between the person and the device (see Listing 4.2).

```
    {
        "@id": "kb:Relationship-D570B93E-B090-455F-9DF1-17D5BCC88CE8",
        "@type": "uco-core:Relationship",
        "uco-core:source": {
            "@id": "kb:Person-D3F91CFD-7920-4763-887C-F81B0E4C2732"
        },
        "uco-core:target": {
            "@id": "kb:Photo-315D842B-3283-4942-B307-DE4DFB0364DA"
        },
        "uco-core:kindOfRelationship": "Depicted_In",
        "uco-core:isDirectional": true,
        "uco-core:hasFacet": [
```

Listing 4.10 Investigative action using hypothesis test results in Listing 4.9 to evaluate the potential relationship between the person (Eoghan Casey) depicted within the selfie taken using the Samsung device.

```
                    {
                        "@type": "uco-core:ConfidenceFacet",
                        "uco-core:confidence": {
                            "@type": "xsd:nonNegativeInteger",
                            "@value": "99"
                        }
                    }
                ]
            },
            {
                "@id": "kb:Relationship-D570B93E-B090-455F-9DF1-17D5BCC88CE8",
                "@type": "uco-core:Relationship",
                "uco-core:source": {
                    "@id": "kb:Photo-315D842B-3283-4942-B307-DE4DFB0364DA"
                },
                "uco-core:target": {
                    "@id": "kb:Device-0ADD0214-D495-4418-B43A-A1CDD3455D71"
                },
                "uco-core:kindOfRelationship": "Taken_With",
                "uco-core:isDirectional": true,
                "uco-core:hasFacet": [
                    {
                        "@type": "uco-core:ConfidenceFacet",
                        "uco-core:confidence": {
                            "@type": "xsd:nonNegativeInteger",
                            "@value": "99"
                        }
                    }
                ]
            },
            {
                "@id": "kb:Photo-315D842B-3283-4942-B307-DE4DFB0364DA",
                "@type": "uco-observable:File",
                "uco-core:tag": [
                    "Image"
                ],
                "uco-core:hasFacet": [
                    {
                        "@type": "uco-observable:RasterPictureFacet",
                        "uco-observable:pictureType": "jpg",
                        "uco-observable:pictureHeight": 480,
                        "uco-observable:pictureWidth": 640
                    },
                    {
                        "@type": "uco-observable:FileFacet",
                        "uco-observable:fileName": "imgcache.0_25_1543258536",
                        "uco-observable:filePath": "/Root/media/0/Android/data/com.sec.
android.gallery3d/cache/imgcache.0/imgcache.0_25_1543258536",
                        "uco-observable:fileSystemType": "ExtX",
                        "uco-observable:isDirectory": false,
```

Listing 4.10 (Cont'd)

```
                          "uco-observable:allocationStatus": "allocated",
                          "uco-observable:sizeInBytes": 189907,
                          "uco-observable:observableCreatedTime": {
                               "@type": "xsd:dateTime",
                               "@value": "2018-11-26T18:55:36.000Z"
                          }
                     },
                     {
                          "@type": "uco-observable:ContentDataFacet",
                          "uco-observable:hash": [
                               {
                                    "@type": "uco-types:Hash",
                                    "uco-types:hashMethod": {
                                         "@type": "uco-vocabulary:HashNameVocab",
                                         "@value": "MD5"
                                    },
                                    "uco-types:hashValue": {
                                         "@type": "xsd:hexBinary",
                                         "@value": "f618c8868ba6c9ed2fbf01801336c847"
                                    }
                               }
                          ]
                     }
                ]
           },
```

Listing 4.10 (Cont'd)

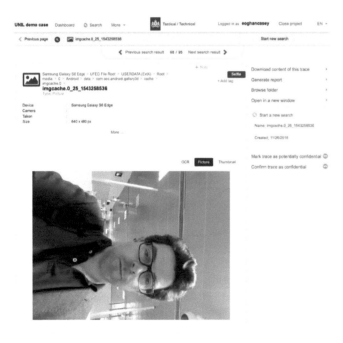

Figure 4.11 Photograph extracted from mobile device and processed using the Hansken DFaaS platform.

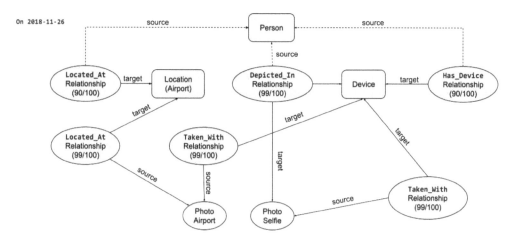

Figure 4.12 Graph of inferred relationships between photo, device, and person based on hypothesis test results.

All of these inferred relationships can be depicted as a graph to visualize the links and to provide transparency into the logic as shown in Figure 4.12. Note that the diagram does not depict direct links between the photo, device, or person. This approach avoids misinterpretation, clarifying that the relationships are the result of hypothesis testing rather than being fixed facts. If there are other hypotheses to be considered in the future, they can be represented in the same manner.

4.8 Effective/Reliable/Responsible Automated Analysis

It is not sufficient to provide decision makers with a conclusion, it is also necessary to explain the logic that led to the conclusion. To this end, forensic science must employ a formalized logical process that is rigorous and repeatable in order to avoid incorrect assumptions (blind spots) and unfounded conclusions. Specifically, to develop clearer understanding and to evaluate observable facts in relation to possible explanations, scientific practices must ascend a path from limited facts and open questions to reach high confidence answers, through a cyclical process of abductive, deductive, and inductive reasoning (Pollitt et al. 2018).

This chapter provides a foundation for developing systems that meet these requirements. When implementing these formalizations, developers will benefit from following the hypothetico-deductive model (Ribaux 2014). Abductive reasoning formulates an inference to the "best" explanation (causal activities) for available observations (traces, analytic results), applying analogous past experiences (knowledge) to eliminate implausible explanations and retain the most plausible explanation.[1] Deductive reasoning tests this most plausible hypothe-sized activities against additional observations, possibly through further study of traces to answer the question "what other traces should be expected for a given hypothesis, with particular scrutiny for contradictory facts (falsification)?". If any contradictory traces are found, the most plausible explanation must be revised. Inductive reasoning can lead to additional knowledge about specific types of activities and/or traces, providing decision-makers with trustworthy understanding of the circumstances to help them make decisions. Inductive reasoning can also lead to a theory generalized from multiple cases or from repeatable experiments, providing new or updated knowledge in forensic science.

Artificial intelligence depends on the ability to understand analytic results and to generate hypothesis test results based on available information and domain specific knowledge. When developing such systems for forensic purposes, there are several considerations for effective automated analysis (Bollé et al. 2020):

1. Is the method fit-for-purpose to address the question being analysed?
   Being able to answer this question requires that the system clearly inform the user on the typical use cases that the system was developed to work on. It also requires that the user knows precisely what they are trying to achieve with this particular tool. Imagine a system designed to detect CSAM. In practice, users of such a system may also want to detect images of young people in bathing suits or underwear. This requirement should be clear from the user perspective and the ability to detect such images should be clear from the system perspective.

2. Is the method reliable to produce an analytic result on the data?
   The reliability of the system is often measured using performance metrics. The choice of the metrics is important as not all of them capture the whole picture. For instance, some metrics may be used to minimize false positives and others to minimize false negatives. Both approaches are valid and choosing one over the other will depend on the context and typical usage of the system. Again, determining that the method is fit-for-purpose is important to assert if the performance measured is adapted to the situation.

3. Is the method understandable to analysts who must evaluate the results?
   This understandability or explainability of a system determines if an analyst is able to understand a particular result and the general functioning of a system. This is particularly important as systems are usually a support in the decision making process made by the analyst. A challenge resides in the fact that the understanding of the user might be subjective. This aspect requires the training needed to appreciate the results to be clearly defined.

4. Is the evaluation of the analytic results consistent, clear, and repeatable?
   The result of the automated system will be a basis for the inferences made dur-ing the evaluation. As explained previously, evaluation requires a set of

---

[1] The term abductive was originally used by Peirce (Eco and Sebeok 1983), and has more recently been described as inference to the best explanation. The original term abductive is used here for compatibility with deductive and inductive terminology.

competing hypotheses. Inferences are made to determine how the observed results are likely to be under each hypothesis. Automated systems should guide the analyst in such a process, which is particularly difficult knowing how versatile the questions that one might want to answer are.

With modern machine learning and deep learning systems, these questions are difficult to answer. The system tends to suggest decisions, for instance by suggesting a possible classification of a particular trace or activity and the mechanisms that lead to this particular suggestion are not accessible to the user (black-box effect). There is a need to develop automated systems that guide the user through the decision process and help them understand the output of the system.

To face that challenge, a new research area emerged in the scientific community, called XAI for eXplainable Artificial Intelligence, which has the following objectives outlined in technical documentation accompanying Google Cloud Explainable AI product (Google 2022):

- Inform and support human decision making
- Improve transparency
- Enable debugging and auditing
- Verify generalization ability and moderate trust

The final idea being to help the user of the system to take better and well informed decisions, and the system developers to improve the system. The discussion between developers and users may often be forgotten but is the cement to the development and usage of effective automated systems.

4.9 Conclusion

Formal representation of digital traces creates a culture of common comprehension, reducing misunderstanding. Formal representation of inferences helps to compare logic, and increases transparency and traceability. This chapter covers both formalizations, providing a foundation for robust reasoning and automated systems supporting forensic analysis.

References

BBC (2018). Chinese AI caught out by face in bus ad, 27 November 2018. https://www.bbc.com/news/technology-46357004 (accessed 23 May 2022).

Biedermann, A. and Kotsoglou, K.N. (2020). Digital evidence exceptionalism? A review and discussion of conceptual hurdles in digital evidence transformation. *Forensic Science International: Synergy* 2 (2020): 262–274. https://doi.org/10.1016/j.fsisyn.2020.08.004 accessed 3 April 2023.

Bollé, T., and Casey, E. (2018). Using computed similarity of distinctive digital traces to evaluate non-obvious links and repetitions in cyber-investigations. *Digital Investigation*, 24, S2–S9. https://doi.org/10.1016/j.diin.2018.01.002 Accessed: 03/04/2023

Bollé, T., Casey, E., and Jacquet, M. (2020). The role of evaluations in reaching decisions using automated systems supporting forensic analysis. *Forensic Science International: Digital Investigation* 34 (2020): 301016. https://doi.org/10.1016/j.fsidi.2020.301016 accessed 5 April 2023.

Caneppele, S., & Aebi, M. F. (2019). Crime Drop or Police Recording Flop? On the Relationship between the Decrease of Offline Crime and the Increase of Online and Hybrid Crimes. *Policing: A Journal of Policy and Practice*, 13(1), 6679. https://doi.org/10.1093/police/pax055 Access date: 03/04/2023

Casey, E. (2020). Standardization of forming and expressing preliminary evaluative opinions on digital evidence. *Forensic Science International: Digital Investigation* 32 (2020): 200888. https://doi.org/10.1016/j.fsidi.2019.200888 April 2023.

Casey, E., Barnum, S., Griffith, R. et al. (2017). Advancing coordinated cyber-investigations and tool interoperability using a community developed specification language. *Digital Investigation* 22: 14–45. https://doi.org/10.1016/j.diin.2017.08.002.

Du, X., Hargreaves, C., Sheppard, J. et al. (2020). SoK: exploring the state of the art and the future potential of artificial intelligence in digital forensic investigation. In: Proceedings of the 15th International Conference on Availability, Reliability and Security (ARES '20). Association for Computing Machinery, New York, NY, USA, Article 46, 1–10. https://doi.org/10.1145/3407023.3407068 April 2023.

Ebrahimi, M., Suen, C.Y., and Ormandjieva, O. (2016). Detecting predatory conversations in social media by deep convolutional neural networks. *Digital Investigation* 18: 33–49. https://doi.org/10.1016/j.diin.2016.07.001 5 April 2023.

Eco, U., and Sebeok, T. A. (Eds.). (1988). *The Sign of Three: Dupin, Holmes, Peirce*. Indiana University Press.

Europol (2021). Internet organised crime threat assessment (IOCTA). https://www.europol. europa.eu/publications-events/main-reports/iocta-report.

Eykholt, K., Evtimov, I., Fernandes, E. et al. (2018). Robust physical-world attacks on deep learning visual classification. CVPR 2018. https://www.gov.uk/government/publications/ development-of-evaluative-opinions April 2023.

Forensic Science Regulator (2021). Codes of practice and conduct development of evaluative opinions. FSR-C-118. Issue 1. https://www.gov.uk/government/publications/development-of-evaluative-opinions April 2023.

Google (2022). AI explanations whitepaper, Google cloud explainable AI. https://storage. googleapis.com/cloud-ai-whitepapers/AI%20Explainability%20Whitepaper.pdf.

Henseler, H. and Hyde, J. (2019). Technology assisted analysis of timeline and connections in digital forensic investigations. 6.

Moutiez, C. (2020). Towards action reconstruction using A.I. techniques. Master's thesis, Batochime, Lausanne: University of Lausanne.

Pollitt, M., Casey, E., Jaquet-Chiffelle, D.-O., and Gladyshev, P. (2018) A framework for harmonizing forensic science practices and digital/multimedia evidence. OSAC Technical Series 0002R1 https://www.nist.gov/organization-scientific-area-committees-forensic-science/framework-harmonizing-forensic-science accessed 5 April 2023.

Ribaux, O. (2014). *Police scientifique: Le renseignement par la trace*. Lausanne: Presses polytechniques et universitaires romandes.

Sanchez, L., Grajeda, C., Baggili, I., and Hall, C. (2019). A practitioner survey exploring the value of forensic tools, AI, filtering, & safer presentation for investigating child sexual abuse material (CSAM). *Digital Investigation* 29 (Supplement, 2019): S124–S142. https://doi.org/10.1016/j.diin.2019.04.005 April 2023.

Ukwen, D.O. and Karabatak, M. (2021). Review of NLP-based systems in digital forensics and cybersecurity. 2021 9th International Symposium on Digital Forensics and Security (ISDFS), 1–9. doi:10.1109/ISDFS52919.2021.9486354.

CHAPTER 5

Servicing Digital Investigations with Artificial Intelligence

Harm van Beek* and Hans Henseler*

Digital and Biometric Traces Division, Netherlands Forensic Institute, Laan van Ypenburg, 6, GB, The Hague, The Netherlands

* Corresponding authors

5.1 Introduction

The importance of digital evidence is rapidly increasing. Analysts expect that the global digital forensics market will have an annual growth rate of 11.2% over the next seven years with a sales forecast reaching US\$ 23.62 Bn in 2030.[1] This field of digital forensics, however, is constantly changing due to the rapid evolution of computers, mobile devices, the internet (of things) and social media. Commercial tool vendors as well as the professional, scientific, and open source communities are doing their best to keep up with new technical challenges. Despite this growth and innovation, most organizations still operate under the traditional paradigm by which experts in the digital forensic lab examine digital evidence and report results to investigators outside the lab.

Organizations are finding that keeping up with new technical challenges in the digital forensic lab is not enough to let investigators benefit from the full potential of digital evidence. This has resulted in the introduction of a new paradigm called digital forensics as a service (DFaaS) (van Baar et al. 2014) in which digital forensic examiners, investigators, innovators, and other stakeholders in the investigation and judicial process can collaborate using a single digital forensic data platform. The UK Forensic Science Regulator stated in her 2019 annual report (Tully 2020) that "How we used to do digital forensics" is no longer fit for purpose. Nowadays, these DFaaS ideas are broadly adopted, amongst others it is part of the Digital Forensic Science Strategy of the UK National Police Chief's Council (NPCC 2020).

---

[1] https://www.futuremarketinsights.com/reports/digital-forensics-market, last visited 7 April 2023.

Artificial Intelligence (AI) in Forensic Sciences, First Edition. Edited by Zeno Geradts and Katrin Franke.
© 2024 John Wiley & Sons Ltd. Published 2024 by John Wiley & Sons Ltd.

One example of such a DFaaS platform is Hansken (van Beek et al. 2015; 2020), a solution that has been built by the Netherlands Forensic Institute. Today, Hansken has been adopted and is being maintained as a closed-source solution by a growing international community of law enforcement and investigating agencies. We foresee that through the big data capabilities of Hansken new AI techniques can be applied supporting users with intelligent assistance when investigating digital evidence. In this chapter we identify various types of intelligent assistance that are either implemented in Hansken or will be in the future and how they benefit from the big data architecture on which Hansken is founded.

We start this chapter by introducing Hansken, its normalized trace model and its forensic tool application process and application programming interfaces in Section 5.2. Next, in Section 5.3, we explain how rule based AI and deep learning AI techniques are currently implemented in Hansken, and how modern deep learning approaches like technology assisted review and semantic search can be added to Hanksen's tool box. We briefly summarize further readings in Section 5.4.

5.2 Introduction To Hansken

Hansken, the DFaaS implementation, is currently developed and maintained by the Netherlands Forensic Institute. A growing number of law-enforcement and intelligence agencies as well as academia have shown interest and joined the Hansken community.

Hansken supports a wide range of users by offering several functions for gaining insight into large amounts of digital evidence. It supports cases with more than a thousand images of seized devices, over 100 terabytes of data and/or over 100 million digital artifacts called *traces* (e.g., emails, chat messages, pictures, and documents). Even such large quantities of data are searchable within seconds. Hansken extracts traces from evidence items (forensic images or reports) by iteratively applying forensic tools. Each trace is processed and enriched, amongst others with digests (for integrity checking as well as identification) and a full keyword index.

All evidence is traceable (chain of evidence), including advanced logging of embedded forensic tools. All handling of the evidence can be audited (chain of custody) and profound judicial reviews took place in several Dutch courts (Court of Amsterdam 2018; Court of Gelderland 2019). These reviews included the support for handling privileged communication. Next to investigative teams, defense lawyers use the platform to access evidence and review investigations.

To handle the growing amount of data, Hansken builds on existing platforms to scale and distribute storage and processing (see van Beek et al. 2020, Table 1). Hansken consists of several services that together implement the DFaaS platform. Key components are the data service built on Hadoop File System and/or Ceph, for storing (seized) data; the extraction service, built on Hadoop MapReduce, for applying forensic tools to the data to extract traces; and the trace service, built on Elasticsearch, for storing these traces and serving them based on querying and filtering.

5.2.1 Normalized Trace Model

A key benefit of Hansken is its normalized *trace model*. All traces identified during the extraction process must be modelled according to this trace model. The trace model defines how digital artifacts must be described in order to be indexed by the Hansken search engine. Each trace is a structured object consisting of data and metadata to describe the data. A trace contains several mandatory intrinsic properties such as *name* and *id*. Furthermore, a trace can have *type*s (e.g., email, file, picture) with per type several typed properties (e.g., email.from, file.name, picture.width). The collection of types and properties form the metadata of a trace. All metadata are categorized (e.g, *extracted* for extracted types/properties or *processed* for properties involving the processing itself). Also, the types have an origin (e.g., system or user) to describe who extracted the metadata from the data.

Each trace in Hansken can be assigned multiple types (e.g., both file and picture, or both document and attachment), which is called duck-typing (Casey et al. 2017). This corresponds to the way humans look at digital artifacts, where the interpretation depends on the perspective and context in which they are being observed. We call a JPEG file a "file" when browsing the file system and a "picture" when discussing its contents, for example.

Depending on the human's perspective, a trace can also have multiple *contents*. The contents of a PDF file for example, can be considered either the raw bytes of the file or the text contained in the document. Some special "types" can be assigned to provide metadata related to these contents, for example the *raw* contents (with properties like the raw size in bytes, mime type and digests) or the *text* contents.

Where traces typically have several types and a few dozen properties, Hanksen's trace model also introduces so-called *tracelets*. These are small, single-typed traces with at most a few properties. Traces typically contain multiple tracelets, like entities (e.g., email addresses, credit card numbers, international bank-account numbers, phone numbers). Because of their frequent occurrence, they are not considered regular traces and follow specific query and filter rules.

5.2.1.1 Modelling AI Results

During extraction, most of the traces result from explainable, deterministic, and validated algorithms. These traces can be reproduced by using alternative tools that also implement the algorithms. In digital forensic investigations, this is the de facto standard for validating extracted traces: two distinct tools produce comparable results. Nowadays, many of the tools applied in any domain, including digital forensics, build on artificial intelligence. As a result, the algorithms applied are not always explainable and results cannot always be reproduced (e.g., due to self-learning properties of the algorithms). In Hansken, we distinguish between these types of traces and properties of such traces by classifying them as *extracted* (by explainable and deterministic algorithms) or *mined* (using artificial intelligence).

A prediction is modelled as a special "type" of tracelet (since they can have high occurrence per trace). Example predictions are objects or faces recognized in pictures and videos. Each prediction comes with the originating machine-learning model (both name and version) and its confidence (value between 0 and 1). Depending on the source artifact and applied model, additional properties can be stored (e.g., the region in the picture where a face is found, or the offset in a video where an object was identified).

Nowadays, the applied models can also produce so-called *embeddings* in a vector space (e.g., photoDNA[2] or face embeddings). Hansken builds on Elasticsearch,[3] which natively supports vectors. As a result, Hansken can dynamically compute query-based similarities (Manhattan distance, Euclidian distance, cosine similarity). Query results can be ordered based on distance (e.g., to find pictures with similar faces, given an earlier found face).

5.2.2 Forensic Tool Application

Hansken implements a framework for applying forensic tools to (seized) data. This so-called *extraction process* builds an index of traces (e.g., email, chat messages, pictures, and documents) and tracelets (e.g., entities, predictions) with all their metadata (types and properties), a full keyword index on all identified pieces of text, and previews when applicable (e.g., picture thumbnails, video key frames).

Hanksen's execution model brings the tools to the data. In general, getting access to the data of any trace are both I/O and CPU intensive: a lot of data is transferred, and a lot of calculations take place. For example, consider a picture that is contained in a compressed file archive that is attached to an email, stored in an email database file, contained in a file system inside a virtual machine, that itself is stored as a file in a file system on a physical hard drive. Getting to this specific picture requires several file system walks, database queries as well as file decompressions (unzipping) and data transformations (base64 decoding). Case investigations typically involve terabytes of data containing millions of such traces. Therefore, Hansken combines both parallel processing with iterative processing (van Beek et al. 2015).

As seen in the example above, traces form a huge tree, where the root of the tree is (a forensic image of) a data carrier (e.g., a hard drive or mobile device). Using distribution technology (Hadoop MapReduce), Hansken distributes the traces on a cluster of compute nodes. Figure 5.1 presents an example Hadoop cluster for an actual Hansken production environment with 23 nodes. The cluster is accessible as a single compute environment with 552 cores with 5.56 terabytes of working memory (RAM).

---

[2] https://www.microsoft.com/PhotoDNA, last visited 7 April 2023.
[3] https://www.elastic.co/elasticsearch, last visited 7 April 2023.

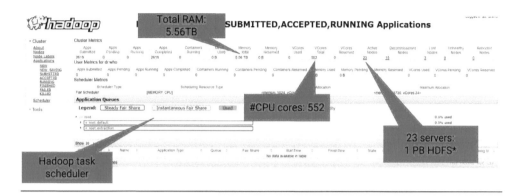

Figure 5.1 Example of a Hansken Hadoop production cluster with a total of 5.56TB RAM, 552 CPU cores, 23 servers with a total of 1 PB HDFS storage and the Hadoop task scheduler.

Once a trace is ready for processing, Hansken offers it to an extraction job, implemented as a Hadoop map task. This task inspects the (partly processed) trace and applies *all* forensic tools as long as tools state that they can process it. In this way, once the data of the example picture is available, forensic tools calculate digests, extract camera details, time stamps and geolocation information, identify objects or text, and calculate face embeddings. Finally, in the Hadoop reduce task, the trace is sent to the Hansken trace service for storing the results.

If, while processing a trace, a tool creates multiple child traces (e.g., files while processing a file system, or emails while processing an email database), these child traces are collected and offered to the distribution process again.

Next to the extracted trace details, the provenance of the actual processing is stored with each trace. For this, traces are extended with so-call *toolrun* details, modelled as tracelets. Each tool application is stored, describing the tool, its version, whether is was successful or failed, and the types and properties extracted by the tool. Like other tracelets, this information can be used for querying and filtering traces (e.g., for summarizing failing tools). Also, Hansken collects an extraction profile, summarizing all applied tools and aggregated details on their use (e.g., number of invocations, total calculation time, and processed number of bytes). In this way, operators and experts can identify bottlenecks and optimize the process.

The extraction process explained above, works well for the majority of tools that process single traces (i.e., single pieces of data). Tools exist, that either combine multiple traces (e.g., for extracting multipart ZIP-files) or require other traces to process a single trace (e.g., decryption tools that require a key). For this, Hansken provides so-called *deferred tools*. These tools are applied to (collections of) traces after the main extraction process is finished. They are implemented as regular tools (with regular matchers on single traces), but have the ability to query and access the earlier processed and stored traces.

5.2.3 Hansken's Application Programming Interfaces

All functions of Hansken are accessible via application programming interfaces (APIs). This enables any user to handle both the platform and the stored data and traces in their preferred way.

To use the APIs, a user first has to authenticate and start a session. Each user is authorized to use specific functions (e.g., only query and filter, or also upload data and start extractions) and specific data (e.g., only assigned cases).

To operate a Hansken platform, it exposes the following functions via its API:
- *case administration*: create/delete/backup/restore cases;
- *image data management*: upload/delete images, validate digests, link images to cases;
- *extraction management*: configure/schedule/order/prioritize extraction tasks, retrieve extraction status/logs/statistics, list available extraction tools, handle additional resource;
- *trace index management*: open/close indexes, (partial) clone indexes, list related images, retrieve index status/statistics, update number of shards;
- *general platform information*: retrieve health status, retrieve platform versions, retrieve release notes, retrieve licenses, retrieve guide.

To use the platform for investigative purposes, Hansken offers the several functions for filtering and selecting traces. A specific query language is defined for this purpose, the Hansken query language (HQL). Hansken offers the following functions via its API:
- *search/filter traces*: filter with HQL, get trace types and properties, get preview data, get text snippets, get chains of evidence and custody details, walk tree structures, download trace data;
- *search/filter tracelets*: filter with HQL, get tracelet types and properties;
- *search/filter values*: filter with HQL, get values for selected properties;
- *keyword suggestions*: autofill keywords;
- *aggregate results*: get summarized details;
- *annotate traces*: add/remove notes, add/remove tags, filter on notes/tags, handle privileged communication.

The HQL is very rich, offering the negation and/or combination of multiple selection criteria on all types and properties of traces, as well as on the indexed texts. Detailed documentation is available in the Hansken guide. The following filter functions, amongst others are available:
- *text queries*: filter on terms anywhere in the data and/or metadata, or only selected types or properties. Terms consist of case-insensitive letters (ignores diacritics) and digits and may include punctuation characters, support for uni-code escape sequences, support for wild cards.
- *phrase queries*: filter on sequences of terms. Support for terms with a close distance.
- *regular expressions*: filter on terms that match a regular expression.

- *date queries*: Filter on dates/times anywhere in the metadata, or only selected types or properties. Support for specific values (year, month, day, etc) or ranges of dates/times.
- *numeric queries*: filter on specific numeric values or ranges of values on selected properties.
- *geolocation queries*: filter on properties defining a location within selected latitude/longitude ranges.

5.3 Large Scale Application of AI Techniques

Digital forensic processing requires a variety of different carvers, parsers, and other techniques to extract traces from information contained in digital devices. Traces are typically extracted from structured data based on well-defined algorithms. Other techniques are required to extract traces and relationships from unstructured data such as picture, document, audio, video, and message contents. This is the area where AI algorithms can be of great value.

In this section we use Hansken as an example to illustrate how AI can assist in structuring unstructured information. In Section 5.3.1 we discuss rule-based AI techniques that are used by Hansken to extract entities. Section 5.3.2 discusses machine learning techniques that Hansken uses for classification of pictures, video, for detecting scene texts and faces in pictures, and how embedding vectors are used to find faces that are similar to a face that has been detected. In Section 5.3.3 we describe more advanced deep learning techniques that have interesting potential for digital forensic investigations. Finally, in Section 5.3.4 we describe the rise of large language models at the end of 2022 and their application to digital forensics.

5.3.1 Rule-based AI Techniques Implemented in Hansken

Rule-based AI techniques can be very effective for extracting entities from unstructured data in case entities having a well defined pattern of symbols (e.g., letters, numbers). Examples are license plates, international bank account numbers (IBANs), email addresses, IP addresses, and credit card numbers. Such patterns can typically be scanned by using a regular expression.[4] The NFI has developed FEEL, a forensic entity extraction library. Entities extracted with FEEL become tracelets in Hansken and have the following properties:
- *type*: the type of entity (e.g., email address, IBAN, URL);
- *value*: the normalized (text) value of the entity;
- *confidence*: the confidence value of the entity, between 0 and 1 inclusive;
- *source*: the property or data stream where the entity was found, (e.g., email.to, data.raw);

---

[4] See for example the community patterns at https://regexr.com/, last visited 7 April 2023.

- *index*: for properties that have a list of values, indicates from which value the entity was extracted (e.g., email.to is a list of values);
- *offset*: the offset within the source property or data stream of the entity;
- *length*: the raw, not normalized length of the entity;
- *encoding*: the character encoding of the entity's raw value.

A regular expression by itself is not necessarily considered an AI technique. However, in digital forensics often binary data is processed containing many random number and character sequences. Consequently, regular expressions in digital forensic applications are known to generate false positives (e.g., a string that matches a regular expression associated with an entity which it is not). Therefore, FEEL implements additional measures to validate the expression and to estimate the confidence based on the context of a string that was matched. A good example are credit card numbers. A number that meets the regular expression for a credit card number should additionally be validated using the Luhn algorithm.[5] Not all entities have a numerical validation algorithm. Therefore, FEEL also performs a confidence estimation based on the context of the string that was matched. For example, a string that matches an email address regular expression is more likely to be an actual email address if it occurs in the context of an email header keyword such as "from", "to" or "cc".

Named entity extraction is another useful application of AI in digital forensics. It refers to the extraction of entities that have names like persons, companies, places. Having entities available in a structured and standardized way helps investigators in their investigation, e.g., to determine who is involved or with linking different digital traces through social network analysis and visualization.

Rule-based extraction of named entities is relatively easy for sources that are known to contain names in a fixed format such as system accounts, document, address books, registry settings, cookies, internet history URLs, and headers from chats, phone calls, and text messages (Henseler et al. 2013; Hofste 2012). Hansken also extracts identities but is currently restricted to identities encountered in email and chat metadata and normalizes their representation (e.g., dashes and spaces are stripped from phone numbers). Hansken stores such identities as tracelets with the following properties:

- *uuid*: the universal unique id of the identity;
- *id*: the unique identifier of the identity, for example an email address, username, or phone number;
- *name*: the name of the identity;
- *first name*: the first name of the identity;
- *last name*: the last name of the identity;
- *username*: the username of the identity;
- *screen name*: the display name of the identity;

---

[5] See ISO/IEC 7812, https://www.iso.org/standard/70484.html, last visited 7 April 2023.

- *email address*: the email address of the identity;
- *phone number*: the phone number of the identity;
- *status*: the social status of the identity (e.g., "being happy", "at the gym");
- *ldapDn*: the ldap distinguished names of the identity;
- *original value*: the original value from which identity was extracted (e.g., "John Doe").

Automatically merging identities into a single identity when they refer to the same person is not easy. For instance, two identities can have different properties (e.g., full name versus email alias) and may suffer from spelling variations (e.g., initials versus first names, spelling errors) .

In a digital investigation it is important to establish the relevance of an identity. The true relevance of an identity in a case is typically only known to the investigator and often not in the beginning but only during the investigation. To assist the investigator, it may be useful to assign (merged) identities a score that is based on the number of times it occurs in the data and in what sources. For example, the importance of a name in a single Windows user account is considered more relevant than a name in a single email (address). Such a ranking score does not provide any information about the relevance of the identity to the investigation but at least it shows the investigator that this identity frequently occurs in the data and/or in important data points.

5.3.2 Deep-learning AI Techniques Currently Implemented in Hansken

Disadvantages of rule-based AI techniques are that they can only be applied to relatively easy pattern recognition tasks, that there must be known rules to detect these patterns, and that these rules need to be maintained which is often a manual task. Using machine learning based AI techniques, it is possible to train statistical models that learn to classify more complex data, such as pictures. They learn this by many examples, using automated procedures, hence, machine learning.

In Hansken currently two types of deep-learning AI techniques are implemented. The first type of techniques is used for predicting labels for pictures and video frames and calculating a confidence level for the predictions:

- ImageNet classification of pictures;
- customized ImageNet trained on specific classes for pictures and video frames;
- scene text prediction;
- recognize barcodes in pictures;
- detect faces in pictures with or without age estimation.

The prediction tools used by Hansken are bundled in FIRE, the forensic image recognition engine library [NFI]. Predictions are stored in the trace model as prediction tracelets similar to *entities* and *identities*. A *prediction* is a statistical prediction about a trace. Hansken supports the following properties for a prediction:

- *type*: the type of the prediction (e.g., a classification, scene text or barcode);
- *model name*: name of the machine learning model that produced this prediction;

- *model version*: version of the machine learning model that produced this prediction;
- *class*: the predicted class;
- *label*: the predicted label;
- *confidence(s)*: the prediction confidence(s), expressed as a value between 0 and 1 (multiple confidences occur in video, for example);
- *embedding*: the calculated embedding (vector) in the model's embedding space;
- *region*: the prediction region as a polygon $[x_1, y_1, x_2, y_2, ...]$ in pixels (without wrapping back to the start position);
- *offset*: offset(s) in seconds from the start of this prediction (for videos).

To search for pictures containing faces that are predicted with a confidence greater than 0.9, for example, can be done using the following HQL query: prediction:{type:face confidence>0.9}. The result is illustrated in Figure 5.2. Not only does the face detection tool in Hansken predict if a face exists in a picture, it also marks the region where the face was detected in the image, as illustrated in Figure 5.3.

Hansken can not only predict classes for pictures, it can also do this for video frames. Since videos can easily contain 25 frames for every second of video, this can be a time consuming task during extraction. Hansken operators, therefore, typically run this tool after standard extractions have finished. The video classification extraction results are then appended to the existing extraction results while investigators can already search the data (for traces that have been extracted in the first run). Figure 5.4 illustrates image classification in videos and lists the results for the following query prediction:{class:firearm confidence>0.9} type:video video.duration>60.

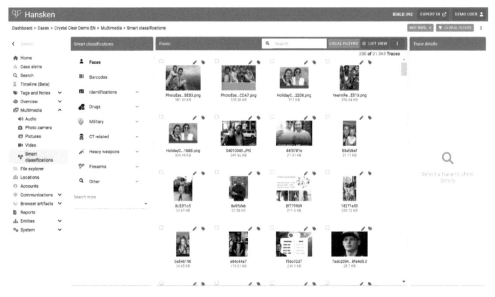

Figure 5.2 Example search result for faces in Hansken.

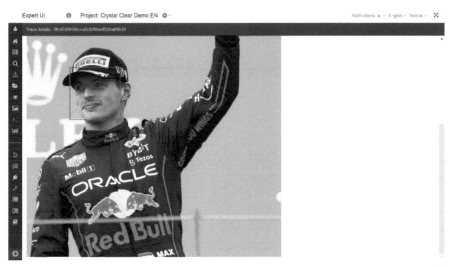

Figure 5.3 Example face found with Hansken.

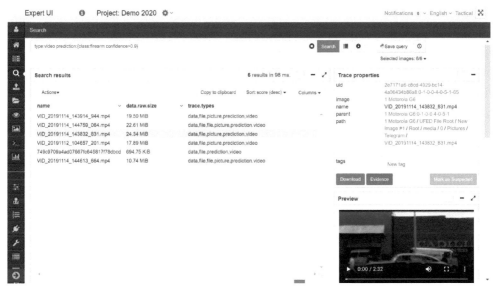

Figure 5.4 Example showing search results in Hansken for videos lasting longer than 60 seconds that contain firearms.

Figure 5.5a The key frame of this video does not contain a firearm but the timeline below the video indicates at what times video frames resulted in a prediction. Most of them are well below 0.9 except for the dark blue line indicating a frame that has been classified as firearm. The user can navigate to that time by clicking the blue line which is illustrated in Figure 5.5b.

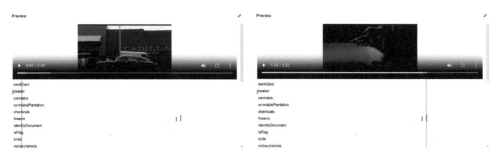

Figure 5.5 Example of (a) video containing firearms found with Hansken and (b) when navigating to the frame classified as firearm.

The classification techniques presented above use a deep-learning model to predict the confidence level of a classification for a picture. This confidence level is a number between 0 and 1 which is typically the activation level of an output node in a classification layer. For some applications it can be interesting to store the feature vector that is constructed by the network before it is classified. The advantage is that this vector can then be used to search for pictures that have similar vectors. In Hansken this is implemented in the face detection engine. When a face is detected, Hansken stores the feature vector representing the face in the *embedding* property of the prediction trace. This property then enables the user to search for pictures containing similar faces. This is illustrated in Figure 5.6.

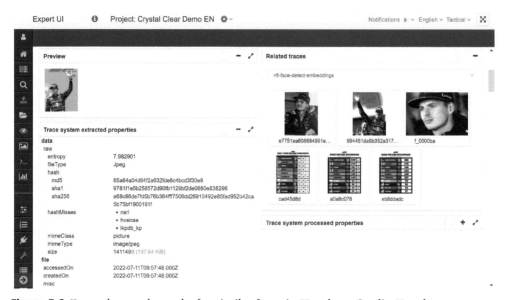

Figure 5.6 Example search results for similar faces in Hansken. Credit: Hansken.

5.3.3 Deep-learning AI Techniques to be Implemented in Hansken

With the rapid advances in deep learning, some of the more traditional digital forensics classification and fuzzy-search algorithms can be replaced using deep learning alternatives. Traditional keyword search and even deep-learning based visual classifiers that were considered state of the art three years ago (e.g., deep convolutional neural networks) are already being replaced by or augmented with new techniques, such as:

- transformer based language models (e.g., BERT (Devlin et al. 2018)) for text-based classification, semantic search, similarity search and visualization of search results through clustering;
- visual transformers such as CLIP,[6] a model for zero shot picture classification, find similar pictures, text based image search;
- entity, topic, event, and relationship extraction for visualization of correlated evidence and building a knowledge graph;
- AI-based malware detection and classification;
- continuous active learning (CAL).

How can transformer-based language models such as multilingual BERT be used in digital forensics? To answer this question it is useful to review a technique from digital forensics called *similaritydigests*, also known as fuzzy hashes. Good examples are SSDEEP, SDHASH and Lempel-Ziv Jaccard Distance (Raff and Nicholas 2018), which create a hash value that can be used to measure the similarity between two binary files. Note that this is different from a cryptographic (or secure) hash (like SHA1) because a cryptographic hash can check exact matches (or non-matches) but not similarity. In fact, the smallest change in the input to a cryptographic hash function will generate a completely different hash value. For binary files, these measures are adequate but for, e.g., documents and pictures, it appears that embedding vectors that have been produced by deep learning provide a better alternative. Embedding vectors not only find similar contents like the feature vectors in the previous paragraph, but they can also find semantically similar contents. This concept is very well illustrated with the *word2vec* model (Mikolov et al. 2013).

The *word2vec* training algorithm is a form of self-supervised learning that learns vector representations for words in a vocabulary based on texts in which these words are used. The neural network is a shallow neural network with one hidden layer. The input to this layer is a bag-of-words representation of a word and the target output is a bag-of-words representation of a word that occurs within a maximum number (e.g., 10) of words. A disadvantage of a bag-of-words vector representation is that they have many dimensions (equal to the size of the dictionary), that a word vector is scarce (just one dimension is 1, the other dimensions are 0) and, consequently, that this representation cannot express if different words are related or

---

[6] Contrastive Language–Image Pre-training, see https://openai.com/blog/clip, last visited 7 April 2023.

have similar meanings. Through this form of self-supervised learning, the network learns to predict for a given word by which other words it is frequently *embedded*. After training, the bag-of-words representation is replaced by the corresponding activity of the hidden layer in the network. This type of vector is called *embedding vector*. The *word2vec* algorithm assigns topologically similar vectors to words with similar embeddings which typically are somehow (semantically) related. This is illustrated by the following example, listing the 10 most similar words to the word *Apple* in the *word2vec* model that was trained on the GoogleNews data set:

```
gensim_model.most_similar(positive=['Apple'])
  [('Apple_AAPL', 0.7456985712051392),
   ('Apple_Nasdaq_AAPL', 0.7300410270690918),
   ('Apple_NASDAQ_AAPL', 0.7175089716911316),
   ('Apple_Computer', 0.7145973443984985),
   ('iPhone', 0.6924266219139099),
   ('Apple_NSDQ_AAPL', 0.6868604421615601),
   ('Steve_Jobs', 0.6758422255516052),
   ('iPad', 0.6580768823623657),
   ('Apple_nasdaq_AAPL', 0.6444970965385437),
   ('Apple_iPad', 0.622774600982666)]
```

The following example illustrates how the meaning of words is captured in the topology of their corresponding vectors. If we take the vector for *Paris,* subtract the vector for *France* and add the vector for *Netherlands* the resulting vector is most similar to *Amsterdam,* the capital city of the Netherlands:

```
gensim_model.most_similar(positive=['Paris', 'Netherlands'],
negative=['France'])
  [('Amsterdam', 0.7488842010498047),
   ('Rotterdam', 0.6150579452514648),
   ('Amsterdam_Netherlands', 0.601604163646698),
   ('Stockholm', 0.5815855264663696),
   ('Utrecht', 0.5681812763214111),
   ('Antwerp', 0.5524181127548218),
   ('Haarlem', 0.5439442992210388),
   ('Rotterdam_Netherlands', 0.528085470199585),
   ('Dutch', 0.5252639055252075),
   ('Eindhoven', 0.5225303173065186)]
```

There are various drawbacks to the *word2vec* algorithm that have been overcome in the past 10 years For instance, there are no vectors for new words (e.g., words that did not occur in the original data set). This problem has been solved by introducing *wordpieces* (Wu et al., 2016). Also, words in natural language can be ambiguous. One drawback, for instance, is that a word like *bank* can have more than one meaning. For example, *bank of the river* or *withdraw money from the bank*. The meaning of *bank* depends on the context in which it occurs. Since *word2vec* can only assign one vector to *bank*, it is not able to represent different meanings. This problem has been solved with the introduction of *transformer networks* such as BERT that create embedding vectors based on a sequence of *wordpieces*.

Modern deep-learning approaches are able to compute multi-modal embedding vectors. For instance, CLIP is trained on pictures and corresponding text captions resulting in multi-modal embedding vectors that represent visual and textual data in the same vector space. This is illustrated in Figure 5.7. In step 1 the CLIP model is trained. Once trained, CLIP embedding vectors can be calculated for all pictures. In Hansken these embedding predictions can be used in two different ways. The user can find similar pictures based on a source picture, or the user can enter a textual query which is then converted into an embedding vector with CLIP which is then used to find pictures with similar CLIP embedding vectors.

5.3.3.1 Technology Assisted Review

Technology assisted review (TAR) is a field in eDiscovery where AI techniques are used to assist users with tagging documents that are relevant for their investigations. In eDiscovery, TAR has been mostly applied to email and document review but it can be easily applied to digital investigations with other types of digital traces.

Initially, TAR was based on predictive coding which uses a machine-learning algorithm that continues to learn and make better decisions while significantly expediting the review process, saving time and money. In predictive coding, humans first need to classify the data set that is used for training a machine model. During the training of this model the users remain passive. The training data sets typically need to be very large and based on a random selection. This

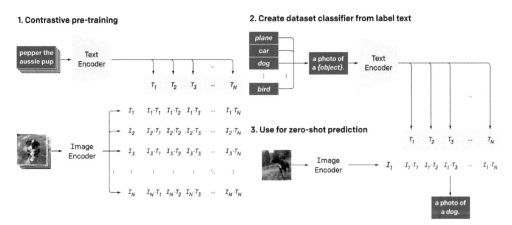

Figure 5.7 How CLIP maps text captions and images in a multimodal embedding-vector space. Credit: OpenAI.

means that subject matter experts are required to also review many irrelevant documents which made the application of predictive coding less popular and also less effective.

To overcome the limitations of predictive coding, a technique called continuous active learning (CAL or or TAR 2.0) was introduced (Cormack and Grossman 2014, 2015). CAL is a form of supervised machine learning but without some of the disadvantages of predictive coding. In CAL, the user is actively participating in the learning process and the model is continuously used for updating the relevance ranking of results that are presented to the user for review.

5.3.3.2 Semantic Search

Earlier, in Section 5.3.1 on rule-based AI techniques, we described how Hansken can extract entities from digital traces which are called tracelets. The expert user interface of Hansken offers a value search feature, allowing users to search and list tracelet values (e.g., extracted entities) as well as trace property values. This is particularly useful for users who are interested in finding facts that are part of traces containing unstructured information like documents or email body texts. With AI techniques, we can further improve this by providing semantic search. Instead of classifying documents and pictures as described earlier in this section, semantic search attempts to assemble tracelets in a meaningful and searchable structure. This structure enables investigators to perform a more exploratory type of search (e.g., by filtering on facets) which is not just powered by traditional metadata but also by semantic concepts and relationships that have been extracted from traces using AI techniques. Van Dijk et al. (2015) describe various text mining methodologies that can be used for enhancing exploratory search. They present a semantic search dashboard that includes entities that are relevant to investigators such as who knew who, what, where and when. Graus (2017) entities build further on these ideas and propose computational methods that aim to support the exploration and sense-making, based on natural language processing and machine learning. Henseler and Hyde (2019) describe how AI techniques such as graph neural networks can assist investigators with the discovery of relationships and patterns in digital forensic evidence.

5.3.4 The application of large language models in digital forensics

The deployment of AI has gained tremendous momentum with the introduction of ChatGPT[7] in November 2022. ChatGPT is a large language model developed by OpenAI that has gained tremendous attention in the months after its introduction for its unique ability to answer questions in a natural dialogue on a wide range of topics it has seen during the learning process. ChatGPT is a fine-tuned version of GPT-3.5. That fine-tuning is based on reinforcement learning from human

---

[7] https://openai.com/blog/chatgpt, last visited 7 April 2023.

feedback (RLHF). That is, ChatGPT has learned, with the help of human reviewers, not to use undesirable language (violent, sexist, racist, etc.) in conversations. Also, ChatGPT has learned what useful answers are, so that conversations flow smoothly. Employing people to review thousands of prompts is costly and seems to be one of ChatGPT's key success factors.

ChatGPT makes mistakes and sometimes hallucinates facts because it is essentially a statistical machine that has learned to predict the next word based on the sequence of preceding words. However, when used as an assistant, and when properly instructed, it appears to be a smart student and may be able to help digital forensic experts more efficiently and effectively investigate cases with digital evidence it has never seen before. For example, by translating natural language investigation questions into structured search queries, detectives can find the right evidence faster without having to learn a sophisticated search language. ChatGPT can also read through digital traces such as emails, instant messages, and browser history and summarize them on demand, allowing investigators to quickly see who, what, where, and/or when something happened. ChatGPT can also analyze links between data, such as repeatedly mentioned email addresses or phone numbers, allowing investigators to interactively and quickly identify key individuals and relevant subjects.

Henseler (2023) experimented with ChatGPT in Hansken and found that with a few examples and explanations of HQL syntax, it is not difficult to get ChatGPT to convert queries in plain language into HQL syntax. For example, the query "Find email traces with attachments sent between July 1 and July 28, 2022 in HQL" is effortlessly translated by ChatGPT as "email.hasAttachment:true email.sentOn>='2022-07-01' email.sentOn<='2022-07-28'". To do that, ChatGPT has read the Hansken HQL manual and read a number of definitions in the trace model, including the email type.

Other researchers in the eDiscovery field also believe that ChatGPT and related techniques can play an important role here. In the article, "What will E-Discovery Lawyers do after ChatGPT?" in LegalTech News and Law[8], the authors outline a number of experiments in which they ask ChatGPT to construct a complex Boolean query based on a fairly simple question. Content-wise, ChatGPT cannot answer queries about information it has not seen before. However, ChatGPT is familiar with the well-known Enron case, which is extensively discussed on the Internet and is also frequently used in eDiscovery education. When asked to provide examples of how Enron violated U.S. Federal Government accounting standards, ChatGPT effortlessly (and, according to the authors, impressively) answers.

The authors suspect that ChatGPT gathered these examples from Wikipedia and countless other online publications that exhaustively analyze Enron's downfall. Such analyses, of course, do not exist in new investigations. The question is

---

[8] https://www.law.com/legaltechnews/2023/01/25/what-will-ediscovery-lawyers-do-after-chatgpt, last visited 7 April 2023.

whether ChatGPT can also analyze documents in new investigations. Based on a limited test, ChatGPT given a specific question appears to be able to determine whether or not an email from the Enron set is relevant and, moreover, can explain why that is so. But this does not work for new cases because the underlying GPT-3 model has not read information about them. Such new information can be learned to GPT-3, and OpenAI offers the ability to fine-tune models in the cloud.

A large language model like GPT is capable of answering questions related to the text used during training. But GPT can also continue to evolve. Through a prompt with a few examples, GPT in many cases intuitively understands what task is meant and can complete new prompts on its own. This is also called few-shot learning and is very useful for getting the model to give an answer with a limited number of examples. But the capacity of this is limited. OpenAI therefore also offers the ability to fine-tune a model with specific data. In doing so, they indicate that the quality of the results is better than with prompt design, that you can train with more data than is possible with prompts, that you end up saving costs because a finetuned model can work with shorter prompts, and that response time improves.

Fine tuning GPT models in the OpenAI playground is costly, and digital forensics labs (at least in Law Enforcement and Intelligence Agencies) cannot upload case documents to public cloud services. That situation is likely to change as alternatives to GPT-3 emerge, that can be trained on proprietary hardware (which is also becoming increasingly powerful). Already in February 2023 Meta announced Llama, a series of large language models with similar or even better capacity than GPT-3 (Touvron et al, 2023). The Llama models are fully documented, are available as open source and the smallest versions of Llama can be fine-tuned on a standalone computer. Meanwhile OpenAI has introduced their more powerful GPT-4 model on March 24 and both Google and Microsoft are rapidly deploying applications of large language models to their users that function as intelligent assistants or *copilots* for tasks that are very close to the work of digital forensics, e.g., programming, documenting, reporting writing, summarizing etc.

5.4 Conclusions and Further Reading

In the last years, several papers have been published on the application of artificial intelligence in the digital-forensic field. In 2010, Mitchell (2010) had already concluded that AI is an ideal approach to deal with many of the problems that still exist in digital forensics. Rughani (2017) presented a high-level approach on how trained models could help in selecting data to acquire, analyze and report, based on earlier defined relevance during forensic investigations. More recently, in 2020, Qadir and Varol (2020) summarized the role that machine learning could play in digital forensics. They also showed how to identify traces of criminal behaviour and intent through learning from previous and historical activities.

Swofford and Champod (2021) presented how such algorithms can support or replace investigators in the evaluation of forensic evidence in general, which can also be applied to the field of digital evidence. Nowadays, most of digital-forensic tools apply AI in varying degrees. With Hansken, we have an open platform that contains all hooks to easily use AI on a large scale, containing the transparency needed in a forensic investigation. It aids case investigators to go through the huge piles of digital evidence. Jarrett and Choo (2021) reviewed the impact of AI on digital forensics. As we see with the use of Hansken, they conclude that AI can speed up the process, reduce the number of (human) errors and reduce the total cost of digital forensic investigations. Hall et al. (2022) researched the use of explainable artificial intelligence (XAI) for digital forensics. They concluded that instead of considering XAI as a replacement for digital forensic examiners, XAI can best be used as a powerful tool to aid investigations, case administration, and prioritization.

Reference

Casey, E., Barnum, S., Griffith, R. et al. (2017). Advancing coordinated cyber-investigations and tool interoperability using a community developed specification language. *Digital Investigation* 22: 14–45. ISSN 1742-2876. https://doi.org/10.1016/j.diin.2017.08.002. accessed 7 April 2023.

Cormack, G.V. and Grossman, M.R. (2014). Evaluation of machine-learning protocols for technology-assisted review in electronic discovery. In: *Proceedings of the 37th International ACM SIGIR Conference on Research & Development in Information Retrieval*, SIGIR '14, 153–162, New York, NY, USA. Association for Computing Machinery. ISBN 9781450322577. https://doi.org/10.1145/2600428.2609601 accessed 7 April 2023.

Cormack, G.V. and Grossman, M.R. (2015). Multi-faceted recall of continuous active learning for technology-assisted review. In: *Proceedings of the 38th International ACM SIGIR Conference on Research and Development in Information Retrieval*, SIGIR '15, 763–766, New York, NY, USA. Association for Computing Machinery. ISBN 9781450336215. https://doi.org/10.1145/2766462.2767771 accessed 7 April 2023.

Court of Amsterdam (2018 April). *Judgment of 19 April 2018, Tandem II, ECLI:NL:RBAMS:2018:2504.* http://deeplink.rechtspraak.nl/uitspraak?id=ECLI:NL:RBAMS:2018:2504 accessed 7 April 2023.

Court of Gelderland (2019 June). *Judgment of 26 June 2019, Bosnië, subs Brandberg, IJshamer, Maan, ECLI:NL:RBGEL:2019:2832.* http://deeplink.rechtspraak.nl/uitspraak?id=ECLI:NL:RBGEL:2019:2832.

David, V.D., Graus, D., Ren, Z. et al. (2015 June). Who is involved? semantic search for e-discovery. In: *ICAIL 2015 Workshop on Using Machine Learning and Other Advanced Techniques to Address Legal Problems in E-Discovery and Information* Governance *(DESI VI Workshop)*. https://www.hsleiden.nl/binaries/content/assets/hsl/lectoraten/digital-forensics-en-e-discovery/publicaties/2015/vandijk-final.pdf accessed 7 April 2023.

Devlin, J., Chang, M.-W., Lee, K., and Toutanova, K. (2018). BERT: pre-training of deep bidirectional transformers for language understanding. *CoRR*, abs/1810.04805. http://arxiv.org/abs/1810.04805 accessed 7 April 2023.

Graus, D. (2017). *Entities of Interest — discovery in Digital Traces*. PhD thesis, Informatics Institute, University of Amsterdam, 6. https://hdl.handle.net/11245.1/51be80bb-1cbf-4633-8ff9-e3128e990bfa accessed 7 April 2023.

Hall, S.W., Sakzad, A., and Raymond Choo, K.-K. (2022). Explainable artificial intelligence for digital forensics. *WIREs Forensic Science* 4 (2): e1434. https://doi.org/10.1002/wfs2.1434. accessed 7 April 2023.

Henseler, H., Hofsté, J., and Maurice, V.K. (2013 August). Digital-forensics based pattern recognition for discovering identities in electronic evidence. In: *Proceedings of the European Intelligence and Security Informatics Conference (EISIC 2013)*, 112–116, United States. IEEE Computer Society. ISBN 978-0-7695-5062-6. doi:10.1109/EISIC.2013.24. null; Conference date: 01- 08-2013.

Henseler, H. and Hyde, J. (2019). Technology assisted analysis of timeline and connections in digital forensic investigations. In: *Proceedings of the First Workshop on AI and Intelligent Assistance for Legal Professionals in the Digital* Workplace *(LegalAIIA 2019) the 17th International Conference on Artificial Intelligence and Law (ICAIL 2019), Montreal, Canada, June 17, 2019* (ed. J.G. Conrad, J. Pickens, A. Jones, et al.), volume 2484 of *CEUR Workshop Proceedings*, 32–37. CEUR-WS. org. http://ceur-ws.org/Vol-2484/paper5.pdf accessed 7 April 2023.

Henseler, H. (2023). ChatGPT: A Digital Sleuth For Detectives? In: ForensicFocus, 21st February 2023. https://www.forensicfocus.com/articles/chatgpt-a-digital-sleuth-for-detectives

Hofste, J. (2012). Scalable identity extraction and ranking in tracks inspector, 11. https://purl. utwente.nl/essays/62780. accessed 30 May 2023.

Jarrett, A. and Raymond Choo, K.-K. (2021). The impact of automation and artificial intelligence on digital forensics. *WIREs Forensic Science* 3 (6): e1418. https://doi.org/10.1002/wfs2.1418. accessed 7 April 2023.

Mikolov, T., Chen, K., Corrado, G., and Dean, J. Efficient estimation of word representations in vector space, 2013. https://arxiv.org/abs/1301.3781.

Mitchell, F. (2010). The use of artificial intelligence in digital forensics: an introduction. *Digital Evidence and Electronic Signature Law Review* 7: 35.

NFI. Smart algorithm lets investigators search through thousands of photographs faster. https:// www.forensicinstitute.nl/news/news/2021/04/01/smart-algorithm-lets-investigators-search -through-thousands-of-photographs-faster. accessed 30 May 2023.

Qadir, A.M. and Varol, A. (2020). The role of machine learning in digital forensics. In: *2020 8th International Symposium on Digital Forensics and Security (ISDFS)*, 1–5. doi:10.1109/ISDFS 49300.2020.9116298.

Raff, E. and Nicholas, C. (2018). Lempel-ziv jaccard distance, an effective alternative to ssdeep and sdhash. *Digital Investigation* 24: 34–49. ISSN 1742-2876. https://doi.org/10.1016/j. diin.2017.12.004. accessed 7 April 2023.

Rughani, P.H. (2017). Artificial intelligence based digital forensics framework. *International Journal of Advanced Research in Computer Science* 8 (8).

Swofford, H. and Champod, C. (2021). Implementation of algorithms in pattern & impression evidence: a responsible and practical roadmap. *Forensic Science International: Synergy* 3: 100142. ISSN 2589-871X. https://doi.org/10.1016/j.fsisyn.2021.100142. https://www.sciencedirect. com/science/article/pii/S2589871X21000103. accessed 7 April 2023.

Touvron, H., Lavril, T., Izacard, G. et al. (2023). LLaMA: open and efficient foundation language models. https://arxiv.org/pdf/2302.13971.pdf.

Tully, G. Forensic science regulator annual report 2019, February 2020. https://www.gov.uk/ government/publications/forensic-science-regulator-annual-report-2019.

UK National Police Chief's Council NPCC. Digital forensic science strategy, July 2020. https:// www.npcc.police.uk/SysSiteAssets/media/downloads/publications/publications-log/2020/ national-digital-forensic-science-strategy.pdf.

van Baar, R.B., van Beek, H.M.A., and van Eijk, E.J. (2014). Digital forensics as a service: a game changer. *Digital Investigation* 11: S54–S62. ISSN 1742-2876. https://doi.org/10.1016/j. diin.2014.03.007. accessed 7 April 2023. Proceedings of the First Annual DFRWS Europe.

van Beek, H.M.A., van den Bos, J., Boztas, A. et al. (2020). Digital forensics as a service: stepping up the game. *Forensic Science International: Digital Investigation* 35: 301021. ISSN 2666-2817. https://doi.org/10.1016/j.fsidi.2020.301021. accessed 7 April 2023.

van Beek, H.M.A., van Eijk, E.J., van Baar, R.B. et al. (2015). Digital forensics as a service: game on. *Digital Investigation* 15: 20–38. ISSN 1742-2876. https://doi.org/10.1016/j.diin.2015.07.004. accessed 7 April 2023. Special Issue: Big Data and Intelligent Data Analysis.

Wu, Y., Schuster, M., Zhifeng Chen, Q.V. et al. (2016). Google's neural machine translation system: bridging the gap between human and machine translation. https://arxiv.org/abs/1609.08144.

CHAPTER 6

On the Feasibility of Social Network Analysis Methods for Investigating Large-scale Criminal Networks

Jan William Johnsen* and Katrin Franke

Department of Information Security and Communication Technology, Norwegian University of Science and Technology, Teknologivegen 22, Gjøvik, Norway

* Corresponding author

Highlights

- We study social network analysis for finding key cybercriminals in hacker forums.
- We prove standard methods to only identify talkative actors such as administrators.
- Identifying talkative actors implies that high profile criminals remain undetected using the standard methods.
- We propose a novel method that removes low-skilled forum users, which results in a 90% reduction of the forum population.
- We present the impact our method has by studying two real-world underground forums.

6.1 Introduction

Cybercriminal underground forums gather like-minded individuals who pursue illicit activities such as malware/exploit development, vulnerability disclosure, hacker tools exchange and distribution, and trading of materials, products and services (Abbasi et al. 2014; Europol 2020; Rosario Fuentes 2020). These underground forums are platforms for the crime as a service (CaaS) business model, where a minority of criminal individuals or groups sell, let, or give away their technical skills to the majority of less experienced cybercriminals (Europol 2014).

Artificial Intelligence (AI) in Forensic Sciences, First Edition. Edited by Zeno Geradts and Katrin Franke.
© 2024 John Wiley & Sons Ltd. Published 2024 by John Wiley & Sons Ltd.

The CaaS significantly reduce buyers' need for knowledge and expertise to conduct successful cyber attacks. To stop the CaaS business model, we need effective methods for targeting key actors within the minority population.

Identifying key actors in small criminal networks can often be done by eye. On the other hand, criminal underground forums are far more complex and involve hundreds of thousands of members and millions of connections. In such cases, forensic investigators and intelligence agents use off-the-shelf tools – which employ social network analysis (SNA) – to obtain a grasp of the members and relationships within the criminal network (Gogolin 2021). SNA-based methods focus on network centrality (Schwartz and Rouselle 2009) to find a criminal's prominence and determine the relative importance or influence that members possess within a network (Gogolin 2021). Network centrality is being used as a way of identifying key actors (e.g., leaders) of criminal organizations (Taha and Yoo 2015).

As seen in Figure 6.1, forensic science (forensics) is the intersection between application, technology, and methodology (Franke and Srihari 2008). Law enforcement applies SNA centrality measures to find the most important or central actors in a network; those actors with more opportunities and fewer constraints. Using centrality measures might have been sufficient when the application was finding key actors in small, physical, and hierarchical criminal networks. However, today's underground forums have several hundred thousand loosely connected actors. The new network characteristics have changed the application domain for SNA, which requires a re-evaluation of the overall investigative methodology (Stoykova 2022). A significant drawback formerly consisted of the lack of scientific work that validated SNA centrality measures methods for the new application of large-scale criminal network analysis.

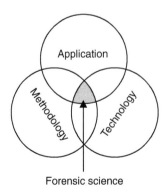

Figure 6.1 Franke and Srihari (2008) define forensic science as the cross section of technology, methodology, and application. This figure is adopted from their paper. The same technology and method will work fine for one application domain, but it might not work for another application domain. Therefore, we need to cross-validate the technology and methodology to solve challenges in other application domains (Stoykova 2022).

Our study addresses this issue, which is urgently required to ensure that law enforcement uses investigative methods correctly. Moreover, the use of unvalidated methods in legal rulings can lead to reduced procedural accuracy and violate the right to a fair trial and human rights (Stoykova 2021). We increase the knowledge of using centrality in forensics by accurately describing how they identify "key" criminal actors. We can validate the results in this study because of our unique access to two real-world criminal underground forum datasets. The complete datasets give us access to some ground truth information, which has rarely been done by other studies (Marin et al. 2018).

This chapter presents two experiments. The first experiment, detailed in Section 6.4.1, conducts a hypothesis testing of the correlation between forum activity and centrality measure ranks. In this part of the chapter, we demonstrate how earlier network centrality research results can misrepresent results in newer research. The second experiment, detailed in Section 6.4.2, is where we present a novel method using Natural Language Processing (NLP) to enable law enforcement and researchers to largely separate the majority and minority population of underground forum users. Our method significantly reduces the number of actors we need to evaluate. The benefits are that: (i) further research can be aimed at better understanding technically skilled members; and (ii) enables law enforcement to focus their limited resources on high-impact cybercriminals.

The rest of the chapter is organized as follows: Section 6.2 explains this work in relation to related and previous work. Section 6.3 details the experimental process model, methods used in our work, and the preprocessing done to the material. Section 6.4 presents the experimental setup, while Section 6.5 discusses the corresponding results. Finally, Section 6.6 recapitulates our study and includes suggestions for further work.

6.2 Previous Work

Existing methods for identifying key actors fall into two main categories: content-based and social network-based analysis. Content-based analysis refers to mining data generated by users of underground forums, such as activity level and content quality. SNA, on the other hand, can model and analyse user interactions in underground forums. Related SNA research targeting critical network actors focuses on the concept of centrality to identify actors who are somehow central, vital, important, key, or pivotal in a criminal network (Schwartz and Rouselle 2009; Sparrow 1991).

Centrality measures have been applied in a diversity of research domains, for instance, analysing the structure of terrorist (Krebs 2002) and criminal networks. Centrality measures are robust in the presence of noise (Ortiz-Arroyo 2010) and empirically measure the structural importance of a single actor in a network. Moreover, researchers believe network centrality leads to an "evidence-based understanding of the overall structure of a criminal network and the positioning of a variety of key actors" (Morselli 2010). Another use of network centrality is the removal of key actors to disrupt criminal networks and underground forums (Pete et al. 2020) and decrease the ability of the criminal network to function normally (Memon 2012; Sparrow 1991).

Pete et al. (2020) identified key actors using network centrality measures and got a similar result to our earlier work (Johnsen and Franke 2018): (i) some actors consistently ranked higher than others in nearly all centrality measures, and (ii) central actors hold administrative positions in the forum and are active forum participants (Grisham et al. 2017). Similar to the work in this chapter, Pete et al. (2020) checked the relationship between actors' ranks and their posting activity using Pearson's correlation test. However, Pearson makes wrong assumptions about the variables when analysing this specific type of problem. In particular, Pearson makes the wrong assumptions that the variables are continuous and their relationship is linear. Therefore, we use Spearman's rank-order correlation to make some assumptions about the data, making it more sensitive to non-linear monotonic relationships and ordinal variables.

Similar to our result in Section 6.5.1, Pete et al. (2020) also showed a significant positive correlation between users' centrality and their posting activity. However, we provide a more in-depth and novel understanding of centrality measures and why the correlation with posting activity is negative from a forensic aspect.

Table 6.1 contains a list of previous works that analyse criminal networks. This table shows that our study is significantly more complex and more extensive when comparing the network sizes; previous work had a median network size of 282 actors. The work of Pastrana et al. (2018) is the only research that comes close in regards to the number of actors studied. The listed research articles use various resources – typically data from the police – to construct the criminal network. On the other hand, we have access to the complete network and the ground truth from leaked underground forums.

Previous work often represents a criminal network by constructing undirected or directed graphs, where vertices are the forum members and edges their interactions. The type of interaction takes on different forms (e.g., forum posts (Johnsen and Franke 2018; Marin et al. 2018; Pastrana et al. 2018; Pete et al. 2020), co-conspirators (Bright et al. 2012; Xu et al. 2004) or other communication forms (Taha and Yoo 2015)) depending on the relationship researchers are trying to model. It is commonly referred to as an interaction network when forum threads and posts are modelled using graphs. Thread starters initiate interactions, and any forum member replying to the thread will take part in the interaction (Pete et al. 2020). More formally, researchers define a (un)directed edge (v,u) if there is a post/reply from member v to thread starter u. Researchers have minor variations in their graph construction to account for different posting times (Marin et al. 2018) or type of data sources (Bright et al. 2012; Lu et al. 2010).

Table 6.1 Comparing network sizes from previous work.

Research article	Nodes	Edges
Krebs (2002)	19	
Lu et al. (2010)	23	
Memon (2012)	62	153
Baker and Faulkner (1993)	78	
Grisham et al. (2017)	100	562
Hardin et al. (2015)	156	
Morselli (2010)	174	
Xu and Chen (2003)	164 – 744	
Diesner and Carley (2005)	227	
Holt et al. (2012)	336	
Décary-Hétu and Dupont (2012)	771	
Xu et al. (2004)	924	
Abbasi et al. (2014)	4576	
Samtani and Chen (2016)	6796	
Pete et al. (2020)	22 – 16401	57 – 624926
Pastrana et al. (2018)	572000	
Johnsen and Franke (2017)	599086	371002
	599085	2672147
Johnsen and Franke (2018)	75416	319935
	33647	98253
	299105	2705578
Johnsen and Franke (2020)	94832	490268
	62933	794868
This work	21432	64938
	299701	2741464
	185806	1794947

6.3 Material and Methods

6.3.1 Real-world Underground Forum Database Dumps

Traditional data collection methods such as web crawling may result in incomplete datasets, because crawlers only collect parts of the forums which they have privileges to access. To analyse complete datasets, we acquired database dumps of real-world underground forums leaked on competing hacker forums. Analysing complete databases reduced the factors that can affect our assessment of centrality measures as a forensic technique.

The leaked underground forums are Nulled.io and Cracked.to (Europol 2020). They are both hacker communities that facilitate the brokering of compromised passwords, provide tools and leaks, and generally act as marketplaces for services, products, and materials. The leaked Nulled database had almost four years of data, while Cracked had over one year of data. See Table 6.2 for a short overview of these two datasets, including the number of users, number of posts, and date and time for the first and last post.

Analysing leaked datasets gives us a unique opportunity with three advantages: (i) we can study real-world and criminal communities with actors of various technical skill levels; (ii) the data is stored in a structured manner, which makes extracting and preprocessing easier compared to other data collection methods; and, more importantly, (iii) we sit on the ground truth with all the user-generated information (such as private and public messages and forum roles), which allows us to assess network centrality measures' results better.

Hacker forums change their top-level domain so frequently that it is difficult to give a permanent link to leaked datasets. Moreover, to access the download links, visitors are required to create an account on the forums. Because of these afore-mentioned difficulties and to allow other researchers to reproduce our findings, we also include the well-known Enron corpus[1] (Shetty and Adibi n.d.) in our experiment.

Comparing the communication between e-mail and underground forums, the content and type of communication are obviously different. For example:

- Forums facilitate different types of interactions and discussions, so users more often reply to thread starters, while e-mail communication are typically received.
- Public forum posts are one-to-many or many-to-one, while e-mail communication is more similar to one-to-one direct messages.

Despite these minor differences, we can interpret and compare network centrality results in a similar manner because they both represent an interaction graph *structure*. Additionally, because the result of network centrality measures are similar in all three datasets, it strengthens our critique of using network centrality to find "key" criminal actors in Section 6.5.1.

Table 6.2 Statistics over dataset users and public posts.

Dataset	Users	Posts	First post	Last post
Enron	75416	252759	30 Oct 1998	3 Feb 2004
Nulled	599085	3495596	26 Nov 2012	6 May 2016
Cracked	321444	2459543	19 Mar 2018	21 Jul 2019

---

[1] https://www.cs.cmu.edu/enron.

6.3.2 Network Centrality Measures

Centrality measures highlight important actors differently, because there are many ways of interpreting "important". The commonality with all the measures is that they rank actors from high to low, where important actors tend to have high centrality scores (Abbasi et al. 2014; Marin et al. 2018). The most considered centrality measures for directed graphs (digraphs) are in-degree (C_{D^-}), out-degree (C_{D^+}), betweenness (C_B), closeness (C_C), and eigenvector (C_E) (Prell 2012). We include these five measures in our analysis because they are the most common centrality measures, and also on account of their use in off-the-shelf forensic investigation tools such as IMB i2 Analyst's Notebook (IBM software n.d.).

Degree centrality is an indicator of importance, influence, control, and can signify visibility (Bright et al. 2012; Morselli 2010). Actors with a high degree of centrality are considered to influence a large number of people and are capable of communicating quickly with actors in their neighbourhood (Ortiz-Arroyo 2010). Moreover, actors with a high degree of centrality are more likely to be arrested (Morselli 2010), found guilty, receive longer sentences, and larger fines (Baker and Faulkner 1993). Therefore, actors with a high degree of centrality are often considered leaders, experts, or hubs in a criminal network (Xu and Chen 2003). Degree centrality is split into two measures for digraphs, where in-degree is often seen as a measure of prestige or popularity, while out-degree captures the outreach of a user to the community.

Betweenness centrality measures information flow through individuals. It is an indicator to show whether an actor plays the role of a broker or gatekeeper in a network. Broker exchanges between two other actors, and a gatekeeper controls (e.g., withhold or distort) information passing between actors (Lu et al. 2010). Actors with high betweenness centrality were less likely to be arrested because they were less likely to be part of the criminal network (Morselli 2010). Closeness centrality measures how easy it is for one actor to be able to communicate with others in the network (Lu et al. 2010). Thus, actors with high closeness centrality can reach most or all other actors in the network (Bright et al. 2012).

6.3.3 Measuring Association Using Bi-variate Analysis

The related work by Pete et al. (2020) used Pearson's correlation test to check the association between the two variables: network centrality and forum post activity. However, Pearson makes wrong assumptions about the variables when analysing this specific type of problem. In particular, Pearson makes the wrong assumptions that the variables are continuous and their relationship is linear. Therefore, we use Spearman's rank-order correlation to make some assumptions about the data, making it more sensitive to non-linear monotonic relationships and ordinal variables. The Spearman's assumptions better fit our experimental data as seen in the scatter plots of Figures 6.4, 6.5, and 6.6.

6.3.4 Topic Modelling Algorithms

6.3.4.1 Latent Dirichlet Allocation

Latent Dirichlet allocation (LDA) is a generative model which learns the joint probability distribution $P(x, y)$. More specifically, LDA tries to solve a general problem with an intermediate step by modelling how a particular topic y would generate input data x. The model can subsequently pick the most likely topic by calculating the conditional probability $P(y \mid x)$. That is, what is the probability of topic y given the input values of x? In the case for LDA, the inputs x is latent variables aimed to capture abstract notions such as topics (Blei et al. 2003). The result is a set of human-interpretative topics, which explain why some parts of the data are similar.

The creation of a LDA model is controlled by three hyper-parameters k, α, and β. The hyper-parameters control the number of topics (k) and two Dirichlet distributions for the document-topic (α) and topic-word (β) density. Thus, LDA allow for a nuanced way of "soft clustering" documents into k topics, as documents can belong to multiple topics.

6.3.4.2 Gibbs Sampling Algorithm for the Dirichlet Multinomial Mixture

LDA makes the sensible assumption that longer texts contain multiple topics. However, the increasing popularity of micro-blogging websites such as Twitter and Facebook challenges this assumption. The topic modelling algorithm Gibbs Sampling algorithm for the Dirichlet Multinomial Mixture (GSDMM) (Yin and Wang 2014) assumes that a document can only belong to a single topic, which makes it better suited for topic modelling of shorter text. The other difference is that LDA requires the k number of topics to be set in advance, whereas GSDMM only requires an upper bound of k number of topics to infer the number of topics from the data. These changes has shown that GSDMM generally outperforms LDA on short text (Mazarura and de Waal 2016).

6.4 Experimental Setup

The two experiments detailed in this chapter require separate process models for data preprocessing, structuring, analyses, and result interpretation. Sections 6.4.1 and 6.4.2 show the experimental process model for (i) hypothesis testing, and (ii) using communication contents to eliminate low-skilled forum users, respectively.

6.4.1 Evaluating Network Centrality Measures for Forensics

Figure 6.2 illustrates the process model for testing our hypothesis: that there is a correlation between the number of replies thread starters receive and how important network centrality measures assess them.

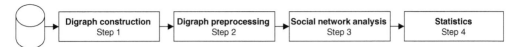

Figure 6.2 Process model for evaluating centrality measures.

Step 1. Digraph construction
In this experiment, we construct a digraph by extracting information from all three datasets about users and how they interact with each other. We carefully handle irregularities in the extracted data, such as some users being identified by the same user identification (ID) or e-mail alias, as the case for the Enron dataset. This step is crucial for correct results because it ensures a vertex uniquely identifies every user in the digraph.

Irregularities in the data are things like e-mail aliases, which are one or more alternative e-mail addresses that forward messages to another address. It is out of this study's scope to account for all the e-mail aliases inside the Enron corpus. This is better addressed in other research articles or when it is mission-critical for the application, such as in police investigations.

We found 97 out of 149 known employees had one or more e-mail aliases, which were normalized so all 149 known employees were represented by a unique address. Then a subgraph containing those 149 employees (as senders or receivers of e-mail messages) and their recipients was extracted. Concentrating on a smaller subset of vertices is analogous to police investigations, where the focus is on a few primary suspects, and the complete network structure is unknown.

Nulled and Cracked datasets contain instances where multiple vertices can represent individuals. For example, individuals can register multiple user accounts on the forum, or the database has conflicting entries. Identifying actors who have registered or are using multiple forum accounts is outside this chapter's scope and should be addressed by other researchers. We focused our attention on the latter case, as some users had non-unique combinations of user ID numbers and usernames. These conflicting database entries happened for fifteen users in Nulled and three in Cracked. Although database conflicts were low, they had to be addressed to uniquely identify individuals in the social network. We achieved uniqueness by replacing the ID numbers on duplicated database entries.

Creating accurate digraphs are essential to avoid meaningless centrality scores and attribute incorrect significance to users (Abbasi et al. 2014). Thus, deciding how to construct the digraph and what vertices and edges represent are crucial when modelling the underground forum interactions. For these reasons and to allow us to discuss our result with that of others, we use a construction approach that is identical to how previous works have constructed their graphs.

We denote a set of users V and a set of posts E, as the vertices and edges in a digraph $G = (V, E)$. The set E contains ordered (v, u) pairs of edge elements, where user v makes a post (i.e., reply) to a forum thread started by user u, and $\{v, u\} \in V$.

Similarly for the Enron corpus, the set E contains ordered (v, u) pairs, where address v sends an e-mail message to the address u. An edge is created for every u if v send the e-mail message to multiple recipients.

Step 2. Digraph preprocessing
Self-loop edges and isolated vertices are not of interest when analysing a network because users' relationship with themselves are uninteresting and isolated vertices have an infinite distance to other vertices (Prell 2012). Self-loop edges and isolated vertices are, therefore, removed before the analysis without affecting the result (Kumar and Sinha 2021). Table 6.3 shows the reduction in the number of vertices and edges when removing self-loops and isolates.

Table 6.3 shows that 597 vertices become isolated after removing 33 134 self-loop edges from the Nulled dataset, while 456 vertices were isolated after removing 14 091 self-loop edges from the Cracked dataset. These vertices were disconnected from the larger network component because they started forum threads which did not receive any reply and they had no other interaction on the forum. However, they only become isolated (defined as a vertex without edges) after removing their self-loop edge.

A word of warning: removing self-loop edges and isolated vertices are fine in this situation because we could manually control that it did not remove skilled cybercriminals. Other researchers and investigators must be cautious when following this exact approach because proficient cybercriminals can use this preprocessing against them. For example, cybercriminals can create a scenario where they only generate self-loop edges by creating forum threads and then exclusively reply to their own threads. This is how proficient cybercriminals can sell their services to other underground forum users yet remain hidden during the forensic analysis because removing self-loops make them isolates (as per the definition) and then subsequently removes them from the graph. However, forum administrators must assist by blocking other users' attempts at replying to those threads, because vertices will not be isolates if others make a reply.

Step 3. Social network analysis
In this step we analyse graphs that were constructed and preprocessed as described in the two previous steps. The analysis here involves network centrality measures

Table 6.3 Comparing the reduction in vertices and edges.

	Before preprocessing		After preprocessing	
Dataset	Vertices	Edges	Vertices	Edges
Enron	21 432	64 938	21 432	64 845 (−0.1%)
Nulled	299 701	2 741 464	299 104 (−0.2%)	2 708 330 (−1.2%)
Cracked	185 806	1 794 947	185 350 (−0.3%)	1 780 856 (−0.8%)

from SNA to identify important and influential individuals. Section 6.3.2 provides details on the five centrality measures used in this study. Centrality measures give vertices a score that reflects their importance for a particular centrality measure. Sorting these scores will rank nodes against each other, with some having higher scores than others. If an actor has a high centrality score, they are relatively more important or influential than others with lower scores (Abbasi et al. 2014; Marin et al. 2018).

Step 4. Bi-variate analysis
This is the last step for this part of the experiment, where we find the association between actors' centrality ranks and the number of replies they receive on their forum threads. To test our hypothesis that there is a relationship between these two variables, we use bi-variate analysis which can determine a statistical association exists between two variables, the degree of association, and whether one variable may predict the other variable (Sandilands 2014). Here we use Spearman's rank-order correlation as described in Section 6.3.3.

The experimental data is created by collecting two variables. The first variable x is the centrality score sorted in descending order (collected in Step 3), and this arrangement illustrates the rank users receive from centrality measures. For example, rank 1 contains the user with the highest score for a particular centrality measure; rank 2 contains the second-highest score; and so forth. Thus, the x-axis is the users' rank order $(1,2,3,...,n)$, sorted from higher centrality to lower centrality. The second variable y is the number of replies users received to their forum threads. The x and y variables explained here are found in the scatter plots of Figures 6.4, 6.5, and 6.6.

It is important to note that bi-variate analysis cannot statistically account for or control variables other than the two studied variables. Consequently, bi-variate correlations alone do not necessarily imply causation (Sandilands 2014) because both variables can be associated with a different casual variable. We discuss this in more detail in Section 6.5.1.

6.4.2 Our Novel Approach for Analysing Cybercriminal's Technical Skills

Figure 6.3 illustrates the iterative process model for our proposed approach to removing low-skilled users from the dataset. In this experiment, we focus on analysing the two underground forums, Nulled and Cracked (Europol 2020). We begin the process with standard text preprocessing steps, as well as replacing repeating words and characters to normalize the text further (Johnsen and Franke 2020). We generate topic models with LDA or GSDMM depending on the iteration. The process continues by identifying users' topic distribution, attained by calculating the similarity between topics and users' posts. The final step is to identify appreciation topic(s) by evaluating topic keywords and users' topic distribution and remove users who have primarily posted in those selected topics before

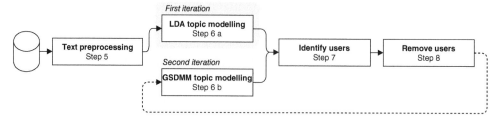

Figure 6.3 Process model for our novel approach.

continuing to the next iteration. This section explains every step of this process in more detail.

Step 5. Text preprocessing
The text must be preprocessed before it can be analysed by topic models such as LDA or GSDMM. Thus, we conduct a series of standard and original text preprocessing steps tailored for the online communication-type of data found in Nulled and Cracked datasets. Importantly, we ensure anything removed from the text is replaced with white space. This white space replacement is necessary to guarantee that words are not unintentionally combined and cause the text (or topics) to become unintelligible. The following is a list of our preprocessing steps and their order:

(a) Convert text to lowercase.
(b) Remove special newline, tabular, and return characters.
(c) Remove BBcode tags.
   • BBcode tags format messages in online forums, usually indicated by a keyword surrounding square brackets.
(d) Remove URLs.
(e) Remove HTML tags (including most content) and HTML entities.
(f) Remove forum-specific text.
   • Leaking credentials is one primary focus for Nulled and Cracked, which means they contain posts with large dumps of e-mail and passwords. We remove any "e-mail:password"-combination, e-mail addresses and emojis.
(g) Remove symbols and numbers (anything non-alphabetic).
(h) Use lemmatization to transform inflected words to be analysed as a single item.
(i) Remove stopwords, around 700 of the most common English stopwords.
(j) Search and replace repeating words and characters.

Users frequently express exaggeration and other emotions by repeating characters (e.g., "thaaaaanks") and words (e.g., "thxthx"). This way of writing creates many unnecessary words that have the same meaning (e.g., "thanks"). Thus, this step, together with lemmatization, greatly reduces the number of word variations and, consequently, improves the topic models. We refer readers to our previous research article (Johnsen and Franke 2020) for more details about this step.

Step 6. Topic modelling

Researchers commonly build topic models to automatically organize, understand, search, and summarize large document corpora. Where each document is one message or a combination of messages. The topic model is subsequently used to find the topic for unseen data. In this experiment, however, we use the model to identify groups of similar users and use this knowledge to separate low-skilled users from presumably medium-/high-skilled users.

We use the two topic modelling algorithms LDA and GSDMM to learn the contents of our large document corpora. These algorithms have distinct advantages when modelling long and short text documents, where LDA has better performance on long documents, and GSDMM performs better on shorter text. In this step, we explain the different document construction approaches required by the algorithms while referring readers to our previous research article (Johnsen and Franke 2019) for other document construction approaches.

a. LDA topic modelling

For the first iteration, we construct the documents by combining all messages from a user into a single document. The number of documents is equal to the number of users. The documents were used to train a LDA model controlled by low hyper-parameter values ($k = 10$, $\alpha = 0.05$, and $\beta = 0.05$), which we had found works better for our proposed method (Johnsen and Franke 2019). A low k is sufficient because the aim is to create a coarse grouping of topics instead of identifying all possible topics. While low α and β values assume that documents contain fewer topics and topics are composed of few words.

With a low number of k, the topics in a LDA model are likely to contain mixed categories of text. Analysts would normally want one category per topic, however, this mix is fine for our use-case. We utilize this to find topics with uniform content, i.e., users who exclusively post a certain type of message, in this case it is appreciation messages. See Step 8 for our definition of "appreciation messages". The LDA algorithm groups users posting mixed category contents and those who exclusively post appreciation messages. This group separation allow us to selectively remove users found in the latter group, which turned out to be the majority of the underground forum population.

b. GSDMM topic modelling

Continuing using LDA for the second iteration proved difficult for two reasons: (i) the concatenated document construction does not distinguish users with mixed posts/topics because messages are merged, and (ii) LDA works poorly on short text (predominantly appearing in our corpus datasets). Thus, the concatenated document construction lacked the nuanced ways for distinguishing users further.

This could be solved by changing the document construction and treating each message as a separate document. However, we would encounter the common LDA issues with learning from short texts. Another approach can be increasing the α hyper-parameter to identify documents with more than one topic.

Ultimately we chose to use the GSDMM algorithm, which is better suited for short text because it assumes that documents only belong to one topic. Changing topic model for the second iteration also required us to use a different document construction approach, where we consider each user's message as a separate document. We keep the hyper-parameters the same as for the first iteration, where $k = 10$, $\alpha = 0.05$, $\beta = 0.05$, and $i = 30$ number of iterations.

Step 7. Identify users

This intermediary step is necessary to (i) infer the categories for topics, and users' association to topics. To identify the topics' category, we list out the $m = 20$ top keywords per topic and then interpret the keywords to infer the category. To then find the users' association to topics, we calculate the similarity between users' messages and every topic in the LDA or GSDMM model, depending on the iteration. Notably, users' messages must be constructed similarly to the document construction which generated the model.

We use the following process to find the similarity/association between users' messages and topics. We calculate the conditional probability $P(y \mid x)$ to find the similarity between a document y given a topic x, which results in a k-length vector of floating-point values between 0.0 and 1.0 for every user. This approach only works when each user has a single vector, i.e., one document per user such as in the case of the first iteration. The second iteration, however, resulted in multiple vectors (one per document) for each user. To represent every user with a single vector, we summed the vectors for each user and divided it by the number of messages they sent.

Finally, we want to avoid working with floating-point vectors because this requires us to define threshold values for when to remove users. We see threshold values as a potential weakness because the values may change depending on the dataset being analysed. Additionally, threshold values must be defined after further studies. We perform binarization on the vectors by replacing the highest topic(s) score(s) with a one, while the other topics are replaced by zeros.

Step 8. Remove users

Now we can remove users based on the content they produce with the knowledge we gained in the previous step. More specifically, in this step we remove users who post messages with appreciation content, i.e., posters who use keywords that recognise the good quality of shared content, approving actions of others, and similar. Examples of appreciation messages are: "good work, man", "tested, it works well", "nice share, thank you", etc.

The removal process is: (i) identify topics with semantically coherent appreciation words, and (ii) remove users who predominantly write messages on these topics. For example, let there be $k = 10$ topics numbered from $0 - 9$ since tagging them is unnecessary. Assume a human analyst evaluates the top m keywords for every k topics, and assign topics 4 and 7 to contain appreciation keywords. Then the analyst remove all users who have a binary value of one in topic 4 or 7 (or both) from the dataset. We follow this step for both iterations and the results of this process are found in Section 6.5.2.

6.5 Experimental Results and Discussion

This section details the results of our experiments and discusses their significance. It is divided into two subsections, which detail and discuss the two primary goals of our research separately. More specifically, the subsections concentrate on: (i) hypothesis testing the correlation between centrality ranks and number of replies thread starters receive, and (ii) a novel method for discarding uninteresting users from underground forums.

Section 6.5.1 details the correlation we found between the two previously discussed variables. Additionally, this subsection elaborates on the adverse effect the correlation can have on police investigations into underground forums and other groups of criminals (e.g., gangs, organized crime, and so forth).

Although our findings demonstrate why investigators cannot rely on network centrality measures for finding "key criminal actors", they still need to identify a small group of more prominent criminals to focus their investigations on them. Section 6.5.2 details our novel method of discarding low-skilled forum users, which leaves a smaller group of cybercriminals that can be the targets of law enforcement investigations.

6.5.1 Correlation Testing

Our research hypothesis is that there is a correlation (i.e., a relationship) between the two variables: (1) the order of centrality ranks, and (2) the number of replies thread starters receive. In other words, users who start popular threads (i.e., threads with more replies and attention) will be more central in the social network and, consequently, obtain higher centrality ranks. We begin scrutinizing our hypothesis by investigating the relationship between the two variables using scatter plots, as seen in Figures 6.4, 6.5, and 6.6 for the datasets Enron, Nulled, and Cracked, respectively.

The first sub-figure in Figures 6.4, 6.5, and 6.6 shows the raw data curve where the users are ranked (in descending order) according to the number of received e-mail and forum thread replies. Users with more popular forum threads are found on the left side of the scatter plot, while the popularity quickly reduces towards the right. The Enron dataset has a similar interpretation, where the popularity in this dataset is the number of received e-mail messages.

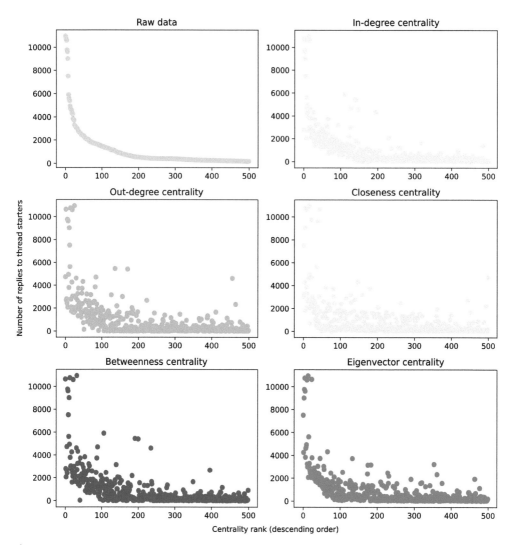

Figure 6.4 Enron statistics.

More importantly, Figures 6.4, 6.5, and 6.6 also show the scatter plots for the relationship between various centrality measures and the number of replies to e-mail messages/thread starters. These scatter plots show that the relationship between the two variables follows a similar non-linear relationship as the raw data sub-figure. Notably, users with more replies rank higher in in-degree, closeness, betweenness, and eigenvector centrality. We perform a Spearman rank-order correlation test to determine the strength and direction of the relationship between the two variables. The Spearman test is appropriate due to the ordinal variable of centrality ranks and the non-linear monotonic relationship revealed by the scatter plots.

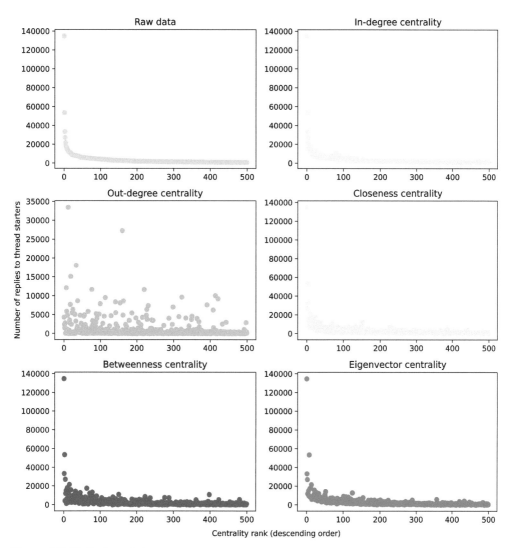

Figure 6.5 Nulled statistics.

Table 6.4 shows the results of the Spearman rank-order correlation test. Spearman's r_s value indicates the strength of the relationship between two variables to change in tandem. The relationship strength is typically categorized in five levels: very strong $(1.0 - 0.9)$, strong $(0.89 - 0.7)$, moderate $(0.69 - 0.4)$, weak $(0.39 - 0.1)$ and no correlation $(0.39 - 0.1)$. Table 6.4 demonstrates a moderate/strong correlation between the two variables for closeness, betweenness, and eigenvector centrality, while in-degree centrality has a very strong correlation. Moreover, the r_s value indicates a positive relationship, as users with more replies tend to coincide with high network centrality ranks. The strong positive relationships are clearly visible in Figures 6.4, 6.5, and 6.6.

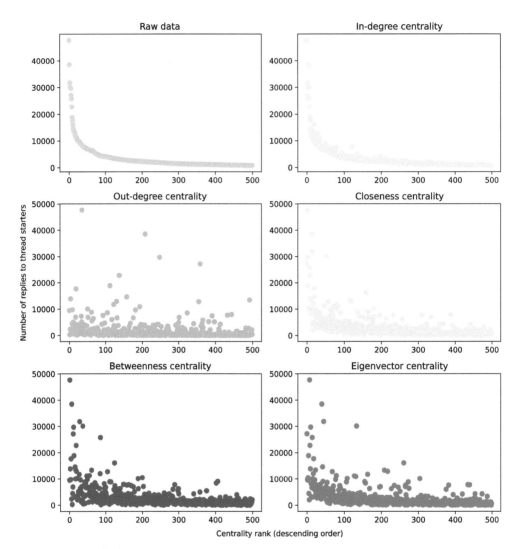

Figure 6.6 Cracked statistics.

The p-value is used for hypothesis testing. The default null hypothesis (H_0) says there is no correlation between the two variables, while the alternate hypothesis (H_1) says there is a correlation between them. The p-value provides statistical evidence to reject or accept the H_0 if the p-value is below or above the $\alpha = 0.05$ threshold of probability.

The p-values in Table 6.4 have many leading zeros behind the decimal point, but the values are not zero. The low p-values ($p < \alpha$) provide very strong evidence against the null hypothesis being true. The test result is statistically significant and we can, therefore, reject the H_0 with a low probability of making a Type I error (i.e., null hypothesis is actually true).

Table 6.4 Spearman rank-order correlation.

Dataset	Centrality	r_s	p-value
	C_{D^-}	0.6711	0.00
	C_{D^+}	0.5042	0.00
	C_C	0.4601	0.00
	C_B	0.5004	0.00
Enron	C_E	0.4620	0.00
	C_{D^-}	0.9956	0.00
	C_{D^+}	0.3841	0.00
	C_C	0.6218	0.00
	C_B	0.7142	0.00
Nulled	C_E	0.6518	0.00
	C_{D^-}	0.9969	0.00
	C_{D^+}	0.2934	0.00
	C_C	0.4633	0.00
	C_B	0.5665	0.00
Cracked	C_E	0.4549	0.00

Note that a weak correlation r_s value can have a significant p-value, which means that the weak correlation is not due to chance factors but is representative of the population. Based on our observations of the data, we claim that there is a relationship between the number of replies and centrality ranks. In other words, central criminal actors are those users with more replies to e-mails or forum threads.

It is important to note that an observed correlation/association does not assure that the relationship between two variables is casual (Schober et al. 2018). A casual relationship can be established with well-designed empirical research. Our research shows that the top central "criminal" actors can be those actors who receive the most attention because of the similar curves seen in Figures 6.4, 6.5, and 6.6. Publicly active actors indeed receive attention from other peers; however, high-skilled actors do not need to be publicly active.

Let us illustrate the issue with an example from related work. Baker and Faulkner (Baker and Faulkner 1993) reviewed sworn testimonies citing actors who participated directly in price-fixing conspiracies. They find that "the more direct contacts a conspirator has, the greater the likelihood of a guilty verdict" (Baker and Faulkner 1993). Unsurprisingly, having a higher degree of centrality is a legal vulnerability because eyewitnesses to crimes can testify against suspects (i.e., "fingered by eyewitnesses").

Baker and Faulkner (1993) analysed a graph constructed from reviewing testimonies, where central actors are those being fingered by the most eyewitnesses. While we analyse a graph constructed from underground forum communications, where central actors are those who receive the most replies. Although Baker and Faulkner (1993) only looked at degree centrality, the Enron corpus in this study show an identical result to the analysis of underground forums (see Figures 6.4, 6.5, and 6.6). In both their (Baker and Faulkner 1993) and our research, network centrality measures find actors with the most of something, where the interpretation of "something" depends on the underlying graph.

Centrality measures are simple algorithms and our work demonstrates how forensic investigators and other researchers must be careful when applying network centrality to identify "key" actors in criminal networks. The notion of "key" must be interpreted within the graph's context, and that "key" only refers to a vertex's position in the network structure (depending on the centrality measure used). For example, our digraph is modelled after those who send and receive posts, and the most central actors will be those users with more replies to their threads.

Centrality is not a "criminal score" nor an indicator of an important actor, such as a highly-skilled CaaS cybercriminal or criminal network leaders. Forensic investigators risk identifying non-key actors with high activity, such as secretaries and military staff with numerous contacts or connections but without any authority or influence when uncritically using network centrality measures. Therefore, the use of centrality measures is not forensically sound because results can easily be misinterpreted.

6.5.2 Our Newly Proposed Method

Although researchers and investigators cannot rely on network centrality measures for identifying interesting criminals in a network, they still need to differentiate between high- and low-skilled criminals. This section shows the results of our proposed method, which can identify and remove low-skilled criminal actors on a large scale. Our method uniquely identifies actors who predominantly post appreciation messages and removes them from the dataset, thereby reducing the number of criminal actors to consider.

Tables 6.5 and 6.6 show the result of our process after the first iteration, as described in Section 6.4.2. These tables show the ten topics, the number of posts, and the keywords associated with each topic. The result obtained in Tables 6.5 and 6.6 uses an LDA model learned on documents constructed by concatenating users' messages into individual larger documents. The LDA model creates ten "clusters" that contain users posting similar content. We can see that topics 1 and 9 from Table 6.5, and topics 5, 6, and 8 from Table 6.6 contains words that express appreciation.

The next step is to remove users who have posted on these topics, as explained previously in Section 6.4.2, Step 8. We removed 199 786 and 133 454 users from

Table 6.5 Nulled first iteration (LDA).

Topic #	# of posts	Keywords
0	35715	file set add function enemy type bot attack
1	113068	nice good man work brother test job share wow
2	34037	php inurl http qwerty asp game product cumsot
3	34537	game origin sims email battlefield unknown
4	72924	work account share post check game hope time
5	34335	qwerty qwe xx lol try wsx abc thanks wso kid
6	34043	http site password php username capture point
7	35678	account pm skin sell level bump email price rp
8	43826	script bol work kappa lol update help test thanks
9	151050	thanks test share brother man work nice mate

Table 6.6 Cracked first iteration (LDA).

Topic #	# of posts	Keywords
0	37343	yeah account leech leave post work thread link
1	15722	combo premium subscription status recur
2	16266	premium country family credit spotify false plan
3	17815	pour le file partage je asd de ce da la deep mon
4	15549	game lil platform php cry assassin creed fortnite
5	104954	work man good nice hope great brother mate
6	35985	share brother lot combo man work hope men
7	15867	true rar sb txt xnr php pdf account lik asba
8	33777	thanks dude brother friend much you por best
9	16318	live checked unknown account state united

Nulled and Cracked, respectively. An additional 32166 (10.73%) and 13754 (7.40%) users were removed because the rigorous text preprocessing had taken out all of their content and LDA could not assign empty users' documents to topics. The first iteration removed a very large portion of the forum users, as 67767 and 38602 users remained in the datasets. Thus, this iteration reduced the number of users by 77.39% and 79.23%.

Tables 6.7 and 6.8 contain the results for the second iteration. The process is identical to the first iteration: identify appreciation expression topics and remove users who predominantly post such messages. The distinction between these iterations is that we use a GSDMM model for the second iteration, which was learned by treating each public post as a separate document. We can see that topics 0 and 8 in Table 6.7 and topic 6 in Table 6.8 show appreciation keywords.

Table 6.7 Nulled second iteration (GSDMM).

Topic #	# of posts	Keywords
0	25976	thanks share test man check brother nice bump
1	1248	de thanks por account eu se da aporte friend para
2	4712	post ban account rep leech help work forum
3	2182	script good vayne best play work well game
4	2903	game good play well love time lol guy kappa best
5	7003	work download update file crack bol link version
6	2836	account pm sell work email paypal buy free skype
7	707	skin account level te ekk key rler rp champion
8	20904	work thanks good nice hope share man test
9	206	php game http password account email site key

Table 6.8 Cracked second iteration (GSDMM).

Topic #	# of posts	Keywords
0	7895	quote work post good time vouch forum thread
1	2637	proxy checker download work combo link
2	1818	sdf point df sd dfg awd fd gf dd key fg ng er rt
3	2420	leech leave account post report enjoy thread ban
4	2523	thanks pour le partage je te de asd ekk rler ce
5	1448	commercial obrigado muito ich gim da bom por
6	17739	share brother work bump good thanks man hope
7	813	expires leech bol leave war de ii quote ik fire
8	2698	account discord free work sell buy add link
9	294	premium yeah game lil country account live php

The second and final iteration is where we remove users who have predominantly posted messages in topics identified in the Tables 6.7 and 6.8. We removed an additional 46 678 and 17 552 users from Nulled and Cracked, respectively, and 101 and 187 users we could not assign to any topic. Thus, the second iteration reduced the number of users by 69.03% and 45.95%, resulting in 20 988 and 20 863 remaining users, as seen in Table 6.9.

The Nulled and Cracked datasets initially had 299 719 and 185 810 users. While we ensured to set up the experiment to remove specific low-skilled users, we also rigorously checked our results against the datasets. This ensured that our method removed lower-skilled forum users instead of users such as reverse engineers and administrators. Our method consistently removed lower-ranked members (such as active members, banned users, and users with bought ranks) from the dataset.

Table 6.9 Reduction in underground forum users.

Dataset	Original size	Reduced size
Nulled	299 719	20 988 (−93.00%)
Cracked	185 810	20 863 (−88.77%)

The final result after two iterations – as seen in Table 6.9 – is a reduction of 93.00% and 88.77%. The design of the user removal method ensures that higher-skilled individuals are kept for further analysis.

Our method is limited to the two iterations as described in this chapter. Any attempts using GSDMM models for a third iteration resulted in unintelligible topic models, which could not be used to distinguish individuals further and remove additional users.

6.6 Conclusion

Law enforcement, intelligence, and researchers employ off-the-shelf tools to be more efficient at identifying key actors in large-scale criminal networks. These tools make use of SNA centrality methods, which past researchers have used to identify leaders and other key actors in small criminal networks. This chapter addresses the need to evaluate and validate centrality measures as a forensic technique for identifying key actors in large criminal networks and to increase our understanding of using centrality in forensics.

We created three interaction networks – where two of them model the communication found in real-world criminal underground forums – and analysed them using five centrality measures. We evaluated the result using bi-variate analysis to understand better which individuals they identify as more important. Our findings show that network centrality measures strongly correlate with the number of replies thread starter users receive. Thus, centrality measures identify actors with more popular forum threads rather than network leaders or other key CaaS/criminal actors. Although centrality measures give an evidence-based quantification of actors' positions within the *network structure*, they are not an indicator for leaders or highly skilled CaaS actors. Consequently, law enforcement resources may be wasted on non-key actors with popular forum threads.

We propose a novel method of separating less skilled forum users from underground forum datasets using topic modelling. This method removes 93.00% and 88.77% of an underground forum population, enabling law enforcement to focus on the remaining (and arguably more interesting) actors. We suggest that future researchers, law enforcement, and intelligence use other analyses to extract knowledge further and gain insight from the remaining actors to target offenders for removal or develop strategies to disrupt criminal networks.

Acknowledgements

The research leading to these results has received funding from the Research Council of Norway programme IKTPLUSS, under the R&D project "Ars Forensica - Computational Forensics for Large-scale Fraud Detection, Crime Investigation & Prevention", grant agreement 248094/O70. We want to thank Dr. Stefan Axelsson and Dr. Patrick Bours for their effort in reading and providing feedback to this chapter.

Preprint submitted to Forensic Science International: Digital Investigation February 15, 2023

References

Abbasi, A., Li, W., Benjamin, V. et al. (2014). Descriptive analytics: examining expert hackers in web forums. In: *2014 IEEE Joint Intelligence and Security Informatics Conference*, 56–63. The Hague, Netherlands: IEEE. doi:10.1109/JISIC.2014.18. http://ieeexplore.ieee.org/document/6975554 accessed 21 November 2022.

Baker, W.E. and Faulkner, R.R. (1993). The social organization of conspiracy: illegal networks in the heavy electrical equipment industry. *American Sociological Review* 58 (6): 837. doi:10.2307/2095954. http://www.jstor.org/stable/2095954?origin=crossref accessed 21 November 2022.

Blei, D.M., Ng, A.Y., and Jordan, M.I. (2003). *Latent Dirichlet Allocation* 30.

Bright, D.A., Hughes, C.E., and Chalmers, J. (2012). Illuminating dark networks: a social network analysis of an Australian drug trafficking syndicate. *Crime, Law and Social Change* 57 (2): 151–176. doi:10.1007/s10611-011-9336-z. http://link.springer.com/10.1007/s10611-011-9336-z accessed 21 November 2022.

Décary-Hétu, D. and Dupont, B. (2012). The social network of hackers. *Global Crime* 13 (3): 160–175. doi:10.1080/17440572.2012.702523. http://www.tandfonline.com/doi/abs/10.1080/17440572.2012.702523 accessed 21 November 2022.

Diesner, J. and Carley, K.M. (2005). Exploration of communication networks from the enron email corpus. In: *SIAM International Conference on Data Mining: Workshop on Link Analysis, Counterterrorism and Security*, Newport Beach, CA.

Europol (2014). The internet organised crime threat assessment (IOCTA) 2014. Tech. rep. https://www.europol.europa.eu/sites/default/files/documents/europol_iocta_web.pdf

Europol (2020). The internet organised crime threat assessment (IOCTA) 2020, Tech. rep.

Franke, K. and Srihari, S.N. (2008). Computational forensics: an overview. In: *Proceedings of the 2nd International Workshop on Computational Forensics, IWCF '08*. Springer-Verlag, Berlin, Heidelberg, 1–10. doi:10.1007/978-3-540-85303-9_1. http://dx.doi.org/10.1007/978-3-540-85303-9_1 accessed 21 November 2022.

Gogolin, G. (2021). *Digital Forensics Explained*. CRC Press. https://books.google.no/books?id=YMIZEAAAQBAJ accessed 21 November 2022.

Grisham, J., Samtani, S., Patton, M., and Chen, H. (2017). Identifying mobile malware and key threat actors in online hacker forums for proactive cyber threat intelligence. In: *2017 IEEE International Conference on Intelligence and Security Informatics (ISI)*. IEEE, Beijing, China, 13–18. doi:10.1109/ISI.2017.8004867. http://ieeexplore.ieee.org/document/8004867 accessed 21 November 2022.

Hardin, J.S., Sarkis, G., and Urc, P.C. (2015). Network analysis with the enron email corpus. *Journal of Statistics Education* 23 (2).

Holt, T.J., Strumsky, D., Smirnova, O., and Kilger, M. (2012). Examining the social networks of malware writers and hackers. *International Journal of Cyber Criminology* 6 (1): 891.

IBM software (2013). IBM i2 analyst's notebook social network analysis. https://cryptome. wikileaks.org/2013/12/ibm-i2-sna.pdf

Johnsen, J.W. and Franke, K. (2017). Feasibility study of social network analysis on loosely structured communication networks. *Procedia Computer Science* 108: 2388–2392. doi:10.1016/j. procs.2017.05.172. http://linkinghub.elsevier.com/retrieve/pii/S1877050917307561 accessed 21 November 2022.

Johnsen, J.W. and Franke, K. (2018). Identifying central individuals in organised criminal groups and underground marketplaces. In: *Computational Science – ICCS 2018*, 10862. Springer International Publishing, Cham, 379–386. doi:10.1007/978-3-319-93713-7_31. http://link. springer.com/10.1007/978-3-319-93713-7_31 accessed 21 November 2022.

Johnsen, J.W. and Franke, K. (2019). The impact of preprocessing in natural language for open source intelligence and criminal investigation. In: *2019 IEEE International Conference on Big Data (Big Data)*. IEEE, Los Angeles, CA, USA, 4248–4254. doi:10.1109/BigData47090.2019.9006006. https://ieeexplore.ieee.org/document/9006006.

Johnsen, J.W. and Franke, K. (2020). Identifying proficient cybercriminals through text and network analysis. In: *2020 IEEE International Conference on Intelligence and Security Informatics (ISI)*. IEEE, 1–7. doi:10.1109/ISI49825.2020.9280523. https://ieeexplore.ieee.org/abstract/document/9280523

Krebs, V. (2002). Uncloaking terrorist networks. *First Monday* 7: 4. https://doi.org/10.5210/fm. v7i4.941. http://journals.uic.edu/ojs/index.php/fm/article/view/941 accessed 21 November 2022.

Kumar, P. and Sinha, A. (2021). Information diffusion modeling and analysis for socially interacting networks. *Social Network Analysis and Mining* 11 (1): 11. doi:10.1007/s13278-020-00719-7. http://link.springer.com/10.1007/s13278-020-00719-7 accessed 21 November 2022.

Lu, Y., Luo, X., Polgar, M., and Cao, Y. (2010). Social network analysis of a criminal hacker community. *Journal of Computer Information Systems* 12.

Marin, E., Shakarian, J., and Shakarian, P. (2018). Mining key-hackers on darkweb forums. In: *2018 1st International Conference on Data Intelligence and Security (ICDIS)*. IEEE, South Padre Island, TX, 73–80. doi:10.1109/ICDIS.2018.00018. https://ieeexplore.ieee.org/document/8367642.

Mazarura, J. and de Waal, A. (2016). A comparison of the performance of latent Dirichlet allocation and the Dirichlet multinomial mixture model on short text. In: *2016 Pattern Recognition Association of South Africa and Robotics and Mechatronics International Conference (PRASA-RobMech)*. IEEE, Stellenbosch, South Africa, 1–6. doi:10.1109/RoboMech.2016.7813155. http://ieeexplore.ieee.org/document/7813155

Memon, B.R. (2012). Identifying important nodes in weighted covert networks using generalized centrality measures. In: *2012 European Intelligence and Security Informatics Conference*. IEEE, Odense, Denmark, 131–140. doi:10.1109/EISIC.2012.65. http://ieeexplore.ieee.org/document/6298823.

Morselli, C. (2010). Assessing vulnerable and strategic positions in a criminal network. *Journal of Contemporary Criminal Justice* 26 (4): 382–392. doi:10.1177/1043986210377105. http://journals.sagepub.com/doi/10.1177/1043986210377105 accessed 21 November 2022.

Ortiz-Arroyo, D. (2010). Discovering sets of key players in social networks. In: *Computational Social Network Analysis: Trends, Tools and Research Advances* (ed. A. Abraham, A.-E. Hassanien, and V. Sná¿el), 27–47. London: Springer London. doi:10.1007/978-1-84882-229-0_2. https://doi.org/10.1007/978-1-84882-229-0_2 accessed 21 November 2022.

Pastrana, S., Hutchings, A., Caines, A., and Buttery, P. (2018). Characterizing eve: analysing cybercrime actors in a large underground forum. In: *Research in Attacks, Intrusions, and Defenses* (ed. M. Bailey, T. Holz, M. Stamatogiannakis, and S. Ioannidis), 207–227. Cham: Springer International Publishing.

Pete, I., Hughes, J., Chua, Y.T., and Bada, M. (2020). A social network analysis and comparison of six dark web forums. In: *2020 IEEE European Symposium on Security and Privacy Workshops (EuroS&PW)*. IEEE, Genoa, Italy, 484–493. doi:10.1109/EuroSPW51379.2020.00071. https://ieeexplore.ieee.org/document/9229679.

Prell, C. (2012). *Social Network Analysis: History, Theory and Methodology*. SAGE Publications. https://books.google.com/books?id=p4iTo566nAMC accessed 21 November 2022.

Rosario Fuentes, M. (2020 May). Shifts in underground markets: past, present, and future. Tech. rep. Trend Micro Research.

Samtani, S. and Chen, H. (2016). Using social network analysis to identify key hackers for keylogging tools in hacker forums. In: *2016 IEEE Conference on Intelligence and Security Informatics (ISI)*. IEEE, Tucson, AZ, USA, 319–321. doi:10.1109/ISI.2016.7745500. http://ieeexplore. ieee.org/document/7745500.

Sandilands, D.D. (2014). Bivariate analysis. In: *Encyclopedia of Quality of Life and Well-Being Research* (ed. A.C. Michalos), 416–418. Dordrecht: Springer Netherlands. doi:10.1007/978-94-007-0753-5. https://doi.org/10.1007/978-94-007-0753-5 accessed 21 November 2022.

Schober, P., Boer, C., and Schwarte, L.A. (2018). Correlation coefficients: appropriate use and interpretation. *Anesthesia & Analgesia* 126 (5): 1763–1768. doi:10.1213/ANE.0000000000002864. http://journals.lww.com/00000539-201805000-00050 accessed 21 November 2022.

Schwartz, D.M. and Rouselle, T.D. (2009). Using social network analysis to target criminal networks. *Trends in Organized Crime* 12 (2): 188–207. publisher: Springer.

Shetty, J. and Adibi, J. (n.d.). The enron email dataset database schema and brief statistical report 4. http://citeseerx.ist.psu.edu/viewdoc/download?doi=10.1.1.296.9477&rep=rep1&type=pdf.

Sparrow, M.K. (1991). The application of network analysis to criminal intelligence: an assessment of the prospects. *Social Networks* 13 (3): 251–274. http://www.sciencedirect.com/science/article/pii/037887339190008H.

Stoykova, R. (2021). Digital evidence: unaddressed threats to fairness and the presumption of innocence. *Computer Law & Security Review* 42: 105575. doi:10.1016/j.clsr.2021.105575. https://linkinghub.elsevier.com/retrieve/pii/S0267364921000480 accessed 21 November 2022.

Stoykova, R. (2022). Standards for digital evidence. An inquiry into the opportunities for fair trial safeguards through digital forensics standards in criminal investigations. Ph.D. thesis, Dual PhD University of Groningen and Norwegian University of Science and technology.

Taha, K. and Yoo, P. (2015). SIIMCO: a forensic investigation tool for identifying the influential members of a criminal organization. *IEEE Transactions on Information Forensics and Security* 1–1. doi:10.1109/TIFS.2015.2510826. http://ieeexplore.ieee.org/document/7361998 accessed 21 November 2022.

Xu, J. and Chen, H. (2003). Untangling criminal networks: a case study. In: *Intelligence and Security Informatics* (ed. H. Chen, R. Miranda, D.D. Zeng, et al.), 232–248. Berlin, Heidelberg: Springer Berlin Heidelberg.

Xu, J., Marshall, B., Kaza, S., and Chen, H. (2004). Analyzing and visualizing criminal network dynamics: a case study. In: *Intelligence and Security Informatics* (ed. H. Chen, R. Moore, D.D. Zeng, and J. Leavitt), 359–377. Berlin, Heidelberg: Springer Berlin Heidelberg.

Yin, J. and Wang, J. (2014). A dirichlet multinomial mixture model-based approach for short text clustering. In: *Proceedings of the 20th ACM SIGKDD international conference on Knowledge discovery and data mining*. ACM, New York New York USA, 233–242. doi:10.1145/2623330.2623715. https://dl.acm.org/doi/10.1145/2623330.2623715.

CHAPTER 7

Mapping NLP Techniques to Investigations and Investigative Interviews

Kyle Porter* and Bente Skattør

NTNU, Gjøvik, Norway
* Corresponding author

7.1 Introduction

Criminal investigation is the process of discovering the who, what, where, why, when, and how of a crime, and then supporting this process with evidence. New technology and methods, such as artificial intelligence (AI), have the potential to put investigators in a position to enable them to harness these innovations to gain an edge over the ever-increasing volume of information in our digital era.

Whatever advances in technology are made, investigations are still heavily reliant upon what is said and written. Sources of evidence may be instant messaging logs, text documents, and of course, investigative interviews and their transcriptions. This chapter is concerned with examining how natural language processing (NLP) technologies and the like may be used in an investigation. Through case studies, we have exposed investigator interviewers to NLP technologies and asked them about their unrestricted wants and needs from NLP and how NLP would ideally contribute to their work.

This chapter is an attempt to map what investigators want or need from linguistic technology, and what is available in terms of technology, techniques, and past studies. Our intended audience are digital investigation students or researchers, from the perspectives of law enforcement or computer science. We cover the basics and the state of the art of NLP and automatic speech recognition (ASR), as well as the specific NLP techniques listed in our mapping, and their limitations. We discuss the techniques in the context of digital forensics studies when possible, and conclude with an assessment of their readiness and potential to be

Artificial Intelligence (AI) in Forensic Sciences, First Edition. Edited by Zeno Geradts and Katrin Franke.
© 2024 John Wiley & Sons Ltd. Published 2024 by John Wiley & Sons Ltd.

applied in digital investigations and investigative interviews. We hope that this chapter can act as a roadmap for future research and development regarding linguistic technology and digital investigation.

7.2 Criminal Investigation

The police solve crimes using different methods and techniques, either using them separately or combining them (Bjerknes and Fahsing 2018). The chosen methods and techniques are often selected based on the crime scene. A crime scene is anywhere or anything that can provide evidence of the offence or provide collaboration of a victim's allegation or suspect's defence (Rose 2021; Tiege and Ragde 2021). Forensic technicians utilize many techniques like DNA, lasers, blood tests/spots, damage, physical traces, etc. The different approaches and use of techniques strongly depend on the crime scenes. Assault of a refugee, homicide of a prostitute, robbery of a jeweller, domestic violence, and a terror attack will all be very different crime scenes (Marry 2019; Ragde 2021). The tools and techniques used related to a crime scene, and hence also the investigation, are continually evolving and expanding (Brookman 2020; Hess 2015; Ragde 2021). A good investigation plan made by the chief investigator and the investigation teams is essential during the whole investigation process. Investigative interviews are a part of that plan and are essential to enrich the crime case in many of the steps in the investigation cycle (collect, check, connect, construct, consider, consult), which are used to answer the six investigative questions (what?, where?, when?, who?, why?, how?) (Fahsing 2016).

7.2.1 Investigative Interviews
Even though the police solve crimes using different methods and techniques, crimes are still solved because "somebody talked" (Hess 2015; Marry 2019). Investigative interviews are crucial in all crime investigations and involve human beings, human behaviours, and human rights. Hence, law enforcement must build competent interviewers that will do more to solve crimes (Hess 2015) by using a method that supports investigative interviews (Bjerknes and Fahsing 2018; Hess 2015; Marry 2019; Rachlew et al. 2020).

Our ongoing study uses the investigative interview method used in Norway called KREATIV that builds upon PEACE from the UK (Bjerknes and Fahsing 2018; Police 2020; Rachlew et al. 2020). KREATIV aims to define how the investigator interviews should be carried out professionally, and how they should be structured before, during, and after the interviews. The objective of KREATIV interviews is to gather accurate and reliable information. It is valid whether the interviewee is a suspected criminal, a victim, or a witness. In Norway, the rule of law states that: no threats, no torture nor lies are allowed during interviews (Fahsing 1998) and everyone is innocent until proven guilty (CPT 2002). It is of utmost importance to move away from the confession-driven practice of being accusatory, manipulative, or coercive (Mendez and Areh 2021; Riksadvokaten 2016). The way the interviews are conducted affects society's and citizens' trust in law enforcement and strongly relates to the jurisdictional process (Mendez and Areh 2021; Rachlew et al. 2020; Riksadvokaten 2016). Only the court determines guilt or innocence. A good interrogation contributes to clarifying a criminal act, a bad interrogation can ultimately lead to unnecessary detention or even lead to a wrongful conviction. The investigative interview is evidence, hence not only is the information of importance, but how the information is gathered is also important (Riksadvokaten 2016).

During the interviews, a report is established to contribute to mutual understanding (Gabbert et al. 2021) and ensure sound information gathering (Rachlew et al. 2020). Every year, the Norwegian police manually write thousands of investigative interview reports of different types. Generally, these are a transcription of what is said (dialog reports) in full or partially, or reports are written as a summary of the interviews. In some cases, i.e., interviews of children, the interviews have both a summary report and a dialog report. This is very time-consuming and often tedious work for the investigators and police officers because they write, in total, a substantial number of words. As a consequence, other investigators in the team will read many reports.

7.3 Assessing the Needs of Investigators in an NLP Context

The needs of the investigators in this chapter are based on three different case studies carried out by the police in 2021. The all were carried out with police investigators and police employees with a user centric approach (Beyer and Holtzblatt 1998). All case studies aimed to gather needs and ideas. One of them focused specifically on KREATIV. During two of these case studies the participants were exposed to an ASR-solution. Writing reports manually is very time-consuming and often tedious work for the investigators and police officers. Hence, we noticed that the ASR-solution also inspired the investigator to see other possible AI-solutions, such as NLP. Incoming needs and ideas were prioritized by the participants.

7.3.1 Mapping Interviewer Needs to Existing NLP Tasks

The purpose of this section is to identify and map NLP techniques that sufficiently meet the needs of the surveyed investigative interviewers. We emphasize that the application of NLP techniques to digital forensics and investigations is by no means standard procedure, and thus application of this technology in this section should be seen as a work in progress, or in some cases, future work.

To facilitate a structure of how we discuss the different NLP tasks, we have organized them into three different application categories: extraction, classification, and reduction. At the moment, no standard NLP taxonomy exists, so it is possible that our taxonomy may be improved or refined. An overview of the mapping from an investigator need to a specific NLP tasks can be found in Table 7.1 We note that the list of needs is incomplete, as those listed are those that are most easily addressed by existing technology.

Table 7.1 Mapping between investigator needs and existing NLP techniques.

NLP Application	Investigator Need	Specific NLP Tasks for Support
Extraction	Entity identification Section 7.6.1 Linking entities Section 7.6.4	• Named entity recognition (NER) • NER + market basket analysis • Entity relationship extraction • Entity and Relationship visualization
	Time extraction Section 7.6.1, 7.6.6	• NER • RegEx Temporal Extractors
	Negation detection Section 7.6.6	• Negation detection (RegEx)
	Keyword identification Sections 7.6.1, 7.6.6	• Keyword extraction
	Code Words Section 7.6.6	• NER • Keyword extraction
	Synonym handling Section 7.6.6	• Wordnet • Entity disambiguation
Classification	Text categorization Section 7.7	• Text Classification • Sentiment analysis
	Author profiling Section 7.7.2	• Author profiling classifier • Author attribution • Author verification • Grooming detection
Reduction	Theme extraction Section 7.8.1	• Topic modelling
	Text summarization Section 7.8.4	• Text summarizer

The subsequent sections are organized in the following manner. We first briefly discuss ASR, how it is evaluated, and what state-of-the-art performance looks like. We then cover some background information that is common for NLP tasks, such as how human written text is encoded and how it is preprocessed. Afterwards we discuss the specific NLP techniques identified in the mappings in depth.

7.4 Automatic Speech Recognition

ASR is a similar but different language technology to NLP. A primary difference in this technology versus traditional NLP is that the inputs for ASR are audio files files where a major objective is to transcribe the audio to text.

7.4.1 ASR Basics

To evaluate the performance of an ASR solution, human written transcripts of the audio are compared with the transcripts produced by the ASR models. There are three kinds of transcription errors that can be made. A word can be deleted (the machine transcription is missing a word), a word can be inserted (the machine transcription added an extra word), or a word can be substituted (the machine transcription misheard a word). When comparing the performance of ASR models, the standard evaluation metric used is the word error rate (WER), which is the sum of all transcription errors divided by number of words in the reference script, producing a percentage (Ali and Renals 2018).

There are a number of different audio factors that can decrease the effectiveness of ASR tasks, and at the personal level they can be divided into inter-speaker variation and intra-speaker variation (McTear et al. 2016). Inter-speaker variation refers to effects caused by the different ways of speaking between different speakers. This includes aspects such as accent, age, and sex. Intra-speaker variation refers to the effects that are caused by aspects of an individual speaker. This includes things such as health, tiredness, emotional state, and whether text is read or freely spoken. Other sources of error may be contributed from recording quality, spoken distance to the microphone, and audio file fidelity.

7.4.2 ASR, Digital Investigation, and the State of the Art

Very few recent works have studied ASR in the context of digital investigation. Negrão and Domingues (2021) used open source engines to create a third party module for autopsy that performs both voice activity detection (VAD) from audio or video files, as well as ASR. Using INA's inaSpeechSegmenter engine for VAD and Mozilla's DeepSpeech engine they identified all files with human voices, obtained a 27.2% WER for non-native English speakers, and a 7.8% WER for high fidelity voice files from native English speakers. They note the benefits of using opensource engines, as opposed to commercial solutions, in that they do not have to rely upon cloud solutions, thereby having full custody over potentially sensitive data.

The performance achieved by Negrao and Domingues is not far from state-of-the-art speech recognition research,[1] and performed nearly as well as human transcribers. Studying human transcribers on the English read Librispeech dataset,[2] Amodei et al. (2016) noted human transcription obtaining a 5.83% WER for transcribing clean data, and 12.69% WER for transcribing more difficult sound files. The highest performing ASR results on the same dataset achieved 1.8% WER with clean data, and 2.9% WER with more difficult sound files (Hsu et al. 2021).

Despite the impressive performance of modern ASR solutions on read benchmark datasets, ASR still has areas with significant limitations. For instance, ASR for young children is still inadequate (Yeung and Alwan 2018), and not all languages, dialects, or accents may be equally supported (Feng et al. 2021; Koenecke et al. 2020; Solberg and Ortiz 2022). Notably, applying ASR to spontaneous speech is considered much more difficult than read speech.

---

[1] https://github.com/syhw/wer_are_we.
[2] https://www.openslr.org/12.

Thus, direct application of transcribed audio via ASR to analytical techniques such as NLP would not be advised due to the likelihood of erroneous text. Instead, using ASR as a means to expedite human transcription has been found to be significantly faster than transcriptions performed solely by a human. Some state-of-the-art ASR models worth mentioning due to their performance and relative ease of use are Wav2Vec 2.0 and Whisper. Wav2Vec 2.0 requires very little data to fine-tune the model (10 minutes of transcribed audio) to see state-of-the-art results (4.8% WER on the clean Librispeech dataset), thus being effective for "low-resource" languages (Baevski et al. 2020). Whisper on the other hand is intended to be used for state-of-the-art performance "out of the box", where no additional training data is needed (but is still possible). Whisper obtained 2.7% WER on the clean Librispeech dataset (Radford et al. 2022).

7.5 NLP Basics

Before looking at the particular NLP methods and how they may support investigative interviewer needs, we provide a basic background of common NLP concepts and terminology. We provide a running example of text documents to explain these concepts.

7.5.1 Common Terminology

A **corpus** is the term used for a collection or set of documents. If there is more than one corpus, then it is referred to as corpora. Below we provide a small toy corpus, containing two documents.

Document 1: "Fido the dog, Boston bred, had evidence that the quick brown fox didn't jump over the 'lazy dog' at 12:15 p.m."

Document 2: "The fox was actually working for the FBI, and it was evident that he did jump over the lazy dog."

In order for text to be efficiently processed by computers, it must first be normalized. This is part of the **preprocessing** phases. Preprocessing is essentially the steps taken to "clean up" the text in a set of documents, and prepare it for ingestion by a machine learning model. The extent to which text may be preprocessed is also dependent upon the machine learning model being used, as sometimes textual qualities can provide contexts for learning. For some naïve machine learning models, it is preferred that all the text is lower-cased, contractions removed, and that words are standardized to remove redundancy. Our example Document 1 after lowercasing the text, removing and expanding contractions, and punctuation appears as:

Document 1: "fido the dog boston bred had evidence that the quick brown fox did not jump over the lazy dog at 1215 pm"

An extremely important preprocessing step is **tokenization**. Tokenization refers to how one splits up the **tokens** (typically words) in the given documents. A typical method of tokenization is to split documents on spaces, commas, periods, and other similar punctuation. This results in the document being split into an array of tokens. However, tokenization does not always need to occur with respect to spaces and full words. Tokens can be words, syllables, a consecutive set of characters, or characters themselves. Some special tokens may be added to the list of tokens that consider special context to text input, such as the start or end of specific input (Devlin et al. 2018). Below, we show white space and punctuation tokenization applied to the preprocessed Document 1.

Document 1 (Preprocessed and Tokenized on white spaces): [fido, the, dog, boston, bred, had, evidence, that, the, quick, brown, fox, did, not, jump, over, the, lazy, dog, at, 1215, pm]

Tokenization can be more abstract as well. A popular and simple version of tokenization is referred to as **n-grams**, where a document can be split upon every n words or characters of a text.

An additional preprocessing step to reduce redundancy is word **stemming** or **lemmatization**. Stemming tries to remove the suffix of the word while lemmatization tries to replace a word with its root form (Jurafsky and Martin 2022) (for instance, bred to breed). Document 1 after initial preprocessing, whitespace tokenization, and stemming would appear as so:

Document 1 (Preprocessed, tokenized, and stemmed): [fido, the, dog, boston, bred, had, evid, that, the, quick, brown, fox, did, not, jump, over, the, lazi, dog, at, 1215, pm]

In a similar vein, there are many words in documents that contain very little information. These are known as **stop words**, and the preprocessing step of stop word removal tries to eliminate words of little informative value. Typically speaking, stop words are often extremely common words found throughout a corpus, and also typically include common verbs, pronouns, and grammatical articles ("the", "a", etc.). This is a form of feature reduction. Note, some machine learning models (such as modern NLP models) prefer not stemming words or removing stop words, as it adds context to how they learn. Below, we provide examples of Document 1 and 2 after initial preprocessing, tokenization, stemming, and stop word removal.

Document 1: [fido, dog, boston, bred, evid, quick, brown, fox, jump, lazi, dog, 1215, pm]
Document 2: [fox, actual, work, fbi, evid, jump, lazi, dog]

A **dictionary** represents the set of words known by the NLP model. The dictionary typically does not end up being one-to-one with the words in the raw text, as the preprocessing steps will likely eliminate and change many of the terms.

Dictionary of Document 1 and 2: [1215, actual, boston, bred, brown, dog, evid, fbi, fido, fox, jump, lazi, pm, quick, work].

7.5.2 Vector Space Models and Embeddings

An NLP machine learning model will interpret documents in the context of its dictionary, and in order for a machine learning model to be able to "read" a text document, the document or its words must be converted into a numerical format that ideally captures some of the semantic values of the original word or document. Essentially, we need to extract numerical features from our text documents. This is the purpose of **vector space models** or **embeddings**, wherein a word or document is transformed into a vector such that the distance or similarity between vectors (or words and documents) can be quantitatively calculated and some of the semantic meaning of the document or word is ideally preserved (Jurafsky and Martin 2022). A simple document embedding is known as **bag-of-words**, wherein a document is represented by a vector of the frequency of its terms found in a model's dictionary. Documents 1 and 2 may have the following bag-of-words vectorizations:

Document 1: [1, 0, 1, 1, 1, 2, 1, 0, 1, 1, 1, 1, 1, 1, 0]
Document 2: [0, 1, 0, 0, 0, 1, 1, 1, 0, 1, 1, 1, 0, 0, 1]

At this point, we can treat our documents like any other machine learning problem or calculate the similarity between documents.

Often the bag-of-words approach is too simple, or overly common words have too much influence in NLP tasks. A solution for this is to use the **term frequency inverse document frequency (TF-IDF)**, as it weighs terms in documents such that common terms throughout the corpus are not overly influential (Jurafsky and Martin 2022).

Not only may documents be represented in a vector space model, but so can words. Typically, they are represented as special embeddings, where the vectors are relatively short and dense, as compared to the previously seen long and sparse (meaning often empty) vector space model embeddings. Examples of embedding methods include Word2Vec (Mikolov et al. 2013) or GloVe (Pennington et al. 2014). Dense vectors appear to perform much better overall in NLP tasks than sparse vectors (Jurafsky and Martin 2022). An example of 2-dimensional word embeddings can be seen in Figure 7.1 Note, that more similar words are clustered near each other.

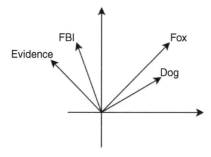

Figure 7.1 Trivial example of possible word embeddings for some of the example terms.

7.5.3 Modern NLP Models

With the introduction of the Transformer deep neural network architecture in 2017 (Vaswani et al. 2017), and the release of Google's BERT (Bidirectional Encoder Representations from Transformers) in 2018 (Devlin et al. 2018), there have been massive advancements in the field of natural language processing. As of 2022, the majority of the research which has performed best on most benchmark NLP tasks use a kind of transformer model.[3]

The workflow of applying modern NLP models usually involves two different steps: pre-training and fine-tuning. Pre-training typically consists of training the model on massive unlabeled language datasets, where the learning objective is more general (Devlin et al. 2018). Pre-training is extremely computationally expensive, and is typically only feasible by large laboratories with sufficient money and hardware. Fine-tuning a BERT-like model begins with the model and its pre-trained parameters, but then the model can be trained on specific downstream NLP tasks, such as NER, where a labeled dataset is used (Devlin et al. 2018). So, it is feasible for non-experts to fine-tune a BERT-like model and achieve comparable state-of-the-art results. Especially since there are user-friendly frameworks for using and fine-tuning pretrained models such as Huggingface's Transformers[4] or spaCy.[5]

We now discuss the particular NLP applications that may be useful for investigative interviewers and digital investigators alike.

7.6 Text Extraction

By "extraction", we are referring to the task of automatically identifying elements from within the text (such as strings). Common examples of extraction include the extraction of proper nouns, keywords, relationships between proper nouns, datetimes, etc. We refer to our NLP application Table 7.1 to look and see which NLP extraction tasks are relevant for our identified investigator needs.

Many of the extraction techniques are dependent on NER, where NER can often be a starting point of the technique. Thus, we discuss NER and its applications to forensics and investigations, followed by techniques which use the extracted entities to obtain more information. We also consider the distinct areas of keyword extraction and regular expression based extraction.

7.6.1 Entity Identification and Named Entity Recognition

The ability to identify dates, names, and other proper nouns of interest is a problem that is somewhat solved using the NER technique. It is, however, not without its caveats. NER is a supervised NLP task which attempts to classify words

---

[3] http://nlpprogress.com.
[4] https://github.com/huggingface/transformers.
[5] https://github.com/explosion/spaCy.

or groups of words into a category that it has been trained on, such as names, places, organizations, or geo-political entities. One exciting benefit of NER is that it is possible to train it to identify words that are not exactly proper nouns, such as dates or names for drugs.

We continue with our running example and apply an idealized NER model on Documents 1 and 2, and show a simplified output.

Document 1: "Fido the dog, Boston bred, had evidence that the quick brown fox didn't jump over the 'lazy dog' at 12:15 p.m."
Fido – PERSON[6]
Boston – LOCATION
Document 2: "The fox was actually working for the FBI, and it was evident that he did jump over the lazy dog."
FBI – ORGANIZATION

Prior to discussing how NER may be applied to digital investigations, we first introduce the metrics used to evaluate NER models.

7.6.2 Named Entity Recognition Metrics

NER is assessed by way of precision, recall, and F1-score. These metrics are useful in instances when measuring the success of searching for "needles in haystacks", where the number of positive samples is much smaller than the number of negative samples. Precision is defined as the percentage of returned results that are items of interest, in the case of NER, proper nouns. Recall is defined as the total percentage of items of interest found. The F1-score is a composition of the two previous metrics, which gives researchers a general idea of how well a machine learning method performs the identification of named entities. We give their mathematical equations below:

$$\text{Precision} = \frac{\text{True Positives}}{\text{True Positives} + \text{False Positives}} \tag{7.1}$$

$$\text{Recall} = \frac{\text{True Positives}}{\text{True Positives} + \text{False Negatives}} \tag{7.2}$$

$$\text{F1} - \text{Score} = 2 * \frac{\text{Precision} * \text{Recall}}{\text{Precision} + \text{Recall}} \tag{7.3}$$

For clarity, positive samples are proper nouns (or elements such as dates if you train the model to identify them), and negative samples are everything else.

NER results may be assessed with respect to all possibly NER categories, or they can be assessed with respect to a specific category. For instance, it is possible for a

---

[6] In the event that a name is not in a model's dictionary, it is possible the output is displayed as a series of tokens. For example, our output for applying a BERT NER model on "Fido" yielded Fi – B-MISC, ##do – I-MISC.

NER model to have an overall 90% F1-score but a 97% F1-score for identifying names.

From our working example, if we identified Boston, and "lazy dog" as named entities from documents 1 and 2, we would have achieved 50% precision and 33% recall. As of the time of writing, Wang et al. (2021) have produced the highest F1-score of 94.6% on the standard CoNLL 2003 dataset.[7]

7.6.3 NER Applied to Investigations

According to past research, the typical use of NER for investigations is to automate the process of extracting metadata information (such as who, what, when, and where) from large sources of unstructured text documents.

At the most generic level, Pollitt (2013) states that by using NER a set of unique entities may be extracted from a dataset, and can be used to identify "subjects or actors" within a digital forensics narrative, warranting further analysis. This not only allows for extraction of entities from an entire set of forensic evidence, but also allows specific files (in his case, emails) to be tagged with specifically named entities.

In order to increase the effectiveness of NER, it is common for researchers and private companies alike to train their NER models with domain-specific datasets. One such approach is to train NER models to identify entities that are of interest to police or investigators. For example, Chau et al. (2002) created a dataset that could also extract words representing personal properties, narcotics, addresses, and vehicles. More recently Wu et al. (2020) trained a deep learning model for proactive crime detection with a specially annotated dataset for the purpose of public opinion monitoring of Chinese text, where they could identify words representing illegal drugs. Such words are given a "CRIME" label. For their given dataset, they achieved an F1-score of 85.24%. Other types of entities may be discovered as well which may benefit investigators, such as the extraction of times, events, or financial terms.

7.6.4 Entity Linking

NER may also just be a preprocessing step prior to conducting further analysis. A common research subject is to first perform NER, followed by methods which try to identify relationships between entities.

A common method used in digital forensics research to link together different entities is to apply a version of the Apriori algorithm (Agrawal et al. 1993). The algorithm essentially attempts to discover items that commonly occur together in a document or database, and provides a level of confidence of an itemset occurring together. Researchers have either applied this to find direct links between entities within documents (Yang and Chow 2015), or indirect links between entities (Al-Zaidy et al. 2012). Applying this technique, Al-Zaidy et al. (2012) identified seven of the eight criminal groupings, with no misidentifications, from

---

[7] https://huggingface.co/datasets/conll2003.

a real Canadian cybercrime investigation. The criminal dataset was a 500 MB chat log from a suspect of a computer hacking case including 220 chat accounts.

Assuming our running example had more documents, it is possible that a grouping of entities may be found via the Apriori algorithm could be (Boston, Fido).

More sophisticated versions of entity relationship can be discovered with a technology known as *Relationship Extraction*, which intends to identify the semantic relationship between pairs of entities. For example, Fido lives in Boston. However, this method has traditionally focused on extracting entity relationships from sentences, rather than documents, and research on document-level relationship extraction is ongoing (Bose et al. 2021).

Iqbal et al. (2019) has demonstrated graph-based visualization methods on *clique-detection*. Due to entity links being transformed into a graph structure, the use of graph theoretical methods, such as centrality measures, can be used to identify important nodes in a graph (Johnsen and Franke 2020). Rodrigues et al. (2022) used a similar method, but rather than constructing networking connections via Apriori-based clique detection, they derive edges from a (sentence-level) relationship extractor on Portuguese text. Batini et al. (2021) also utilized NER as a preprocessing step for visualizing a case where they created a explorable knowledge graph based on the entities and their relationships. In Figure 7.2, we provide a mock example of a possible visualization of relationship extraction performed on our running example of documents, plus some additional documents added to the corpus.

7.6.5 Limitations of Using NER

One would imagine that a primary benefit of applying NER is the ability to identify proper nouns that the machine learning model has not been trained with, including code words. However, research shows that this is a difficult problem for NER models

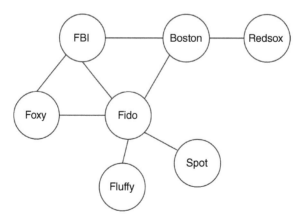

Figure 7.2 Mock visualization of possible relationship extraction (leaving the nature of the relationship undefined) applied to our running example, with some additional documents added to the corpus. Example derived from the works of Iqbal et al. (2019), Rodrigues et al. (2022), and Batini et al. (2021).

(Lin et al. 2020). Fine-tuning pretrained BERT-like language models that consider sentences in a bi-directional fashion, Lin et al. (2020) focused on determining if the context of some given written text was sufficient to guess an entity type correctly. They concluded that if entities are not trained with a regular kind of sentence structure, then the NER performance is greatly diminished. Likewise, if an entity is mentioned too often it weakens the model's ability to learn entity types based on context, thus overfitting onto the actual word. Typical usage of NER models limits its usefulness for identifying terms yet to be encountered, including code words.

7.6.6 Extraction Methods outside NER

NER, although prominent, is not the only method of extraction. Here, we provide some other approaches that investigators may find useful, that do not necessarily rely upon modern AI techniques.

The most basic way of extracting patterns in text is by way of regular expressions. Such rules and tools have been designed for temporal extractors (Strötgen and Gertz 2010), as well as negation detection.[8]

While NER can be used to identify potential keywords, the method of *keyword extraction* may be preferred to identify codewords, because those words may fall outside typical linguistic usage. One such popular unsupervized keyword extractor is known as RAKE (Rapid Automatic Keyword Extractor) (Rose et al. 2010), which is dependent upon the co-occurance of words, wherein the words are tokenized by way of stop words. A newer keyword extractor is YAKE (Yet Another Keyword Extractor), which is corpus and language independent and outperforms RAKE (Campos et al. 2020).

NER also has issues when it comes to synonyms in that a NER model may recognize two entities that in fact refer to the same entity. A solution to manage synonyms has been to use a Wordnet. The original Wordnet (Fellbaum 2010), is a "large electronic database for English", where words are stored in a semantic network such that related words are connected. A similar method of handling synonyms or word ambiguity is through the use of named entity disambiguation, which links identified entities to particular entries in a knowledge database (such as Wikipedia) (Cucerzan 2007).

7.7 Text Classification

Text classification is perhaps one of the more straightforward applications of machine learning and NLP on text. It asks, given some unseen excerpt of text, to which category does it belong? This can be performed with different quantities of text. For example, at the document level, paragraph level, sentence level, or even sub-sentence level (Kowsari et al. 2019).

---

[8] https://code.google.com/archive/p/negex.

Text classification is a broad field, where classification is typically performed at the binary of multi-class level. At the binary level of text classification, text is classified as either a positive or negative class. For example, text could be classified as "fake news" or not. In terms of sentiment analysis, text could be classified quite literally as "positive" or "negative" polarity. At the multi-class level, text may fall under the category of one of several classes. For example, some text may be attributed to one of several possible authors. In terms of sentiment analysis, text may instead be assigned a numerical ranking (such as a number of stars, from 1 to 5), or one of many possible "moods" (happy, sad, angry, etc.) (Zhang et al. 2018).

We emphasize that a classifier is only capable of providing classification labels that it has been trained on. For instance, if you have a news genre classifier and the classes the model was trained on were "sports", "business", and "local", the classifier could only classify unseen documents as one of those three classes. If there was an "international" news article, the classifier would still classify the article as one of the three original genres.

7.7.1 Classification Evaluation Metrics

When evaluating a classification model on a balanced dataset (a roughly equal number of samples per class), and performing either a binary or multi-class classification, the performance of the model will be evaluated with respect to accuracy. For multi-class classification, this is the fraction of the total number of true predictions divided by all samples n (Grandini et al. 2020).

Multi-class classification:

$$\text{Accuracy} = \frac{\text{True Predictions}}{n}$$

The accuracy for binary classification is a similar calculation, only that the "true predictions" is just the sum of true positives and true negatives. In the cases where a binary dataset has an imbalance between positive and negative samples, then the precision, recall, and F1-score are appropriate metrics for evaluation.

7.7.2 Text Classification and Digital Investigation

Past research for text classification being applied to investigative settings appears to be primarily concerned with the following subjects: the classification of predatory text, authorship attribution, authorship verification, authorship profiling, sentiment analysis, and extremism detection.

Predatory text (or grooming) detection is a classification task that searches large corpora for lines of text that are intended to exploit children, for example on conversations in social media (Ebrahimi et al. 2016) or within instant messaging chats (Ngejane et al. 2021). A common dataset used to train and test such models is the PAN-2012 dataset (Inches and Crestani 2012).[9] A typical problem with all

---

[9] https://pan.webis.de/clef12/pan12-web/sexual-predator-identification.html.

imbalanced datasets is that they bias the training of a model and reduce its effectiveness, but recent research trained on the PAN-2012 data achieved a 99% F1-score for identifying predatory lines of text by improving how the data is sampled before training (Borj et al. 2021).

Author verification is a binary classification task that asks, "If we have one or more documents written by author X, can we determine if a document by an unknown author was also written by author X?" Recent results from PAN show that from a dataset of 19 999 pairs of fanfiction documents (Kestemont et al. 2021), Boenninghoff et al. (2021) achieved the highest F1-score of 95.2% for correctly verifying whether the document pairs were written by the same author or not.

Author attribution is a task that asks "given a set of candidate authors, with a finite set of writing samples from the authors, and an unseen document X, can we determine which author wrote document X?" (Kestemont et al. 2021). This task is inherently more difficult than authorship verification due to it being a multiclass classification problem. In a cross-domain authorship attribution task set up by PAN in 2019 (Kestemont et al. 2019), the best obtained results was a macro F1-score (an averaged F1-score across all attribution problems of the dataset) of 69% (Muttenthaler et al. 2019).

Author profiling differs quite a lot from the previous tasks as, rather than creating a model which points to a particular person who wrote a document, author profiling uses models that attempt to determine what kind of person wrote a document. The task asks, "given document X, can we use machine learning to determine the age, gender, or other personal traits of the author?". A PAN profiling competition was also run in 2018, with the focus of determining if text was written by a male or female, where the best results focusing on textual features were above 80% for English (Rangel et al. 2018). A recent competition ran by PAN in 2020 attempted to identify fake news spreaders on Twitter (Rangel et al. 2020). For English tweets, the best results was an accuracy of 75% by Buda and Bolonyai (2020).

Sentiment analysis may be employed by way of a text classification, or by using a sentiment lexicon, which is essentially an index of words which associates words to a positive or negative association (for example, Wordnet). Past research includes the use of sentiment lexicons for identifying radicalism on dark web forums (Al-Rowaily et al. 2015), and for creating an "emotional fingerprint" over a series of short text messages (Andriotis et al. 2014).

A wealth of past work has focused on identifying extremism online using machine learning and deep learning text classifiers with surprisingly high F1-scores and accuracies (often 75%+) (Gaikwad et al. 2021), but a limitation that can be seen is the apparent lack of a benchmark dataset being used to compare results (Aldera et al. 2021).

7.7.3 Classification Limitations

Despite the advancements in text classification, modern techniques have their shortcomings. A long-standing problem for classification has been the difficulty in classifying short texts, in that the accuracies are often low (Song et al. 2014).

Likewise, an issue for modern NLP classification models is also that the text should not be too long. The majority of modern BERT-like transformer models have the limitation that their input is only 512 tokens (Gao et al. 2021), which is less than 512 actual written words. There is currently research being done on transformers for long-form text documents (Beltagy et al. 2020). And like all other machine learning models, classifiers are prone to bias due to dataset imbalances, in that classifiers will tend to prefer the dominant class (Tanha et al. 2020).

7.8 Text Reduction

By text reduction, we refer to NLP tasks that provide the reader of a text with a quick bird's eye view on either a single large text excerpt, or a corpus of documents. The methods in which a text can be "reduced" vary considerably in terms of their methodology and evaluation, and can even rely on previously mentioned extraction methods (Iqbal et al. 2019) or classification methods (Wagh et al. 2021). Here, we focus on methods that are uniquely used for the purpose of data reduction: text summarization and topic modelling, as referenced in Table 7.1.

We begin our discussion with topic modelling, as this is more often found in the digital investigative literature.

7.8.1 Thematic Extraction and Topic Modelling

Topic modelling includes a family of algorithms which apply unsupervised learning to large corpora to extract some user defined k number of topics of which a corpus of documents are composed, as well as the the document-topic compositions. The two most popular topic modelling techniques are latent semantic indexing (LSI) (Hofmann 1999) and latent Dirichlet allocation (LDA) (Blei et al. 2003), the latter being the most popular. The latent, or hidden, elements being learned in these methods are the document-topic, and topic-word compositions.

Topics are essentially the dictionary of a corpus of terms such that they are organized from most relevant to least relevant per topic. In Table 7.2, we give some examples of potential topics which could potentially have been extracted

Table 7.2 LDA topic modelling example.

Topic 1	Topic 2
dog	evidence
cat	law
fox	guilty
nest	innocent
hunt	burden
jump	proof

from a corpus that included our example Documents 1 and 2, where we let the number of topics be $k = 2$. Unlike classification, it is up to the user to interpret what the themes of topics are actually concerned with. When looking at the example topics, the first topic appears to be about animals or hunting, and the second topic seems to be about some legal aspects. A common issue for any topics derived from a topic model is that they are not always readily interpretable or coherent according to actual humans (Chang et al. 2009).

As mentioned before, topic models not only learn the potential topics of a series of documents, but they also learn how much of each particular document is composed of each topic. This feature allows LSI and LDA to be useful for the purpose of unsupervised document categorization (at least with respect to the other documents the models were trained with).

Topic models are often qualitatively judged by human users, but a common quantitative metric used to determine the appropriate number of topics is the perplexity. This metric scores how well a topic model represents data it has not seen before. The k with the lowest perplexity is ideally the appropriate number of topics to choose (Anupriya and Karpagavalli 2015). However, it is still advisable to manually inspect topics to ensure interpretable topics are being derived (Jacobi et al. 2016). There are other metrics as well, such as topic coherence, which scores individual topics based the conditional probability of a word given the other words in a topic (Boyd-Graber et al. 2017), or topic diversity, which measures "how diverse the top-k words of a topic are to each other" (Terragni et al. 2021).

7.8.2 Topic Modelling and Digital Investigations

One of the simplest use-cases of topic modelling is to generate topic models over a large corpus of documents to get a bird's eye view of the content. Porter (2018) applied this to all the extracted posts from the DarknetMarket subreddit over a year to see how topics changed from month to month, and also to identify topically relevant keywords that were previously unknown. For example, if a generated topic was about darknet market vendors, many of the highly relevant terms may be other vendors or administrators that may have not been in an investigator's keyword list.

Another use-case of topic models is identify to semantically similar documents, where the document-topic compositions essentially provide a clustering of semantically related documents. Waal et al. (2008) used this approach to understand the relatedness between more than 100 000 documents and files from a real case.

Topic modelling has also been used as a way to enhance search and information retrieval capabilities. For example, Beebe and Liu (2014) applied different clustering algorithms (including LDA) to forensic suite search results. In this way, documents returned to the user based on the search were organized in an unsupervised fashion into clusters. Their results found that by reviewing the documents starting from the centroid and navigating linearly from there yielded faster encounters of relevant documents than traditional searches. Noel and Peterson (2014) also applied LDA as a means for enhancing a keyword search, that relied upon repeated generation of topic models to create subsets of documents of interest, and again applied topic modeling on the subset of documents to narrow their search. An advantage they note was the ability to identify relevant documents that did not include the keyword they were searching for.

7.8.3 Limitations of Topic Modelling

There are typically two different drawbacks of topic modelling: hyperparameter (parameters not learned by training a model) estimation (Panichella 2021), and computational complexity. While frameworks exist in an attempt to optimize these parameter (Terragni et al. 2021), the effect of hyperparameter settings can significantly influence the quality of the produced topic models, and it has been shown that hyperparameter optimization significantly improves topic models over ad-hoc settings. Additionally, while topic modelling is already known for its long processing time, hyperparameter tuning has also been shown to be extremely computationally expensive (Panichella 2021).

In the context of digital forensics and investigations, Noel and Peterson (2014) also experienced long run times for topic model generation. While the study took place in 2014, they noted that the use of topic model based search was much slower than regular expression search, and that generating the models required for search took over 8 hours. They ultimately suggested that LDA should not replace traditional regular expression keyword search.

7.8.4 Text Summarization

Text summarization attempts to re-write a relatively large body of text into a concise handful of sentences, capturing the major points of the larger text. There are two kinds of text summarization methods, *extractive summarization* and *abstractive summarization*. Extractive summarization is tasked with identifying the k most important sentences from a body of text. Abstractive summarization is tasked with writing a larger body of text into its "own concise words." Thus, abstractive summarization may be the more difficult task since it not only has to consider which of the elements of the reference text are important, but it also has to write its summary into human understandable language.

The common metric to measure the performance of text summarization tasks is ROUGE (Recall-Oriented Understudy for Gisting Evaluation) (Lin 2004). This is essentially a set of statistics that calculates the similarity between between a human written summary and a machine written summary. Sub-types of ROUGE that are typically used are ROUGE-n and ROUGE-L. All definitions for these metrics are derived from Allahyari et al. (2017).

ROUGE-n counts the common number of n-grams (sequences of n words) between the automatically produced text summary and the reference summary. Let q be the number of n-grams in the reference summary and p be the number of common n-grams between between the generated and reference summary. ROUGE-n is the calculated value of $\frac{p}{q}$. ROUGE-1 and ROUGE-2 in particular are commonly measured.

ROUGE-L returns the value of the *longest common subsequence* (LCS) between the produced summary and the reference summary. In other words, the method looks for the longest sequence of words that are shared between the generated summary and the reference summary.

It is often noted that ROUGE may not be representative of the true quality of the summary because the method of evaluation may be too simple (Ganesan 2018).

7.8.5 Text Summarization and Digital Investigations

Text summarization has rarely been applied to digital forensics or investigation research, with the exception of the application of an ad-hoc method of extractive summarization (Pollitt 2013). In Pollitt's experiments, he extracted verb-noun pairs from each sentence, but he noted that some of the derived summaries were "meaningless".

The state-of-the-art results with respect to text summarization has advanced significantly in the last decade, and while many different techniques exist, deep learning methods have proven to provide the most substantial improvements (Mridha et al. 2021). MatchSum by (Zhong et al. 2020) achieved some of the highest ROUGE results for English extractive summaries with ROUGE-1: 44.41, ROUGE-2: 20.86, and ROUGE-L: 40.55. For abstractive summaries, Liu et al. (2022) achieved ROUGE-1: 47.78, ROUGE-2: 23.55, and ROUGE-L: 44.57.[10]

7.8.6 Summarization Limitations

Like other BERT-based models, summarization models are typically limited by their input restrictions, the standard being 512 tokens and 4096 tokens for longer documents. There is also a lack of diversity in the training dataset used to train summarization models, where the data is often composed of news articles and their headline summaries (Mridha et al. 2021).

Lastly, we reiterate that it is worth being skeptical of the summary evaluative metrics, as they do not necessarily correlate well with human evaluation of comparing reference summaries and automatically generated summaries.

7.9 Discussion and Conclusion

In the previous sections, we have shown the capabilities of different linguistic technologies that have the potential to be applied to digital investigation and investigative interviews. We now attempt to synthesize these findings to draw a conclusion on their readiness to be practically applied.

---

[10] http://nlpprogress.com/english/summarization.html.

The best automatic speech recognition (ASR) technology has better word error rates (WER) than human transcribers for transcribing benchmark English datasets of read audio, but other studies have shown a number of limitations regarding performance bias towards ideal conditions. For instance, studies have shown WER performance is worse on audio with spontaneous speech (Solberg and Ortiz 2022), non-standard accents (Koenecke et al. 2020), and children (Yeung and Alwan 2018).

But it is not only the accuracy of the ASR systems that is important, but also the speed of automatic transcriptions. Our preliminary studies have noted a significant increase in speed of audio transcriptions when having a human-in-the-loop to correct an ASR transcription. However, more studies need to be conducted to determine the extent of the effectiveness of ASR for investigative interviews.

The extent to which NLP methods can be applied on ASR transcribed text still needs to be studied, but in general, assuming the text is sufficiently clean, past studies have shown some success in applying NLP to investigative text.

Tools for entity extraction, such as NER, appear to be most commonly researched in the context of investigation. In particular, past studies have shown that NER models can be trained to a particular investigative domain. While the highest performing F1-score for a NER model obtained 94.6% for a benchmark dataset (Wang et al. 2021), more studies need to be conducted on investigative specific NER models. Furthermore, NER is often only a preprocessing step before applying further analytical methods to identify connections between different entities, which also appears to be a work in progress. However, past researchers have noted the benefits in expediting the investigative process by visualizing such connections (Batini et al. 2021; Iqbal et al. 2019). We also stress that older methods such as regular expression based string searches, or keyword extraction tools, still have their place for text extraction. In particular, for the extraction of code-words, keywords, or terms of negation.

NLP for text classification tasks that are concerned with binary classification of imbalanced data, such as grooming detection, extremism detection, and author verification have very high F1-scores. This indicates that such models have the potential to handle the majority of filtering-out of irrelevant information on such topics, or at least expediting the process of doing so. Text classification tasks that focus on making multi-class predictions on text such as author profiling or attribution appear to have less reliable accuracies and F1-scores. Furthermore, while such methods could expedite an investigation, they may also introduce bias. Classification may also assist the KREATIV interviewing methodology, expediting the evaluative step to identify questions from the interviewer with negative sentiment.

Tools for text reduction appear to be the least reliable, and in particular there are next to no studies of applying text summarization to investigation. The creation of topic models is not only a time-consuming process, but even the analysis of the generated topics is both time-consuming and prone to randomness. Lastly, both summarization and topic modelling have fairly heuristic evaluation metrics, which makes the understanding of how well a model is performing quantitatively difficult. Despite their drawbacks, topic modelling still appears to be useful for exploring large corpora, and summarization might be helpful for summarizing interview transcriptions.

Limitations for most modern NLP models are the maximum input size of models of either 512 or 4096 tokens, or the the the fact that many models are assessed with out-of-domain data, or relatively old datsets.

7.9.1 Future Work

In summary, many of the referenced ASR and NLP tools have potential to expedite aspects of an investigation given their state-of-the-art performance, despite their limitations. Although we have provided a mapping between some items that investigators want and the technologies that might support them, there still needs to be a stronger understanding of how well these technologies work within the realm of investigations, and furthermore, how they might be worked into the investigative cycle.

Thus, a potential research direction would be the creation of datasets for ASR and NLP tools that could satisfy a particular investigative context. Furthermore, studies need to be conducted to study the effectiveness of such tools in an investigative context.

Another item that needs to be researched is the effectiveness of OpenAI's large language model chat bot, ChatGPT, for investigations and investigative interviews. ChatGPT took the world by storm in late 2022, so while there have been relatively few studies explicitly exploring how it can be applied to a law enforcement context, the technology appears promising (Scanlon et al. 2023). ChatGPT is essentially a chat bot that can perform a plethora of different NLP tasks listed in this chapter, where the user can write a human understandable prompt to ChatGPT. ChatGPT version 3.5, at least anecdotally speaking, can summarize, answer classification questions, note contradictions in text, and note relevant entities from text excerpts in a variety of languages. Furthermore, improvements to ChatGPT are currently being made, where larger amounts of text input will be allowed, and the correctness statements by ChatGPT are being improved (Nolan B. 2023). The extent that these abilities are useful for investigations and investigative interviews, ignoring any current legal or ethical issues, still needs to be explored.

References

Agrawal, R., Imieliński, T., and Swami, A. (1993). Mining association rules between sets of items in large databases. In: *Proceedings of the 1993 ACM SIGMOD international conference on Management of data*, 207–216.

Aldera, S., Emam, A., Al-Qurishi, M. et al. (2021). Online extremism detection in textual content: a systematic literature review. *IEEE Access* 9: 42384–42396.

Ali, A. and Renals, S. (2018). Word error rate estimation for speech recognition: e-wer. In: *Proceedings of the 56th Annual Meeting of the Association for Computational Linguistics (Volume 2: Short Papers)*, 20–24.

Allahyari, M., Pouriyeh, S., Assefi, M. et al. (2017). Text summarization techniques: a brief survey. arXiv preprint arXiv:1707.02268.

Al-Rowaily, K., Abulaish, M., Haldar, N.A.-H., and Al-Rubaian, M. (2015). Bisal–a bilingual sentiment analysis lexicon to analyze dark web forums for cyber security. *Digital Investigation* 14: 53–62.

Alta, D.W., Venter, J., and Barnard, E. (2008). Applying topic modeling to forensic data. In: *IFIP International Conference on Digital Forensics*, 115–126. Springer.

Al-Zaidy, R., Fung, B.C.M., Youssef, A.M., and Fortin, F. (2012). Mining criminal networks from unstructured text documents. *Digital Investigation* 8 (3–4): 147–160.

Amodei, D., Ananthanarayanan, S., Anubhai, R. et al. (2016). Deep speech 2: end-to-end speech recognition in english and mandarin. In: *International conference on machine learning*, 173–182. PMLR.

Andriotis, P., Takasu, A., and Tryfonas, T. (2014). Smartphone message sentiment analysis. In: *IFIP International Conference on Digital Forensics*, 253–265. Springer.

Anupriya, P. and Karpagavalli, S. (2015). Lda based topic modeling of journal abstracts. In: *2015 International Conference on Advanced Computing and Communication Systems*, 1–5. IEEE.

Baevski, A., Zhou, Y., Mohamed, A., and Auli, M. (2020). wav2vec 2.0: a framework for self-supervised learning of speech representations. *Advances in Neural Information Processing Systems* 33: 12449–12460.

Batini, C., Bellandi, V., Ceravolo, P. et al. (2021). Semantic data integration for investigations: lessons learned and open challenges. In: *2021 IEEE International Conference on Smart Data Services (SMDS)*, 173–183. IEEE.

Beebe, N.L. and Liu, L. (2014). Clustering digital forensic string search output. *Digital Investigation* 11 (4): 314–322.

Beltagy, I., Peters, M.E., and Cohan, A. (2020). Longformer: the long-document transformer. *arXiv preprint arXiv:2004.05150*.

Bjerknes, O.T. and Fahsing, I.A. (2018). *Etterforskning: Prinsipper, metoder og praksis*. Fagbokforlaget.

Beyer, H, Holtzblatt K, (1998) "Contextual Design: Defining Customer-Centered Systems". Morgan Kaufman Publisher, ISBN 1558604111.

Blei, D.M., Ng, A.Y., and Jordan, M.I. (2003). Latent dirichlet allocation. *Journal of Machine Learning Research* 3 (Jan): 993–1022.

Boenninghoff, B., Nickel, R.M., and Kolossa, D. (2021). O2d2: out-of-distribution detector to capture undecidable trials in authorship verification. *arXiv preprint arXiv:2106.15825*.

Borj, P.R., Raja, K., and Bours, P. (2021). Detecting sexual predatory chats by perturbed data and balanced ensembles. In: *2021 International Conference of the Biometrics Special Interest Group (BIOSIG)*, 1–5. IEEE.

Bose, P., Srinivasan, S., Sleeman IV, W.C. et al. (2021). A survey on recent named entity recognition and relationship extraction techniques on clinical texts. *Applied Sciences* 110 (18): 0 8319.

Boyd-Graber, J., Yuening, H., Mimno, D. et al. (2017). Applications of topic models. *Foundations and Trends® in Information Retrieval* 110 (2–3): 0143–296.

Buda, J. and Bolonyai, F. (2020). An ensemble model using n-grams and statistical features to identify fake news spreaders on twitter. In: *CLEF (Working Notes)*.

Campos, R., Mangaravite, V., Pasquali, A. et al. (2020). Yake! keyword extraction from single documents using multiple local features. *Information Sciences* 509: 257–289.

Chang, J., Gerrish, S., Wang, C. et al. (2009). Reading tea leaves: how humans interpret topic models. *Advances in Neural Information Processing Systems* 22.

Chau, M., Xu, J.J., and Chen, H. (2002). Extracting meaningful entities from police narrative reports. In: *Proceedings of the 2002 annual national conference on Digital government research*, 1–5.

CPT (2002). 12th general report on the cpt's activities (european committee for the prevention of torture and inhuman or degrading treatment of punishment).

Cucerzan, S. (2007). Large-scale named entity disambiguation based on wikipedia data. In: *Proceedings of the 2007 joint conference on empirical methods in natural language processing and computational natural language learning (EMNLP-CoNLL)*, 708–716.

Devlin, J., Chang, M.-W., Lee, K., and Toutanova, K. (2018). Bert: pre-training of deep bidirectional transformers for language understanding. *arXiv preprint arXiv:1810.04805*.

Ebrahimi, M., Suen, C.Y., and Ormandjieva, O. (2016). Detecting predatory conversations in social media by deep convolutional neural networks. *Digital Investigation* 18: 33–49.

Fahsing, I.A. (1998). "konvensjon mot tortur og annen grusom, umenneskelig eller nedverdigende behandling eller straff" (convention against torture and other cruel, inhuman or degrading treatment or punishment).

Fahsing, I.A. The making of an expert detective: Thinking and deciding in criminal investigations. 2016.

Fellbaum, C. (2010). Wordnet. In: *Theory and Applications of Ontology: Computer Applications*, 231–243. Springer.

Feng, S., Kudina, O., Halpern, B.M., and Scharenborg, O. (2021). Quantifying bias in automatic speech recognition. *arXiv preprint arXiv:2103.15122*.

Gabbert, F., Hope, L., Luther, K. et al. (2021). Exploring the use of rapport in professional information-gathering contexts by systematically mapping the evidence base. *Applied Cognitive Psychology* 35 (2): 329–341.

Gaikwad, M., Ahirrao, S., Phansalkar, S., and Kotecha, K. (2021). Online extremism detection: a systematic literature review with emphasis on datasets, classification techniques, validation methods, and tools. *IEEE Access* 9: 48364–48404.

Gao, S., Alawad, M., Todd Young, M. et al. (2021). Limitations of transformers on clinical text classification. *IEEE Journal of Biomedical and Health Informatics* 25 (9): 3596–3607.

Grandini, M., Bagli, E., and Visani, G. (2020). Metrics for multi-class classification: an overview. *arXiv preprint arXiv:2008.05756*.

Hess, J. (2015). *Interviewing and Interrogation for Law Enforcement*. Routledge.

Hofmann, T. (1999). Probabilistic latent semantic indexing. In: *Proceedings of the 22nd annual international ACM SIGIR conference on Research and development in information retrieval*, 50–57.

Hsu, W.-N., Bolte, B., Hubert Tsai, Y.-H. et al. (2021). Hubert: self-supervised speech representation learning by masked prediction of hidden units. *IEEE/ACM Transactions on Audio, Speech, and Language Processing* 29: 3451–3460.

Inches, G. and Crestani, F. (2012). Overview of the international sexual predator identification competition at pan-2012. In: *CLEF (Online working notes/labs/workshop)*, 30.

Iqbal, F., Fung, B.C.M., Debbabi, M. et al. (2019). Wordnet-based criminal networks mining for cybercrime investigation. *IEEE Access* 7: 22740–22755.

Jacobi, C., Wouter, V.A., and Welbers, K. (2016). Quantitative analysis of large amounts of journalistic texts using topic modelling. *Digital Journalism* 4 (1): 89–106.

Johnsen, J.W. and Franke, K. (2020). Identifying proficient cybercriminals through text and network analysis. In: *2020 IEEE International Conference on Intelligence and Security Informatics (ISI)*, 1–7. IEEE.

Brookman, F. Jones, H. Williams R., and Fraser J. (2020). The use of cctv during homicide investigations: challenges and risks.

Jurafsky, D. and Martin, J.H. (2022). Speech and language processing. 3rd.

Kavita, G. (2018). Rouge 2.0: updated and improved measures for evaluation of summarization tasks. *arXiv preprint arXiv:1803.01937*.

Kestemont, M., Manjavacas, E., Markov, I. et al. (2021). Overview of the cross-domain authorship verification task at pan 2021. In: *CLEF (Working Notes)*.

Kestemont, M., Stamatatos, E., Manjavacas, E. et al. (2019). Overview of the cross-domain authorship attribution task at {PAN} 2019. In: *Working Notes of CLEF 2019-Conference and Labs of the Evaluation Forum, Lugano, Switzerland, September 9- 12,2019*, 1–15.

Koenecke, A., Nam, A., Lake, E. et al. (2020). Racial disparities in automated speech recognition. *Proceedings of the National Academy of Sciences* 117 (14): 7684–7689.

Kowsari, K., Meimandi, K.J., Heidarysafa, M. et al. (2019). Text classification algorithms: a survey. *Information* 100 (4): 0 150.

Lin, C.-Y. (2004). Rouge: a package for automatic evaluation of summaries. In: *Text Summarization Branches Out*, 74–81.

Lin, H., Yaojie, L., Tang, J. et al. (2020). A rigorous study on named entity recognition: can fine-tuning pretrained model lead to the promised land? *arXiv preprint arXiv:2004.12126*.

Liu, Y., Liu, P., Radev, D., and Neubig, G. (2022). Brio: bringing order to abstractive summarization. *arXiv preprint arXiv:2203.16804*.

Marry, P. (2019). *The Making of A Detective – A Garda's Story of Investigation Some of Ireland's Most Notorious Crimes*. Penguin Books.

McTear, M.F., Callejas, Z., and Griol, D. (2016). *The Conversational Interface*, vol. 6. Springer.

Mendez, J.E. and Areh, I. (2021). *Principles on Effective Interviewing for Investigations and Information Gathering*. APT, Association pour la prévention de la torture.

Mikolov, T., Chen, K., Corrado, G., and Dean, J. (2013). Efficient estimation of word representations in vector space. *arXiv preprint arXiv:1301.3781*.

Mridha, M.F., Lima, A.A., Nur, K. et al. (2021). A survey of automatic text summarization: progress, process and challenges. *IEEE Access* 9: 156043–156070.

Muttenthaler, L., Lucas, G., and Amann, A. (2019). Authorship attribution in fan-fictional texts given variable length character and word n-grams. In: *CLEF 2019 Labs and Workshops, Notebook Papers*. CEUR-WS.org.

Negrão, M. and Domingues, P. (2021). Speechtotext: an open-source software for automatic detection and transcription of voice recordings in digital forensics. *Forensic Science International: Digital Investigation* 38: 301223.

Ngejane, C.H., Eloff, J.H.P., Sefara, T.J., and Marivate, V.N. (2021). Digital forensics supported by machine learning for the detection of online sexual predatory chats. *Forensic Science International: Digital Investigation* 36 (301109).

Noel, G.E. and Peterson, G.L. (2014). Applicability of latent dirichlet allocation to multi-disk search. *Digital Investigation* 11 (1): 43–56.

Nolan, B. (2023). 5 ways GPT-4 is better than older versions of OpenAI's ChatGPT. *Business Insider*. Available at: https://www.businessinsider.com/gpt4-openai-chatgpt-everything-you-need-to-know-4-2023-3 (Accessed: 2 June, 2023).

Norwegian Police (2020). Politiets e-læring for avhør/ police investigative interviews e-learning.

Panichella, A. (2021). A systematic comparison of search-based approaches for lda hyperparameter tuning. *Information and Software Technology* 130:0: 106411.

Pennington, J., Socher, R., and Manning, C.D. (2014). Glove: global vectors for word representation. In *Proceedings of the 2014 conference on empirical methods in natural language processing (EMNLP)*, 1532–1543.

Pollitt, M. (2013). The hermeneutics of the hard drive: using narratology, natural language processing, and knowledge management to improve the effectiveness of the digital forensic process.

Porter, K. (2018). Analyzing the darknetmarkets subreddit for evolutions of tools and trends using lda topic modeling. *Digital Investigation* 26: S87–S97.

Rachlew, A., Løken, G.-E., and Bergestuen, S.T. (2020). *Den profesjonelle samtalen: En forskningsbasert intervjumetodikk for alle som stiller spørsmål*. Universitetsforlaget.

Radford, A., Kim, J.W., Tao, X. et al. (2022). Robust speech recognition via large-scale weak supervision. Technical report, Tech. Rep., OpenAI.

Rangel, F., Giachanou, A., Ghanem, B.H.H., and Rosso, P. (2020). Overview of the 8th author profiling task at pan 2020: profiling fake news spreaders on twitter. In: *CEUR Workshop Proceedings*, 2696, 1–18. Sun SITE Central Europe.

Rangel, F., Rosso, P., Gómez, M.M.-Y. et al., (2018). Overview of the 6th author profiling task at pan 2018: multimodal gender identification in twitter. *Working Notes Papers of the CLEF*, 1–38.

Riksadvokaten, A.G. (2016). Politiavhør", rundskriv nr.2/2016.

Rodrigues, F.B., Giozza, W.F., de Oliveira Albuquerque, R., and Villalba, L.J.G. (2022). Natural language processing applied to forensics information extraction with transformers and graph visualization. *IEEE Transactions on Computational Social Systems*. Digital Object Identifier 10.1109/TCSS.2022.3159677

Rose, A. (2021). Forensics: the golden hour. In: *Modern Police Leadership*, 223–233. Springer https://doi.org/10.1007/978-3-030-63930-3_18.

Rose, S., Engel, D., Cramer, N., and Cowley, W. (2010). Automatic keyword extraction from individual documents. *Text Mining: Applications and Theory* 1 (1–20): 10–1002.

Scanlon, M., Nikkel, B., and Geradts, Z. (2023). Digital forensic investigation in the age of ChatGPT. *Forensic Science International: Digital Investigation* 44: 301543.

Solberg, P.E. and Ortiz, P. (2022). The norwegian parliamentary speech corpus. *arXiv preprint arXiv:2201.10881*.

Song, G., Yunming, Y., Xiaolin, D. et al. (2014). Short text classification: a survey. *Journal of Multimedia* 9 (5).

Strötgen, J. and Gertz, M. (2010). Heideltime: high quality rule-based extraction and normalization of temporal expressions. In: *Proceedings of the 5th international workshop on semantic evaluation*, 321–324.

Tanha, J., Abdi, Y., Samadi, N. et al. (2020). Boosting methods for multi-class imbalanced data classification: an experimental review. *Journal of Big Data* 7 (1): 1–47.

Teige, T. and Ragde, E.B. (2021). *På åstedet, jakten på bevisene spørsmål*. Aschehoug.

Terragni, S., Fersini, E., Galuzzi, B.G. et al. (2021). Octis: comparing and optimizing topic models is simple! In: *Proceedings of the 16th Conference of the European Chapter of the Association for Computational Linguistics: System Demonstrations*, 263–270.

Vaswani, A., Shazeer, N., Parmar, N. et al. (2017). Attention is all you need. *Advances in Neural Information Processing Systems* 30.

Wagh, V., Khandve, S., Joshi, I. et al. (2021). Comparative study of long document classification. In: *TENCON 2021-2021 IEEE Region 10 Conference (TENCON)*, 732–737. IEEE.

Wang, X., Jiang, Y., Bach, N. et al. (2021 Aug). Automated concatenation of embeddings for structured prediction. In: *the Joint Conference of the 59th Annual Meeting of the Association for Computational Linguistics and the 11th International Joint Conference on Natural Language Processing (ACL-IJCNLP 2021)*. Association for Computational Linguistics.

Wencan, W., Chow, K.-P., Mai, Y., and Zhang, J. (2020). Public opinion monitoring for proactive crime detection using named entity recognition. In: *IFIP International Conference on Digital Forensics*, 203–214. Springer.

Yang, M. and Chow, K.-P. (2015). An information extraction framework for digital forensic investigations. In *IFIP international conference on digital forensics*, 61–76. Springer.

Yeung, G. and Alwan, A. (2018). On the difficulties of automatic speech recognition for kindergarten-aged children. *Interspeech 2018*10.21347/Interspeech.2018-2297.

Zhang, L., Wang, S., and Liu, B. (2018). Deep learning for sentiment analysis: a survey. *Wiley Interdisciplinary Reviews: Data Mining and Knowledge Discovery* 8 (4): e1253.

Zhong, M., Liu, P., Chen, Y. et al. (2020). Extractive summarization as text matching. *arXiv preprint arXiv:2004.08795*.

CHAPTER 8

The Influence of Compression on the Detection of Deepfake Videos

Meike Kombrink* and Zeno Geradts

Netherlands Forensic Institute, Ministry of Justice and Security, Hague, Netherlands
* Corresponding author

8.1 Introduction

Many videos are shared on online platforms every day. Yet, it is becoming increasingly difficult to determine the authenticity of these videos due to the increased popularity and availability of deepfake creation software (Dolhansky et al. 2020). Deepfake videos are videos that have been manipulated using deep learning. Although many different types of deepfakes exist, the current most popular type of deepfake is a face swap between a target person and an individual in a video (Rossler et al. 2019). The quality of deepfake videos has improved significantly, to the point where deepfake videos and genuine videos are becoming harder to distinguish with the human eye. While the analysis of single, high-impact videos for evidence of manipulation is possible (Dolhansky et al. 2020), this can only be performed properly by experts (making this method of detection limited in its applicability), for whom the process is time consuming. The limited number of experts available to distinguish between deepfakes and genuine videos, means that we cannot analyse all videos that are uploaded daily given the current speed of detection. In order to review each of the hundreds of thousands of videos uploaded to the Internet or social media platforms every day, automation of the process is needed.

Although the techniques used to create deepfakes can be used in a non-harmful way, the advances in deepfake creation has also lead to the possibility of misuse. When we look at society, Rossler et al. (2019) stated: "At best, this [increase in quality of deepfake material] leads to a loss of trust in digital content but could potentially cause further harm by spreading false information or fake news.". These detrimental effects can be minimized by automated deepfake detection, allowing individuals to determine the authenticity of a video themselves.

Artificial Intelligence (AI) in Forensic Sciences, First Edition. Edited by Zeno Geradts and Katrin Franke.
© 2024 John Wiley & Sons Ltd. Published 2024 by John Wiley & Sons Ltd.

Apart from the harmful effects on society, deepfakes can also be abused by criminals. As a deepfake allows a person to change appearance – and thus identity – criminals are able to exploit the deepfake software to exchange identity with an innocent citizen. If this goes undetected it could lead to innocent citizens being found guilty while the actual offender walks free. Therefore, it is vital to be able to distinguish between deepfake videos and genuine videos to limit the harm they could inflict on society and the criminal justice system. The distinction between genuine and deepfake videos should be made in realistic settings (e.g., currently only high-quality videos are used, whereas a wide range of different qualities can be expected in real cases), where the amount of abstraction put upon deepfakes is limited as much as possible. Any abstraction used to train and test algorithms can cause an overstatement of the performance of the model, limiting the usefulness of said model to society.

In recent years the automated distinction between deepfake and genuine videos has seen a surge of interest from scientists, leading to considerable progress within the field Lyu (2020). Both the construction of detection algorithms (Afchar et al. 2018, Chollet 2017, Rahmouni et al. 2017, Cozzolino et al. 2017) and the construction of more realistic deepfake databases (Dolhansky et al. 2020, Rossler et al. 2019, Bojia et al. 2020, Jiang et al. 2020, Yuezun et al. 2020) have seen great improvement. Previously, one of the biggest bottlenecks was the level of abstraction (e.g., compression, occlusion, etc.) present in the deepfake datasets, where the number of realistic deepfakes in datasets was very small. Recently, more datasets have been developed that contain such realistic deepfakes, though some still apply a level of abstraction. For example: the DFDC (Dolhansky et al. 2020) dataset does not apply any augmentation to the dataset and thus it consists of only high quality deepfakes. Any accuracy reported on this dataset is, therefore, likely to be an overstatement of the accuracy in realistic settings.

Recently created databases for deepfake detection have become more and more realistic (Rossler et al. 2019, Bojia et al. 2020, Jiang et al. 2020). These databases contain different types of augmentations, amongst which: compression (Rossler et al. 2019), Bojia et al. 2020, Jiang et al. 2020), changes in colour (Jiang et al. 2020), blurring (Jiang et al. 2020), resolution (Bojia et al. 2020), and more. These databases come closer to real life scenarios through the bigger diversity in the permutations and augmentations they contain. Yet, one of the problems that two of the datasets have (Bojia et al. 2020, Jiang et al. 2020) is that they do not provide annotations with these permutations. Because of this, no analysis can be performed to assess how close the dataset is to real life scenarios (e.g., if only 1% of the dataset is compressed, it is less realistic than if 99% of the dataset is compressed). Another drawback is the lack of annotations currently present in datasets. As a result, this keeps researchers from properly analysing their results on the database. This makes improving the algorithms more challenging as it can be informative to the creator to know that, for example, on heavily compressed images the network performs poorly whereas largely occluded images pose no problem.

The absence of annotated scenarios that are representative of real world scenarios is what this research aims to – partly – solve. This research will focus on one of the real world scenarios that any deepfake video shared online will be subject to: compression. Compression is one of the major steps within a process called social media laundering (Lyu 2020) which is performed on any image uploaded to social media. Compression is the part of the social media laundering process which intuitively can be described as the reduction in size of a target file (Bhaskaran and Konstantinides 1997). Understanding the influence of compression on deepfake video detection is vital to allow deepfake video detection in real-life scenarios. A difference should be made between lossy and lossless compression. While lossy compression allows for the irreversible loss of information upon compression, lossless compression does not lose any information within a file during or after compression. Lossy compression is mostly used to compress multimedia data such as audio, video, and images, whereas lossless compression is most commonly required for text and data files, as losing part of the information in, for example, a bank record is not desired. This study will use deepfake videos and thus make use of lossy compression, as this is the most commonly used form of compression for this datatype. It can be expected that lossy compression has an influence on the detection of deepfake videos, as it has been shown to (1) cause a huge loss of information (Afchar et al. 2018) and (2) launder manipulation traces from a video (Rossler et al. 2019).

Previous research has shown that compression has an influence on the detection ability of deepfake video detection algorithms (Rossler et al. 2019). Rossler et al.'s research constructed a dataset of deepfake videos that had been compressed to three different levels – non, moderate and high – resulting in different quality subsets of the data. They showed that compression had a negative influence on the detection of deepfake videos, though not all algorithms showed the same decrease in accuracy. Some of the tested algorithms achieved reasonable scores even on the lowest quality set (Afchar et al. 2018, Chollet 2017) for which the accuracy on all three quality sets stayed above or around 90% (Rossler et al. 2019). The accuraciy of other algorithms were decreased severely with the addition of compression (Rahmouni et al. 2017, Cozzolino et al. 2017) where the highest quality set reached 95–100% accuracy, while the low quality set only reached between 65% and 75% (Rossler et al. 2019). Rossler et al. (2019) showed that compression has an influence on the detection of deepfakes, yet that the exact influence of compression differs per algorithm.

However, several shortcomings were found within this research (Rossler et al. 2019). Most importantly, the research used an older standard for compression (H.264) that has since been succeeded by a new standard (H.265/HEVC) Koumaras et al. (2012). The difference between these standards is quite substantial, where almost all aspects of compression have been improved in H.265/HEVC. It was shown that H.265 is more cost effective, has optimized videos quality as well as compression efficiency, spatial resolution, temporal resolution and computational complexity when compared to H.264 Koumaras et al. (2012). Yet, H.265 is at least as applicable as H.264, for the aim of developing H.265 was explicitly to continue the applicability of the compression standard to almost all use cases that H.264 was applicable to (Grois et al. 2016). It can therefore be expected that the effect that compression has on the detection of deepfake videos using the H.264 standard will not be the same as the effect compression has on the detection of deepfake videos using the H.265 standard. The newer standard (H.265) is currently used by most social media platforms, while the older standard (H.264) is still used in most hardware products (e.g., cameras). It is, therefore, of vital importance to understand the effects of this newer standard on the detection of deepfake videos alongside the effect of the older standard.

However, H.265 is no longer the newest standard available. At the time of this research, a newer standard, AV1, is being developed by AOMedia AOMedia (2021) and is being adopted by more and more online companies. AV1 promises to yield higher compression rates without loss of quality compared to H.265. It is also specifically designed to be open source and royalty free, which has caused over 30 major companies to become official members of the development of this standard (amongst which are: Netflix, Microsoft, and Google (Grois et al. 2016)). The standard has not been fully launched yet, but beta versions are available. The biggest change AV1 brings is that its encoder has a two-pass coding option, improving the rate-distortion performance (Grois et al. 2016). However, the greatest drawback is the time it takes to encode a video, e.g., a one hour movie takes no less than 40 hours to compress when using AV1. In comparison, when using H.265 a 1 hour movie would take only 80 minutes to compress (Sims 2021). Due to the vast support for this standard it is important to understand the influence of AV1 on the detection of deepfakes. However, due to the scope of this research and due to the time constraints of AV1, no full comparison can be made. Nevertheless, a preliminary investigation into its effects will be performed which can provide an indication of the effects of AV1 on the detection of deepfake videos.

Rossler et al. (2019) have shown that compression using H.264 has a negative influence on the detection of deepfakes, whereas Verdoliva (2020) has shown that compression can also be used as an artefact. This research stated that JPEG-compressed deepfake images can be distinguished from genuine images using compression as a method (Verdoliva 2020). This approach has shown that JPEG-compressed images that undergo manipulation and are then compressed again, show compression artefacts all over the image, except for where the manipulation occurred. Verdoliva (2020) stated that the exploitation of compression artefacts within video material is also possible, though more complicated compared to its use with images. This added difficulty is posed by the higher complexity of video encoding algorithms when compared to image encoding algorithms. Consequently, even though compression seems to make detection of deepfake videos by neural network-based methods more difficult (due to the laundering of manipulation traces), it can also be exploited as an artefact to detect deepfake videos. Thus, while compression can make deepfake detection more difficult, it also shows possibilities for being exploited for the purpose of detecting deepfakes. Although this research will not focus on the detection of deepfakes through compression, it is important to acknowledge the twofold role of compression in deepfake detection.

8.2 Method

8.2.1 Dataset

To understand the influence of compression on the detection of deepfake videos, it was necessary to create a large dataset which holds different levels of compression. In order to fully analyse the effect of compression on its own, no other augmentation had to be present in the dataset. The selected database has recently (2020) been published and is, to the best of the author's knowledge, the largest dataset available to date (Dolhansky et al. 2020). Due to the size of the deepfake detection challenge (DFDC) dataset (Dolhansky et al. 2020), it was only necessary to use the publicly available training set since it contained sufficient data to constitute all the subsets (training, validation, and test), without causing a too limited number of videos in the dataset. The DFDC dataset holds a total of 119 154 videos in its training set, in which each video is exactly 10 seconds (Dolhansky et al. 2020). A total of 486 unique actors appear in the training set. In total, 83.9% of the DFDC training set is labelled as deepfake video by the creators.

Given the scope of this research, a dataset of around 15 000 training videos was needed. The DFDC dataset (Dolhansky et al. 2020) is much larger than this, which is why many of the training videos in the original dataset were not used. In order to create a more applicable dataset for the problem at hand, the dataset was preprocessed. First, the percentage of deepfake videos in the dataset was reduced to 60%, causing a reduction in size of the dataset. The alteration of the percentage of deepfakes was made to ensure limited bias within the network to predict deepfake over genuine. However, this was still not within the scope of this research. Therefore, the dataset was further reduced in size, resulting in 15 000 training videos and 3 000 validation videos, where 50% of the training and validation set is composed of deepfakes. The resulting test set would also have to conform to the 50/50 deepfake/genuine ratio to not create a distortion between validation set accuracy and test set accuracy.

8.2.1.1 H.265

In order to analyse the performance of deepfake detection algorithms on videos with compression, the resulting dataset had to be compressed to different extents. Five different sets were constructed, of which four would be subject to compression. Previous research used three different sets, of which two were subject to compression. Based on only two sets with compression, it is difficult to properly analyse the effects of compression as it does not show a trend, but merely an increase in accuracy or a decrease in accuracy. Therefore, it was chosen to increase the amount of sets to five for this research. The four sets that will be subject to compression will each be compressed to a different extent in order to be able to accurately analyse the effect of different levels of compression.

Compression was performed using a publicly available GUI for ffmpeg batch compression[1] on Windows. This allowed for a single upload of each subset which would consequently all be compressed to the same extent. The H.265 compression standard was used to compress all subsets. H.265 allows users to set the constant rate factor (CRF) to any number between 0 and 51, where the amount of compression increases along with the CRF value (making 51 the highest compression possible with H.265). It was later found that any number below 20 would enlarge the file, rather than reduce it. It was also discovered that the reduction in size is not linearly correlated with the increase in CRF. After testing compression on an original video of 6.52 MB, it was decided that the four subsets that had to undergo compression would be subject to CRFs of 20, 25, 32, and 51 respectively. These four values led to the following sized videos after compression: a 4.67MB video, a 1.89MB video, a 540KB video, and a 165KB video respectively. An overview of the CRF set for the different subsets can also be seen in Table 8.1

8.2.1.2 AV1

The newest compression method – AV1 – was also used to evaluate the performance of deepfake detection algorithms on compressed videos. The same principle was used for this standard. Again, five subsets were created each with a different level of compression. However, the number of videos in this set was vastly different. In total 100 videos were in the AV1 test set, with a 50/50 deepfake/genuine ratio. Five subparts of 20 videos were created and each was compressed to a different extent. The CRF of the

Table 8.1 CRF (constant rate factor) set for each subset of the dataset. For H.265 the maximum possible CRF was 51, while for AV1 the maximum possible CRF was 63.

Setset	H.265	AV1
0	No	No
1	20	20
2	25	25
3	32	40
4	51	63

---

[1] https://sourceforge.net/projects/ffmpeg-batch.

sets that underwent compression within this set were: 20, 25, 40, and 63, as shown in Table 8.1. The minimum CRF found was 20 to not increase the size of a video, while 63 was the maximum CRF that could be set for this standard.

When trying to read the AV1 compressed videos within Python, it was found that they were regarded as empty videos (no frames) by the program. To solve this problem, a workaround was found. This workaround included an extra lossless compression to be put over the AV1 videos, allowing for non-empty input within the program. This lossless compression, using the H.264 standard, was applied to all videos within the set, including originally non-compressed videos. To verify whether this method would be applicable, the change in pixelvalues before and after lossless H.264 was determined. It was shown that the pixelvalues of both the AV1 file and the H.264 file were identical. Therefore, it can be assumed that no influence of the added H.264 compression will be seen in the results.

Due to the much smaller size of this dataset, the difficulty level of individual videos is a lot more influential on the results reported than it is in the larger (H.265) set. To ensure that the results found truly reflect the influence of AV1, the 100 videos used for the AV1 set were also compressed using H.265. This created two identical sets, one which was compressed using different extents of AV1 and one that was compressed using different extents of H.265. To ensure the largest similarity between these two sets, both of the smaller sets were losslessly compressed using H.264, although this step was not necessary for H.265 as those videos could be read by Python without alterations. The construction of both these sets allows comparison between H.265 and AV1 regardless of the 100 videos and their specific properties.

8.2.2 Deepfake Detection

To test the influence of compression on the ability of algorithms to detect deepfake videos, different deepfake detection algorithms needed to be (re)implemented and trained on the newly created dataset. A total of two algorithms were implemented and trained. These two algorithms both showed very promising results with previous research into the influence of compression using the H.264 standard (Rossler et al. 2019). The first algorithm that was trained and tested on the new dataset was MesoNet (Afchar et al. 2018), which aims to distinguish between deepfakes and genuine videos by looking at mesolevel artefacts (between micro and macro). The second algorithm was XceptionNet (Chollet 2017), which aims to classify images by using inception modules in the architecture.

Although both of the trained and tested networks used in this study have different architectures, the process of training the networks was, for the most part, identical. This process is graphically shown in Figure 8.1 The process shown has been performed on the larger dataset with H.265 compression, no training has been performed on AV1 compressed data.

First, all the training data was collected, including both the videos and their corresponding labels. This collection can easily be changed from the smaller set to the bigger set, and vice versa. These videos – and their corresponding labels – were

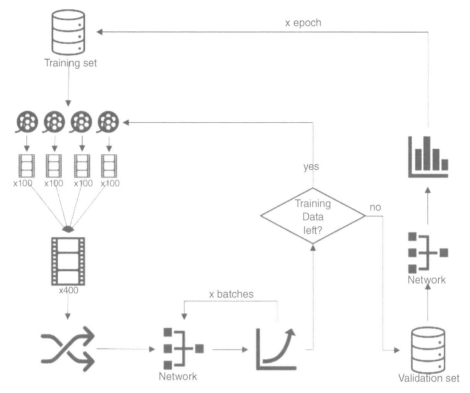

Figure 8.1 Flowchart showing the training process for both networks. The architecture of the networks differs, but the training process is (almost) identical for both.

then shuffled to ensure the networks are trained on videos in random order and cannot use the order of the presented data as a learning feature. Then, the next four videos within the training set were selected, and of these four videos the first 100 frames were extracted. The reason why frames were used over entire videos was because neither of the algorithms considered for this research uses the temporal aspect of a deepfake to classify the video. These frames were then all added together and again shuffled to ensure that each batch of these 400 frames has different frames and different labels within it, limiting the influence of the order of data-points. These 400 frames were then divided into four batches for Mesonet and 16 batches for XceptionNet, and the networks were trained sequentially on these smaller batches. The batch sizes were chosen such that they would fit the memory capacity for this research. This entire process was repeated until all training videos were iterated through. Any code used within this study will be available on GitHub[2]

After all videos dedicated to the training set were optimized, the validation set was loaded. All frames from the videos in this set were extracted for validation

---

[2] https://github.com.

purposes, after which the output of all frames was considered. An accuracy is computed based on these outputs and reported as the validation accuracy. The training and validation process was then repeated a total of 54 times for MesoNet and a total of 46 times for XceptionNet. The training process should have been repeated until the networks showed no further improvement, indicating they reached their optimal settings. However, one of the networks, XceptionNet, could not be trained this far within the scope of this research. Therefore, the training of both networks either continued until the validation accuracy stabilised, or until no continuation of training was possible.

8.2.2.1 MesoNet

MesoNet is an artificial neural network that was published in 2018 (Afchar et al. 2018) for the explicit purpose of deepfake detection. The aim of Afchar et al. (2018) was to achieve high detection scores through analysis at mesoscopic level, rather than at the microscopic level more commonly found in other neural networks. They motivated this choice by stating that microscopic analysis cannot be applied on compressed videos, as the noise within the images will be strongly degraded due to compression, while analysis at microscopic level is based on this noise within images. To achieve the mesoscopic level of analysis, MesoNet was constructed as a deep neural network, consisting only of a small number of layers.

The network consists of a sequence of four layers that successively convolve and pool. After these four layers the architecture finishes with utilizing a dense network with one hidden layer. The network uses ReLu activation within the convolution layers to improve generalization. Finally the network uses a sigmoid function to ensure output between 0 and 1.

In the original implementation of MesoNet (Afchar et al. 2018), the authors did not use the constructed architecture on entire videos, nor on entire frames. They first extracted all faces in videos through the Viola Jones (Viola and Jones 2001) face detection algorithm and performed deepfake detection on these faces only. Viola Jones is the currently most used commercial face detection algorithm, yet it has been shown to work poorly on images/videos where an individual's head is not in an upright and frontal position (Chen et al. 2020). The original set-up of MesoNet, including the Viola Jones face detection, was tested on the dataset used for this research. Within the first 10 videos the Viola Jones face recognition algorithm did not find any faces in a video, whereas two faces were present. In this original implementation from Afchar et al. (2018) this led to an error and killed the deepfake detection process altogether. Because of the demonstrated inability of Viola Jones to handle faces that are anything other than frontal and upright, and knowing the wide variety of poses of the actors in the dataset, it was decided to use the architecture constructed by Afchar et al. (2018) on entire frames, leaving out face detection as a step.

8.2.2.2 XceptionNet

XceptionNet (Chollet 2017) was first published in 2017, with the goal of delivering a well performing image analysis network. This network has not been made specifically for the purpose of deepfake video detection, yet it has been shown to perform very well at this task (Rossler et al. 2019).

XceptionNet (Chollet 2017) uses inception modules within its architecture, which were first introduced in 2014 (Szegedy et al. 2015), and have since proven to perform better than many other algorithms in image analysis tasks (Chollet 2017). The idea of inception modules is to solve a problem that all convolutional neural networks face: that convolutional layers in a network are tasked with learning to filter in a 3D space, with only two dimensions (width and height) and a channel dimension to account for the third. Therefore, a single convolutional filter has to learn both spatial correlations and cross-channel correlations at the same time. The hypothesis behind inception modules is that the cross-channel correlations and the spatial correlations are sufficiently decoupled so that it is preferable to not map them jointly. Through this, they make the process of learning two different correlations at the same time easier and more efficient. Inception modules work by explicitly factoring both types of correlations into a series of operations that would independently look at cross-channel correlations and spatial correlations. Specifically, most inception modules first factor in cross-channel correlations by applying a set of 1 × 1 convolutions, mapping these convolutions into several separate spaces. After which regular convolutions are applied to learn spatial correlations.

The creators of XceptionNet go one step further: their hypothesis is that the two types of correlations within the features maps of CNN's are *entirely* decoupled, rather than sufficiently (Chollet 2017). Therefore, their architecture is based entirely on depthwise separable convolution layers, where they structured a total of 36 convolutional layers into 14 modules.

8.3 Results

8.3.1 Compressed Dataset

Compression was applied to the DFDC dataset (Dolhansky et al. 2020), which resulted in the subsets that can be seen in Table 8.2.

These sets were then combined together and divided into training, validation, and test sets again. The training set contains 30 179 videos and has a size of 59.1 GB. The validation set contains 3 353 videos and has a size of 6.6 GB. The test set contains 14 364 videos and has a size of 28.2 GB. All sets are approximately 60% deepfake videos and 40% genuine videos. An equal share of each subset's videos was used for the construction of the different sets.

A smaller training and validation set was later constructed to limit the time necessary for one training epoch. These smaller sets contained 15 000 and 1 500

Table 8.2 Properties of the different subsets created for this research. Each individual subset has approximately 60% deepfake videos and 40% original videos.

Subset	Number of videos	Original size	CRF	Final size	Compression ratio
0	9617	42.2 GB	N/A	42.2 GB	100%
1	9600	42.2 GB	20	31.4 GB	74.41%
2	9580	42.2 GB	25	14.0 GB	33.18%
3	9559	41.8 GB	32	4.9 GB	11.72%
4	9538	41.7 GB	51	1.5 GB	3.6%

Table 8.3 Properties of the different subsets created for this research using the AV1 standard. The final size reported was determined after the lossless H.264 compression was applied as well as AV1.

Subset	Number of videos	Original size	CRF	Final size	Compression ratio
0	20	100 MB	N/A	100 MB	100%
1	20	103 MB	20	63.2 MB	61.4%
2	20	94.9 MB	25	41.9 MB	44.2%
3	20	103 MB	40	15.1 MB	14.7%
4	20	75.6 MB	63	4.11 MB	5.4%

videos respectively, where the deepfake/genuine ratio was set to 50/50. The test set was also further reduced in size, which resulted in 11 000 videos with a deepfake/genuine ratio of 50/50.

The resulting dataset with AV1 is considerably smaller than the one constructed using H.265. The division of this dataset's compression ratios can be seen in Table 8.3.

8.3.2 Algorithms

8.3.2.1 Previous Results
When Afchar et al. (2018) reported their results of MesoNet (Afchar et al. 2018), the network was trained and tested on the precursor of FaceForensics++ (Rossler et al. 2019), FaceForensics (Rössler et al. 2018). The method performed well on this dataset at detecting face swaps, even though the accuracy of the network does decrease when a higher level of compression is applied, where the initial accuracy, without compression, was 0.946 (Afchar et al. 2018). With light compression the accuracy decreased to 0.924 and with high

compression it further decreased to 0.832 (Afchar et al. 2018). These results suggest that MesoNet is capable of handling compression to some extent. The method showed a slightly lower accuracy of 0.891 in detecting deepfake videos (Afchar et al. 2018). On the FaceForensics++ (Rossler et al. 2019) dataset, however, MesoNet was shown to perform well at detecting deepfakes under different levels of compression. In this study the accuracy never dropped lower than approximately 0.9 for deepfake detection. Yet, when looking at the performance for FaceSwaps, the accuracy is inversely correlated with the amount of compression added.

XceptionNet's (Chollet 2017) creators never tested their own model for the purpose of deepfake detection. After the construction of FaceForensics++ Rossler et al. (Rossler et al. 2019) tested XceptionNet for this pupose. FaceForensics++ is a dataset with three different subsets, each with a different level of compression. Of the six detection algorithms this research tested, XceptionNet scored best on all three different compression subsets. The decrease in accuracy of XceptionNet when more compression is added is the lowest of the examined algorithms. The accuracy of this network never dropped below approximately 0.94. Yet, another research claims that the accuracy of XceptionNet (Chollet 2017) on FaceForensics++ (Rossler et al. 2019) dropped significantly more, where they claim XceptionNet scored 99.26% accuracy on raw videos, 95.73% accuracy of slightly compressed videos and 81.00% accuracy on severely compressed videos (Bojia et al. 2020).

8.3.2.2 Training and Validation Results

While training both networks, it was observed that the vastness of the resulting data set was confirmed by the amount of time each of the networks needed to complete one epoch of training and validation. For MesoNet, one full training epoch (training + validation) would take about 11 hours and 54 minutes on average, while XceptionNet needed 20 hours and 36 minutes to complete one training epoch. The training progress over several epochs can be seen in Figure 8.2, which depicts the accuracy on the validation set after each epoch.

A few noticeable differences can be observed between MesoNet and XceptionNet. First, all the differences in initial accuracy are particularly high. After the first epoch MesoNet already reached an accuracy of 72.8% on the validation set and did not drop below this value afterwards. On the other hand XceptionNet's first accuracy was only 47.3%, which is a lot lower. Beside this initial accuracy difference, MesoNet shows a very smooth line that increases in the beginning and stabilizes over time, while XceptionNet's line is a lot more rigid, with multiple declines and climbs in accuracy over time. XceptionNet's accuracy did not stabilize within the number of epochs that could be done within the scope of this research. It should be noted that the validation set accuracy of XceptionNet never surpasses the valididation set accuracy of MesoNet.

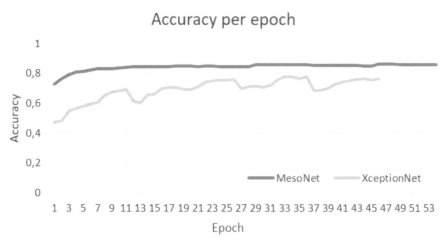

Figure 8.2 Progress of training both networks, in which the accuracy on the validation set is depicted for each epoch.

8.3.2.3 Test Results H.265

MesoNet achieved an overall accuracy of approximately 85% on the constructed validation set and 74.3% on the constructed test set. Per subset this accuracy differs, as one can see in Figure 8.3, which shows that MesoNet's accuracy increases when heavier compressed sets are used at first, with an increase of approximately 1.3% over the first three subsets. However, the third and fourth subsets show a decrease in accuracy again where both of these subsets' accuracies are below the

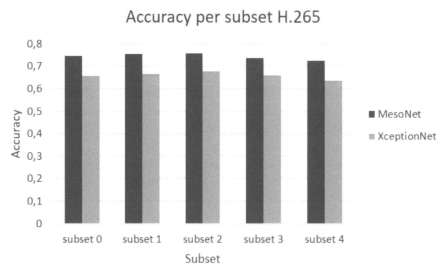

Figure 8.3 The accuracy MesoNet and XceptionNet achieved on the constructed test set. The figure shows the accuracy for each separate subset, where the amount of compression increases from left to right.

accuracy of the subset with no compression (subset 0). The same trend can be observed for XceptionNet's accuracies over the different subsets, where the accuracy initially increases when more compression is added, and starts decreasing between subset 2 and subset 3. Although the shift seems less immediate than it is for MesoNet, as MesoNet's accuracy on subset 3 is below its acccuracy without compression (subset 0) but this is not yet the case for XceptionNet on subset 3. One notable discrepancy between the two trained networks is the difference in accuracy, where MesoNet achieved an average accuracy of 74.3% over all sets, XceptionNet reached 65.9% accuracy on average over all sets.

The accuracies shown in Figure 8.3 have been calculated using the number of correctly classified frames per subset that have been classified correctly by the networks. The exact accuracies per subset can also be seen in Table 8.4

The results show the MesoNet detects fewer deepfake frames than present within the test set, as shown in Table 8.5. It should be noted that the slight difference in number of frames for deepfake videos and genuine videos is caused by the number of frames per video. Although there are equal numbers of videos per subset and each video is always 10 seconds, the number of frames can differ between some videos, leading to a different number of frames per subset. Therefore, an even division in the number of videos does not equal an even number of frames. Table 8.3 shows that MesoNet predicts a lot of deepfake frames as genuine frames. This comes down to the fact that more genuine frames are predicted to be genuine frames than there are genuine frames present in the test set, yet less deepfake frames were predicted than there are present in the test set.

Table 8.4 Accuracy of both MesoNet and XceptionNet on each subset of the test set.

	Subset 0	Subset 1	Subset 2	Subset 3	Subset 4
MesoNet	74.4%	75.3%	75.7%	73.5%	72.6%
XceptionNet	65.6%	66.6%	67.9%	66.0%	63.5%

Table 8.5 The actual number of deepfake and genuine videos in the test set, as well as the predicted amount of deepfake and genuine videos from both networks.

	Deepfakes	Real
Test set	1 616 647 (49.6%)	1 642 477 (50.4%)
MesoNet (%)	1 271 459 (−10.6%)	1 987 665 (+10.6%)
XceptionNet (%)	753 184 (−26.2%)	2 461 796 (+26.2%)

The same observation can be made for XceptionNet, except that the amount of deepfake frames predicted by XceptionNet is even lower than that by MesoNet. XceptionNet's final model (for this research) predicted less than 50% of the deepfake frames to be a deepfake frame.

8.3.2.4 Test Results AV1

MesoNet achieved an overall accuracy of 50.9% on the constructed AV1 test set, which is the same rounded accuracy as MesoNet achieved on the smaller H.265 set. The accuracy for MesoNet shows that it follows the same trend as on this smaller set, regardless of compression method, as it did on the larger test set, as shown in Figure 8.4. For XceptionNet the overall accuracy on the smaller test set compressed using AV1 was 47.7%, while the same set with H.265 as a compression method achieved an overall accuracy of 47.3%. This difference in accuracy is explained by the difference in accuracy on the last subset, as all other subsets achieve the same rounded accuracy. XceptionNet does not show the same trend previously visible for this model within the smaller test set. On this set, XceptionNet shows a decrease in accuracy when more compression is added to the set. Only when using AV1 as a compression method does this decline in accuracy turn around on the last set, where a slight improvement can be seen again.

Figure 8.4 also shows the accuracies of the same models on the H.265 version of the smaller dataset. The comparison between MesoNet and XceptionNet's performance on the smaller H.265 set and the larger H.265 set shows that the smaller set is a lot more challenging, which is shown by the decrease in overall

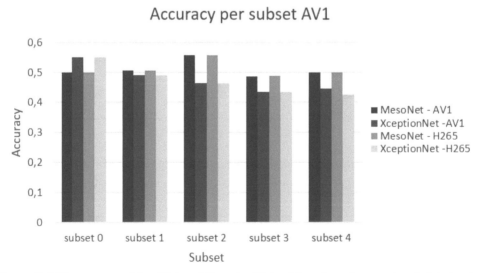

Figure 8.4 The accuracy MesoNet and XceptionNet achieved on the constructed test set using AV1 as a compression method. Each subset is depicted as a separate column for which an accuracy is shown for MesoNet (dark blue) and XceptionNet (light blue).

accuracy of approximately 20% compared to the larger set previously discussed. Despite this increased difficulty, the trend that was visible for MesoNet on the large H.265 set is also visible on this smaller set, regardless of which compression method is applied. However, XceptionNet shows a very different trend, where the accuracy decreases with each time more compression is applied to the set. Apart from the accuracy of XceptionNet on the last subset, the accuracy does not change when a different compression method is applied to the same data.

The accuracies shown in Figure 8.4 have been calculated using the number of frames each network predicted correctly per subset. The exact accuracies per subset for both networks (MesoNet and XceptionNet) can be seen in Table 8.6. The table depicts the accuracies for both the smaller H.265 set and the AV1 set.

For the AV1 set, it has also been analysed how many deepfakes and genuine videos were predicted. Table 8.7 shows that the percentage of predicted deepfakes for both MesoNet and XceptionNet is below 100%. Thus, both networks predict a video to be a deepfake less often than it predicts a video to be a genuine one. Consequently, both networks show a bias towards predicting videos to be real, rather than deepfake. This bias within the predictions of both networks is likely to be larger for XceptionNet than it is for MesoNet, which is shown by the larger

Table 8.6 Accuracies per subset for the smaller set created for this study. The results are shown for both networks (MesoNet and XceptionNet) on both versions of the smaller dataset (H.265 and AV1).

	Subset	Subset	Subset	Subset	Subset
	0	1	2	3	4
MesoNet – AV1	49.9%	50.5%	55.6%	48.6%	49.9%
XceptionNet – AV1	55.1%	49.1%	46.2%	43.3%	44.5%
MesoNet – H.265	49.9%	50.5%	55.6%	48.7%	49.9%
XceptionNet – H.265	55.1%	49.1%	46.2%	43.3%	42.6%

Table 8.7 Actual number of deepfake and genuine videos in the test set created using AV1 as a compression method, as well as the predicted amount of deepfake and genuine videos from both networks.

-	Deepfakes	Real
Test set	14775 (49.7%)	149300 (50.3%)
MesoNet (%)	10356 (−14.8%)	19349 (+14.8%)
XceptionNet (%)	5771 (−30%)	23569 (+30%)

percentage of predicted real frames by the former. For both networks, it can be observed that the percentage of deepfake frames that was predicted to be a deep-fake frame is lower on the AV1 set, than it is on the H.265 set.

8.4 Discussion

The results show that compression with the H.265 standard has an influence on the detection of deepfake videos. This influence is shown to be positive when compression is added at first, but changes to negative when too much compression is present. This effect was seen on both of the networks that were trained for this research. The effect of AV1 was shown less clearly, although the results suggest the effect to be similar to that of H.265.

8.4.1 Deepfake Detection

For the results reported on MesoNet, a few things stand out. First of all, the initial training accuracy is rather unexpectedly high after one epoch. However, the network does not drop below this initial accuracy at any point, indicating that it already learned well during the first epoch and this high initial accuracy was not solely due to well working random settings.

Besides what has just been mentioned, it should be noted that the accuracy on the test set for MesoNet shows something different than expected. Previous research (Rossler et al. 2019) showed that the accuracy of the network dropped upon increasing the compression amount. However, this study shows that the accuracy increases in the first instance, and only drops when the compression rate is increased further, showing two important findings. First, it shows that there is a significant difference between the influence of compression when using H.264 and H.265. Although the research into H.264 used fewer sets, all of the sets showed a (slight) decrease in accuracy, which is contradicted by this research as it shows an increase with fewer compression and a decrease only with larger amounts of compression. Second, MesoNet seems very capable of dealing with compression, while the compression stays under CRF 32. Although the exact CRF value at which the accuracy of MesoNet decreases is unclear, it is known that the accuracy still increases with a CRF of 25 but decreases with a CRF of 32. This suggests that the turning point for MesoNet's accuracy is located between these two values. This ability to handle compression at first could be explained by the architecture of the network itself. It can be suggested that the mesoscopic level at which MesoNet is designed to analyse images is not influenced when little compression is added. Yet that this level is influenced by compression when it surpassed a certain threshold (between CRF 25 and 32).

XceptionNet shows a similar trend to that of MesoNet, where a rise in accuracy can be seen when compression is added at first, but a fall in accuracy is seen when too much compression is added. We cannot be sure were the exact turning point is located for this network, although it is again suggested to lie between CRF 25 and CRF 32 as can be seen in Figure 8.3. The accuracy of XceptionNet does not fall as steeply between CRF 25 and 32 as MesoNet's accuracy does, which suggests that the turning point may be closer to 32 for XceptionNet, while MesoNet's will be closer to 25.

When analysing the results of XceptionNet one notable fact stood out. Previous research (Rossler et al. 2019) suggested that XceptionNet should outperform MesoNet on all levels of compression, and that its accuracy would be likely to be in the 90% regions. Both of these findings were contradicted within this study, where MesoNet outperformed XceptionNet by an accuracy difference of approximately 10% and the accuracy of XceptionNet did not surpass 68% for any of the subsets. This could be due to two factors. First, it is possible that the constructed dataset is a lot more challenging than the dataset previously used to analyse the results of XceptionNet. This would explain the vastly lower score reported in this study, though it does not explain why MesoNet outperformed XceptionNet. Second, it is shown in Figure 8.2 that XceptionNet's validation set accuracy has never stabilized to the extend MesoNet's validation set accuracy stabilized. Which suggests XceptionNet has not been trained to the best of its ability and the reported results are an understatement of XceptionNet's detection accuracy. This explanation is supported by the architecture of XceptionNet, because this network is a lot deeper in design than MesoNet is. This means that many more parameters have to be optimized during a single epoch which results in the fact that more time is needed to optimize XceptionNet than MesoNet. Explaining the lower score for XceptionNet was because too little time was given to XceptionNet to optimize its parameters. However, it is reasonable to assume that a better trained network would change the effect that compression has on the detection ability, therefore, the suggested effects of compression are not undermined by these considerations.

After the construction of the training, validation, and test set, the scope of this research did not permit extensive training of the networks. That is to say, MesoNet has been trained fully and has supposedly reached its peak accuracy. However, it was found to be impossible within this research to extensively tweak the parameters to test their influence on the network. Tweaked parameters could, however, have altered the results of the study, the resulting networks would have been (slightly) different. Due to the time it takes to complete one training and validation epoch, allowing thorough training with many different parameter settings was not feasible, although thorough training with probable yet non-optimized parameters was achieved. For XceptionNet the consideration should be that it is likely to not have been trained to its full potential as the validation accuracy had not yet converged.

8.4.2 Compression

Some caution should, however, be used when interpreting the results, for example, the division of compression amongst the different subsets created for this study. Although these subsets each have a different compression ratio, some compression ratios are closer together than others. For example, the difference in the size reduction between subset 3 and 4 is only approximately 8%, whilst this difference is approximately 41% between subset 1 and 2. These subsets, therefore, are not evenly distributed over the different compression ratios. It should be noted that it is virtually impossible to know the exact compression ratio prior to compression. This is because two different videos of the same size, using CRF, can end up with vastly different compression ratios for the same CRF. Despite this hitch, a better distribution would have strengthened the results.

It should also be noted that any result presented using the AV1 compressed set was only tested on 100 different videos, while neither of the two networks were trained on videos compressed using AV1. This causes a distortion in reporting the performance of MesoNet and XceptionNet on the AV1 compressed set. The results presented for this set should, therefore, be regarded as an indication of whether a difference can be expected between AV1 and H.265 compression standards.

What can be observed from the AV1 test set is that, besides the vastly lower accuracy on this dataset, the trend shown for MesoNet is the same as the trend MesoNet showed on H.265 compressed data, while XceptionNet's trend is vastly different between the smaller test set and the larger test set (for reference see Figure 8.4). The fact that both networks' trends on the smaller set are (almost) identical between the different compression methods that have been performed on the smaller set, indicates that the influence of compression does not alter between compression methods but between detection methods. This would mean that the influence of compression between these two standards is identical, but that the exact effect of this compression is highly dependent on the network itself. Although the results also suggest that with enough datapoints, this effect will – for all compression methods and for all networks – be an initial improvement when more compression is added but a decline in accuracy when compression becomes too much.

The vast difference between the trends of XceptionNet on the larger and smaller set can be explained by the limited size of the smaller set. It is possible that XceptionNet has more difficulty correctly classifying the particular type of video that is present in the smaller. As there are only 20 videos per subset, having more difficulty with only one of these 20 videos will likely show in the results. The fact that MesoNet does not show a similar trend on the smaller set as XceptionNet can be explained through the same principle. Both networks have different classification methods, which are thus likely to be based on different artefacts within a video. The smaller set could be one that, viewed from the way MesoNet classifies images, is very similar to the larger set, while for XceptioNet's point of view these images pose a more significant challenge. Besides this, a consideration that should be taken into account is the fact that neither of the two networks have been trained to handle AV1 as a compression method, they have only been trained on H.265 compressed data. Therefore, any results reported could differ vastly from those that would be reported if the networks have been trained on AV1 compressed data.

8.4.3 Future Work

Future research into the forensic detection of deepfake videos should focus on the type of videos that are most often questioned within the forensic world. This research has aimed to show the effects of compression for the detection of deepfakes, but many more such factors can play a role for the detection of deepfakes. The factors that are found to be most common within the forensic world should be investigated first. Apart from compression (which plays a role in almost all deepfakes), the factors that are seen often should be accounted for before starting with the less common factors.

Future research could also focus on a more thorough analysis of the effects of compression. Currently, no networks other than MesoNet and XceptionNet have been tested on the constructed dataset. However, given the results of this study and the results previously shown, it is possible to hypothesize that other algorithms are likely to show similar effects on a particular compression standard, although the effect of compression changes when a different compression standard is used (Rossler et al. 2019).

It is also expected that many new methods of detection will appear in the literature as well as many new applications to make deepfakes. Often these methods will use new trained networks as well as other designs. A major challenge is to make a deepfake which looks real in a short time based on images and audio of a person, that also has correct lip syncing and also speaks in the same way that a person speaks with all the artefacts that are available in the linguistic properties.

8.5 Conclusion

The results of this study show that in smaller amounts compression has a positive influence on the detection of deepfake videos when using MesoNet as a detection algorithm. However, an increase in compression will result in a decrease in accuracy between CRF values of 25 and 32. Therefore, it can be concluded that MesoNet does not suffer greatly from being exposed to compression, and in smaller amounts it can even benefit from it. However, if too much compression is applied to a video, the ability to accurately detect deepfake videos starts to decrease. The same conclusion can be drawn for the effect of H.265 on XceptionNet's ability to detect deepfakes.

The effect of AV1 on the detection of deepfakes is suggested to be similar to the effect H.265 shows. However, before any definite conclusions can be drawn this hypothesis should be validated on a more substantial dataset.

References

Afchar, D., Nozick, V., Yamagishi, J., and Echizen, I. (2018). Mesonet: a compact facial video forgery detection network. In: *2018 IEEE International Workshop on Information Forensics and Security (WIFS)*. doi: 10.1109/WIFS.2018.8630761.
AOMedia (2021). Aomedia av1 compression. http://aomedia.org/av1 (accessed 10 May 2021).

Bhaskaran, V. and Konstantinides, K. (1997). Image and video compression standards: algorithms and architectures.

Bojia, Z., Chang, M., Chen, J. et al. (2020 October). Wilddeepfake: a challenging real-world dataset for deepfake detection. In: MM '20: *Proceedings of the 28th ACM International Conference on Multimedia*, New York, NY, USA. Association for Computing Machinery. 2382–2390. ISBN 9781450379885. doi: 10.1145/3394171.3413769.

Chen, C.-Y., Ding, J.-J., and Hsu, H.-W. (2020). Prominent facial feature and hybrid learning method-based advanced face detector robust to head-up, head-down, and arbitrary rotation cases. *Signal, Image and Video Processing* 15: 147–154. (2021). ISSN 1863-1703. doi: 10.1007/s11760-020-01729-w.

Chollet, F. (2017). Xception: deep learning with depthwise separable convolutions.

Cozzolino, D., Poggi, G., and Verdoliva, L. (2017 June). Recasting residual-based local descriptors as convolutional neural networks: an application to image forgery detection. In: IH&MMSec '17: Proceedings of the 5th ACM Workshop on Information Hiding and Multimedia Security. 159–164. doi: 10.1145/3082031.3083247.

Dolhansky, B., Bitton, J., Pflaum, B. et al. (2020). The deepfake detection challenge (dfdc) dataset.

Grois, D., Nguyen, T., and Marpe, D. (2016). Coding efficiency comparison of av1/vp9, h.265/mpeg-hevc, and h.264/mpeg-avc encoders. In: *2016 Picture Coding Symposium (PCS)*. doi: 10.1109/PCS.2016.7906321.

Jiang, L., Ren, L., Wayne, W. et al. (2020). Deeperforensics-1.0: a large-scale dataset for real-world face forgery detection. In: *Proceedings of the IEEE/CVF Conference on Computer Vision and Pattern Recognition (CVPR)*.

Koumaras, H., Kourtis, M., and Martakos, D. (2012). Benchmarking the encoding efficiency of h.265/hevc and h.264/avc. In: *2012 Future Network Mobile Summit (FutureNetw)*.

Lyu, S. (2020). Deepfake detection: current challenges and next steps. In: *2020 IEEE International Conference on Multimedia Expo Workshops (ICMEW)*. doi: 10.1109/ICMEW46912.2020.9105991.

Rahmouni, N., Nozick, V., Yamagishi, J., and Echizen, I. (2017). Distinguishing computer graphics from natural images using convolution neural networks. In: *2017 IEEE Workshop on Information Forensics and Security (WIFS)*. doi: 10.1109/WIFS.2017.8267647.

Rössler, A., Cozzolino, D., Verdoliva, L. et al. (2018). Faceforensics: a large-scale video dataset for forgery detection in human faces.

Rossler, A., Cozzolino, D., Verdoliva, L. et al. (2019). Faceforensics++: learning to detect manipulated facial images. In: *Proceedings of the IEEE/CVF International Conference on Computer Vision (ICCV)*.

Sims, G. (2021). MS Windows NT kernel description. https://www.androidauthority.com/av1-codec-1113318 (accessed 23 April 2021).

Szegedy, C., Liu, W., Jia, Y. et al. (2015). Going deeper with convolutions. In: *Proceedings of the IEEE Conference on Computer Vision and Pattern Recognition (CVPR)*.

Verdoliva, L. (2020). Media forensics and deepfakes: an overview. *IEEE Journal of Selected Topics in Signal Processing*. doi:10.1109/JSTSP.2020.3002101.

Viola, P. and Jones, M. (2001). Rapid object detection using a boosted cascade of simple features. In: *Proceedings of the 2001 IEEE computer society conference on computer vision and pattern recognition. CVPR 2001*. IEEE.

Yuezun, L., Sun, P., Qi, H., and Lyu, S. (2020). Celeb-DF: a large-scale challenging dataset for deepfake forensics. In: *IEEE Conference on Computer Vision and Patten Recognition (CVPR)*, Seattle, WA, United States.

CHAPTER 9

Event Log Analysis and Correlation: A Digital Forensic Perspective

Neminath Hubballi[1] and Pratibha Khandait[2]

[1]*Indian Institute of Technology Indore, Simrol, Indore, India*
[2]*Department of Computer Science and Engineering, Indian Institute of Technology Indore, India*

9.1 Introduction

Internet has connected billions of devices and enabled innovative networked applications and services. Applications like e-commerce, online banking, online gaming, and social networking have become part of our daily activity. These applications bring convenience allowing access anywhere and anytime. However, such seamless connectivity has also brought new challenges in the form of cyber attacks, cyber bullying (Al Mutawa et al. 2016), cyber stalking, online fraud, banking fraud, etc. This has necessitated methods for detecting such cyber incidents (https://police.py.gov.in). The cyber security research community has developed several methods for securing applications and systems from cyber attacks. These methods, although successful to a great extent in securing the systems and networked applications, are not foolproof. Every day new vulnerabilities are discovered and exploited to gain undue advantage. Thus, it is always a race between security engineers and cyber criminals with security engineers trying to catch up with new developments. Given that developing foolproof secure systems is not possible, security engineers have adopted methods which can generate information (evidence) when the system is in use. This information is usually in the form of logs written by different applications and systems.

> **Log**: *A chronological time-stamped sequence of event records generated as a result of communication between systems, network devices, users, or applications.*

These logs serve as a useful source of information to assess the functioning of systems. The following are the important use-cases where logs are useful (https://cryptome.org/2014/01/nsa-windows-event.pdf).

Artificial Intelligence (AI) in Forensic Sciences, First Edition. Edited by Zeno Geradts and Katrin Franke.
© 2024 John Wiley & Sons Ltd. Published 2024 by John Wiley & Sons Ltd.

1. **Health Monitoring of Systems:** As today's computer systems are complex and networked, managing these complex systems requires careful planning and, in the event of disruptions or cases which impact the functioning of systems, requires analysis of various things that have happened. In order to assist system and network managers in performing the maintenance task the logs are consulted.

2. **Cyber Attacks and Incidents:** As mentioned previously, cyber attacks and incidents are inevitable. Whenever such incidents occur, these logs serve as a useful source of information to assess the events that have taken place, the damage that has happened, identifying the sources of attacks and finally recovering from the damage.

Log analysis is a technique of reviewing and interpreting logs generated by different systems to gain insight into the internal working of systems, applications, and user behavior. In the case of cyber attacks, these can be used to attribute particular incidents to entities like persons, locations, systems, etc. In this specific case, logs serve as evidence of certain activity. For example, in the investigation of cases involved with the online distribution of banned items like drugs, logs generated by network elements could reveal whether a person's computer had indeed accessed websites selling such banned items. This can be corroborated with other material evidence to establish ground truth.

Traditional forensic investigation techniques have standard methods for collecting, safeguarding, and corroborating the evidence collected from crime scenes. For example, a bank robbery investigation can collect evidence from CCTVs, fingerprints, mobile phones, etc. In the online world, crimes are committed involving digital assets which have similar consequences. In order to deal with the investigation of such cases digital evidence is collected and analyzed. Digital forensic methods help answer questions like: what happened? how did the event happen? when did it happened? and finally, who was involved in the incident? Recently digital forensics methods have been standardized making them sound to collect evidence which can be produced in a court of law. A typical digital forensic investigation involves the following phases (Marshall 2009).

(i) Identification: this involves identifying the sources of digital evidence and also deals with what kind of evidence is collected from where.

(ii) Collection: in this phase actual evidence is collected using sound and proven methods of evidence collection.

(iii) Examination: different applications, systems, and software might write evidence in different formats thus adding disparity to evidence collected. This phase deals with the ability to understand and deal with such diversity.

(iv) Analysis: collected evidence can be either analyzed manually or using some automated tools which can correlate the evidence.

(v) Presentation: in the final phase gathered evidence is presented to support or refute a hypothesis.

Traditional digital forensics methods use evidence collected from memory, computer disk, and also event logs collected from these devices. The techniques to capture and record such evidence are sound. In this chapter, we discuss log analysis and correlation as a digital forensic method. We begin with a discussion of sources and places where logs are generated in Section 9.2, subsequently in Section 9.3 we point out why log correlation is required, and finally we present some techniques to correlate the logs from different sources in Section 9.4.

9.2 Sources of Logs

As mentioned previously, systems, devices, and applications are capable of generating log records. This includes a wide range of programmable technologies, such as network devices, operating systems, software applications, etc. as shown in Figure 9.1. The systems generating logs can be categorized into various types as follows.

1. **Operating System:** An operating system is a complex system software which manages the hardware and facilitates running user applications. The system management and user activities in the system are logged in different places which give insights about system activity.

2. **Networking Devices and Security Systems**: Various networking devices like routers and switches connect computers and facilitate running distributed applications. Monitoring the security of networked systems requires the deployment of security appliances and software like firewalls and intrusion detection systems (IDS), and intrusion prevention systems (IPS). These devices and security monitoring applications come with the capability to generate, store, and offload log records to databases for future analysis.

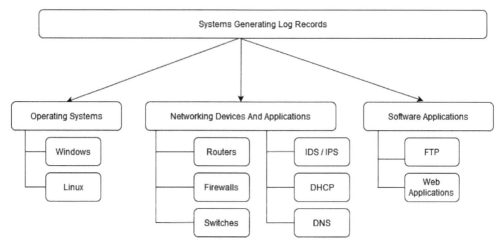

Figure 9.1 Sources of digital logs.

3. **Software Applications**: Several network applications like Web servers, ssh generate logs specific to those applications. For example, connecting to servers hosted on websites, one needs a software application like a web browser that acts as a client on behalf of the user and helps retrieve useful information. Google Chrome, Mozilla Firefox, Safari, and Brave are pupular web browsers used today. The resource requested by clients and whether the request has been served successfully is maintained as part of server logs. Web browsers can remember the events and log them in the form of browsing history and cookies. Cookies contain site preferences and login credentials and can be used to profile user behavior.

9.2.1 End Host System Logs

An operating system is a collection of software that serves as an interface between the user and the underlying hardware. The operating system registers an entry in the log file for each event happening in the system in a time-stamped manner to generate footprints (e.g., memory, CPU utilization, user footprints, etc.). One can use these footprints as pieces of evidence to perform a forensic investigation on an operating system to detect cyber crimes or even a physical attack. To collect such evidence from an operating system, forensic experts need to know where the data resides and how to retrieve and process the data. As the logs are specific to operating systems, are using different formats, and are also stored in different locations within the system, one needs to understand the file systems and formats. In the subsequent paragraphs we provide a brief overview of these logs as found in two popular operating systems.

9.2.1.1 Linux System Logs

Linux generally stores logs in the directory */var/log/*. A possible set of entries in the */var/log/* directory is shown in Figure 9.2. We can see that there are logs related to kernel operations, user login related activities, system boot, new installations done by package managers, etc. All of these logs prove to be valuable when investigating any cyber event. For example from the *auth.log* file, we can see who all have logged in to the system and at what time. Similarly from the *boot.log*, the

```
LinuxSystem:$ cd /var/log
LinuxSystem:/var/log$ ls
alternatives.log       boot.log.2        dmesg.1.gz       journal              syslog
alternatives.log.1     boot.log.3        dpkg.log         kern.log             syslog.1
alternatives.log.2.gz  bootstrap.log     dpkg.log.1       kern.log.1           syslog.2.gz
apache2                btmp              faillog          kern.log.2.gz        ubuntu-
apt                    btmp.1            fontconfig.log   lastlog              advantage.log
auth.log               cups              gdm3             openvpn              unattended-upgrades
auth.log.1             dist-upgrade      gpu-manager.log  Private              vboxadd-install.log
boot.log               dmesg             hp               snort                vboxadd-setup.log
boot.log.1             dmesg.0           installer        speech-dispatcher    wtmp
```

Figure 9.2 List of files in Linux */var/log/* directory.

order in which different components of the operating system have been invoked and whether they have been successful or not can be found. This sequence may be altered if the system is compromised or infected with a boot virus.

In addition to providing the rich information in the form of logs, operating system also keep the meta data information of various files. This can also serve as useful information in a cyber crime forensic investigation. For example, every file on a Linux system has permissions attached to it. Any unusual permissions to specific files and unusual files in specific locations can also serve as indicators of some system compromise. These permissions can be found with the *ls -lha* command. Figure 9.3 shows a sample output after running the *ls -lha* command in the */var/log/* directory. Each file has details of read, write, and execute permissions assigned to it and a timestamp of when the file was created and modified. Some of the cyber attacks/events may change these permissions. Apart from file permissions, other metadata like size of the file, etc can often be useful.

The Linux system also keeps logs about when a user logged in, when the system was shutdown, and when it was started. These events are logged into a log file located within */var/log/* directory. Two files particularly, *utmp* and *wtmp* contain all information of logins, logouts, and system shut down. We can view all login information by executing the *last* command to get the details of login activity. These login details are fetched frWm *wtmp* file which has entries similar to the one shown in Figure 9.4. These details will be helpful in forensic investigation. For example, whether the computer was up and running at the time when some cyber incident happened can be found.

```
LinuxSystem:$ cd /var/log
LinuxSystem:/var/log$ ls -lha
-rw-r--r--     1 root      root      1.3k    Mar 20 23:11    gpu-manager.log
-rw-------     1 root      root      7.8M    Mar 20 23:12    boot.log
-rw-r-----     1 syslog    adm       9.8M    Mar 20 23:16    kern.log
-rw-r-----     1 syslog    adm       8.8K    Mar 20 23:17    auth,log
-rw-r-----     1 syslog    adm       9.9M    Mar 20 23:17    syslog
-rw-rw-r--     1 root      utmp      29K     Mar 20 23:15    wtmp
```

Figure 9.3 A sample output of file permissions.

```
LinuxSystem:$ cd /var/log
LinuxSystem:/var/log$ last
reboot    system boot    5.11.0-34-generic    Wed Oct 13    00:46    still     running
ubuntu    :0             :0                   Thu Oct  7    23:39    down      (01:06)
reboot    system boot    5.11.0-34-generic    Thu Oct  7    23:39    00:46     (01:06)
ubuntu    :0             :0                   wed Oct  6    08:31    down      (03:09)
reboot    system boot    5.11.0-34-generic    wed Oct  6    08:30    11:40     (03:09)
ubuntu    :0             :0                   wed Oct  6    08:22    crash     (00:08)
reboot    system boot    5.11.0-34-generic    wed Oct  6    08:21    11:40     (03:18)
ubuntu    :0             :0                   wed Oct  6    08:14    down      (00:06)
```

Figure 9.4 Output of *last* command showing contents of *var/log/wtmp* file.

9.2.1.2 Windows System Logs

Like Linux and every other operating system, Windows also keeps logs of various events in Windows log. The Windows system supports numerous utilities, tools, and applications to ease tasks for its users. One such tool is Windows Event Viewer that displays Windows event logs. Windows records logs from the operating system, application, and processes running on the server or the client machine. Unlike Linux which allows logs to be viewed through any text editors and command line interface, Windows event viewer provides its users with a graphical user interface to view and navigate the logs. It also includes functionality to filter and export a particular type of log record. This information helps system analysts to provide troubleshooting services and to investigate security issues. Windows event logs are broken and recorded into different sets. Related events are placed in a similar category to make troubleshooting easier for its users. Although there are many categories of logs the major types are Application, System, Security, and Setup. Some sample windows System Logs are shown in Figure 9.5

Logs in each category are assigned an event type, also called an event label, based on the severity of the issue represented by the event. The list includes labels like critical, error, warning, information, verbose, audit success, and audit failure. Users can customize and prioritize events from specific applications in which they are interested. System events labeled as critical are high priority events. Alerts from such logs, if ignored and left unattended, can lead to major issues like unexpected shutdowns, data loss, or system crash. Less severe cases like error messages indicate that a problem has occurred. Every Windows event log shows up some error message even when the system is working fine. This is because Windows usually generates error messages even for small task failures such as unavailability of a driver to execute a printing task or a service failure, which started successfully on subsequent attempts. Such errors can be either ignored or put on hold or resolved later.

Windows Registry Files: The Windows operating system has an additional source of information in the form of a registry database which can serve to be

System	Number of events: 6			
Level	**Date and Time**	**Source**	**Event ID**	**Task Category**
ⓘ Information	30-09-2021 22:41:05	WindowsUpdateClient	19	Windows Update Agent
⚠ Warning	30-09-2021 22:32:06	DNS Client Event	1014	(1014)
ⓘ Error	30-09-2021 17:00:55	Schannel	36871	None
ⓘ Information	30-09-2021 12:20:35	Power-Troubleshooter	1	None
✖ Critical	25-09-2021 14:53:00	Kernel-Power	41	(63)
ⓘ Error	20-09-2021 23:15:06	Ntfs(Ntfs)	55	None

Figure 9.5 Sample windows system log entries from windows event viewer.

useful for a forensic investigator. Registry is an ordered database containing information, settings, options, and other values for all software and hardware installed on all the versions of the Windows operating system. The registry also stores settings, options, and information for the applications that opt to use the registry. Windows registry has two main components: *keys* and *values*. Registry keys are similar to a folder and are referenced with syntax similar to windows pathname to represent the hierarchy. Keys can contain subkeys or values. In the Windows registry subkeys are similar to subfolders, and values are similar to files. New software installation on the system, creates a new subkey in the registry with all the configuration settings specific to that software. This subkey stores all the information relevant to the installed program, such as location, software versions, update details, and executables. The content of the subkeys and values down in the registry key hierarchy is accessed only from a known five key handle. The entire registry is organized into folders or root keys. Five predefined root keys discussed below are named based on their constant handles defined in the Win32 API.

- HKEY LOCAL MACHINE or HKLM: HKLM registry information is organized in six main subkeys/subfolders, namely BCD, HARDWARE, SAM, SECURITY, SOFTWARE, and SYSTEM, depending upon the version of the windows OS. These subkeys contain more subkeys depending upon the applications and software that opt for registry services. All the local machine-related information is stored in these subkeys. The subkey BCD stores boot configuration details while the connected plug and play devices' information is available under the HARDWARE subkey. The SYSTEM subkey contains critical information created by users with administrative privileges. It includes settings for Windows, file system, hardware configuration, etc., which are crucial for running the core system. Keys can have values set or not set. For example, we can identify the application/services that are set to start at the system startup under the key-path HKEY_LOCAL_MACHINE\System\CurrentControlSet\Services. Clicking on the displayed services will open an information window having entries as keyvalue pairs. An example of one such information window is shown in Figure 9.6 for remote registry service. The value associated with the key "start" tells the startup type for the selected service/application. The start value 0 represents boot startup, 1 represents system startup, 2 represents the automatic startup, 3 indicates the manual start, and the value 4 indicates the service is disabled. If any malware is installed on the computer, it typically starts at the system startup and can be caught by the forensic investigators.

Insider attacks are the most popular in corporate industries, where malicious insiders (people inside the company office) steal the company's confidential information to which they do not have access. Attackers often use external flash drives or hard drives for malicious activities and later remove these drives to ensure that they do not leave any traces behind. The attacker performs activities like copying data, installing malicious software (keylogger, malware, etc.).

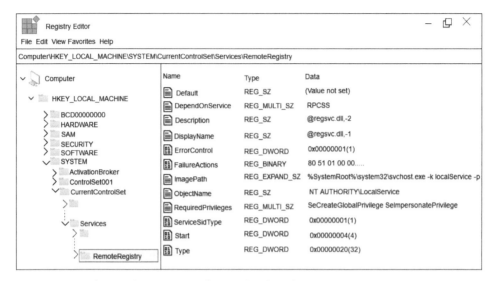

Figure 9.6 Sample Windows registry key and values for remote registry service.

Windows registry logs the detailed list of the external devices connected to the system under the subkey USBSTOR under path HKEY_LOCAL_MACHINE\ SYSTEM\CurrentControlSet\Enum\USBSTOR. Digital forensic experts can catch the suspicious entries for such plug and play USB devices from the list for a detailed analysis.

- HKEY CURRENT USER or HKCU: HKCU contains all the information specific to the currently logged-in user. The information stored in HKCU serves as a roadmap for forensic investigators to track down all user activities in the breach events. For example, the key "RecentDocs" under location HKEY_CURRENT_USER\Software\ Microsoft\ Windows\CurrentVersion\Explorer\RecentDocs keeps track of the most recent documents opened, used, uploaded, or downloaded by the user. The entries are sorted by file extensions. Files with specific extensions like the .tar files could be the suspicious candidates. In the event of malware infection from any internet source, the malware can be traced down from the information recorded at subkey TypedURLs under the path HKEY_CURRENT_USER\Software\Microsoft\ InternetExplorer\ TypedURLs. When a user types a URL in Internet Explorer (IE), the URL entry gets registered in the subkey TypedURLs. When we click on the key TypedURLs it lists last URls visited by the user in IE. Searching suspicious entries in this subkey can reveal the source of malware.
- HKEY USERS or HKU: The registry keys in the HKEY USER contain user-specific settings and information for all the active users who have a login account on the system. Apart from user-specific setting subkeys, HKEY USER contains other subkeys reserved for the system accounts like HKEY_USER\.DEFAULT reserved to be used by the LocalSystem account. Subkey S-1-5-19 is for the LocalService account, and the NetworkService account uses S-1-5-20 as a subkey.

- HKEY CURRENT CONFIG or HKCC: HKEY CURRENT CONFIG does not store any information but instead contains pointer/links to the current software and hardware configuration settings stored in the HKEY LOCAL MACHINE.
- HKEY CLASSES ROOT or HKCR: HKEY CLASSES ROOT is not generic to users but contains helpful information for Windows to know when a user asks it to do something like open a specific file type or view the content of the pen drive. This registry deals with details like file extension association, Program identifiers, class IDs, and interface ID information.

9.2.2 Networking Devices and Security Applications

As mentioned earlier, various networking devices like routers, switches, load balancers, security monitoring appliances and applications like intrusion detection systems, intrusion prevention systems, firewalls, dynamic host configuration servers, domain name servers also generate logs. These logs will also help in forensic investigation. Below we elaborate the logs generated by these systems and applications.

9.2.2.1 Logs from Network Devices

Network devices like Switches and Routers have features to generate information about network connections and data exchanged. This data can be in the form of a packet capture or network trace file generated by tapping to these devices and collected at a host. There are both open source tools like tcpdump (https://www.tcpdump.org), wireshark (https://www.wireshark.org), and also commercial tools available for this purpose. These devices can also generate a summary of data exchange and connection information between two systems in the form of flow records. A flow record generally has the details of two communication end points, the protocol used for communication, and the amount of data exchanged. Figure 9.7 shows a sample output of flow records generated by a device. We can see that along with the communication end points, details like duration of flow and number of packets exchanged, start time of the flow, etc. are also in these logs. This flow level data serves two useful purposes. First, this is much more smaller in size compared to raw network packet data collected as a trace. Second, this data is useful in detecting cyber incidents like botnet, malware, etc. All major networking device manufacturers have provided similar features in their products. For example, CISCO has a

Date	Flow Start	Duration	Protol	Src IP Addr: Port		Dst IP Addr: Port	Packets	Bytes	Flows
2022-01-09	00:00:00:410	0.001	UDP	192.168.0.1:24801	→	192.168.1.1:22901	1	56	1
2022-01-09	00:00:00:383	0.000	UDP	192.168.1.1:22901	→	192.168.0.1:24801	1	82	1
2022-01-09	00:00:00:289	0.001	UDP	192.168.0.2:32801	→	192.168.1.2:32901	1	156	1
2022-01-09	00:00:00:210	0.000	UDP	192.168.1.2:32901	→	192.168.0.2:32801	1	64	1

Figure 9.7 Sample entries in flow record.

feature which they call Netflow (https://www.cisco.com/c/en/us/td/docs/ios-xml/ios/fnetflow/configuration/15-mt/fnf-15-mt-book.html), Junifer network calls it JFlow (https://www.juniper.net/us/en/search.html). Recently open standards like sFlow (https://sflow.org) have emerged. These flow records have been used very extensively to detect different cyber attacks and also for metering purpose. From a forensic investigation point of view, these records can provide details of timing of connection between systems and amount of data exchanged which can be further corroborated with other information to verify a hypothesis.

9.2.2.2 Logs from Security and Network Services

Almost all networks of reasonable size have some security appliances, services, and applications. The security appliances and applications may come in the form of firewalls, intrusion detection systems, and intrusion prevention systems, while the network services can be in the form of dynamic host configuration protocol (DHCP) servers, domain name servers (DNS), etc. These applications and services also generate rich information in the form of logs. We elaborate on the details of logs generated by these devices below.

(i) **Firewall Logs:** A firewall is a device between the internal network and the rest of the Internet. A typical firewall filters traffic or packets in the network and hence acts as a choke point. The actions taken by a firewall include pass and deny. It logs the details of these actions along with the details of traffic/packet on which these actions are applied. These logs also serve as an important source of information for detecting cyber events like a worm or virus outbreak. A sample output of a pfsense (https://www.pfsense.org) firewall logs is shown in Figure 9.8. pfSense is an open-source firewall and a router software distribution that is based on FreeBSD and is entirely managed via a web interface. Each entry in the pfsense firewall log is represented in the following format:

Time-stamp, Hostname, "filterlog:" rule-number, sub-rule-number, anchor, tracker, realinterface, reason, action, direction, ip-version, ip-specific-data, length, source-address, destinationaddress, *protocol-specific-data*

The sample entry in Figure 9.8 represents an outbound packet that hits the interface named

---

Time-stamp Hostname "filterlog:" rule-number, sub-rule-number, anchor, tracker, real interface,
reason, action, direction, ip-version, length, source-address, destination-address,
protocol-specific-data

Jan 09 14:09:02 10.100.100.251 filterlog:61, 16777216, ,1000000552, igb2, match, pass, out, 4, 0x0, ,
64, 21241, 0, DF, 6, tcp, 60, 35.227.227.186, 10.100.57.220, 443, 45084, 0, SA, 2676392704,
347543621, 65535, ,mss;nop; wscale; sackOK; TS

Figure 9.8 Sample firewall log.

"igb2" on Jan 09 at 14:09:02 with a TTL value 64. The entry is logged because the packet is matched against the rule having rule ID "1000000552," and the action taken by the firewall is pass. The packet is sent from source IP 32.227.227.186 with source port no. 443 to a destination machine with IP 10.100.57.220 on port 45084. The field entry for anchor is missing and is represented using an empty space(,,). Anchor is the path/link where the matching rule exists.

(ii) **Intrusion Detection System Logs:** Intrusion detection system (IDS) is a software or a hardware device which monitors the network traffic for any threat and alerts the administrator if anything suspicious is noticed. The alerts generated generally includes the source address of the attacker, address of the victim, along with the type of attack suspected by the IDS. IDS is responsible for scanning both inbound and outbound traffic in the network. Although a firewall may be available to avoid any unauthorized access at the network periphery by blocking and filtering the traffic, an IDS is required to monitor the traffic for any malicious activity or policy violations. There are two primary detection methods used with IDSs: signature based and anomaly detection. Signature based IDS works with a database of signatures of known attack types (Roesch 1999) and anomaly detection systems (Chandola et al. 2009) detect deviations of established normal behavioral patterns of users, applications, network devices, hosts, etc. While the signature based IDS can detect only previously known attacks (for which a signature is available) the anomaly based methods can detect both previously known and new attacks (at least in theory) as well.

IDS logs data about the detected events. The information from the logs are used to verify the alerts generated, and also to investigate the incident. IDS logs are monitored to extract information which can be used to secure the network further. The details like attacks detected, devices/hosts which are vulnerable and targeted, suspicious user behaviors, suspicious system activity, etc. can be found by looking at the IDS logs. Such information can help to get details on the most frequent types of attack over the network, along with the source of the attack. Logs can also be analyzed to know which device which is targeted most often. This information can be used to secure the network from the attacks it is vulnerable to, along with guarding the targeted devices.

Figure 9.9 shows sample entries for Snort (https://www.snort.org). Snort is an open-source intrusion detection system that inspects all incoming and outbound network traffic. The first field in each entry contains the date and the time of the event generated. The following field in the line hints at the intention

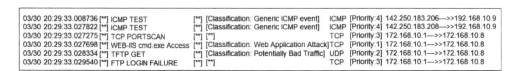

Figure 9.9 Sample log entry of Snort IDS.

of the traffic(ICMP test, TCP Port Scan, malicious content access, FTP logins, failures, etc.). Snort contains predefined rules that assign a fixed class type to specific rules. These class types are represented by the keyword *classification* (e.g., "Classification: Generic ICMP event" in the first entry) in the log entry. The next field in the row indicates the priority assigned to the rule that matches a particular packet. The lower the number, the higher the priority. The last field in the row is the packet's source and destination IP addresses. Sometimes these logs also include references to CVE (https://cve.mitre.org), Bugtracq (https://bugtraq.securityfocus.com/archive) databases from where more details about the attack detected can be found.

Intrusion prevention system (IPS) is a software or appliance which not only detects intrusions but also takes some corrective actions to safeguard the systems. This can be in the form of terminating an existing communication like resetting a TCP connection, placing the source of attack (IP address) on a blacklist, etc.

(iii) **DHCP Logs:** Dynamic host configuration protocol is used by many networks to dynamically assign IP addresses to hosts. Every time an IP address is assigned, it is done with a lease period. The logs generated by DHCP servers can be used to find out which physical machine within the network was given or assigned which IP address in the network at a particular time. The IP address information can be used to identify the user or owner of that system.

The DHCP client and server communicates via series of request-response messages. A sample output of DHCP server logs is shown in Figure 9.10. The first entry in Figure 9.10 is a DHCPDISCOVER(broadcast) packet sent from the client bearing MAC address 00:2a:55:cd:c9:12 using interface eth0. Upon reception of the DHCPDISCOVER message, the DCHP server picks one IP address from the available pool of IP addresses and replies to the client with a DHCPOFFER (IP address 12.10.1.1. in this case) as shown in entry 2. The client sends a DHCPREQUEST requesting the the offered IP address (12.10.1.1) in response to the DHCP offer. The client can request the IP address of its choice (12.10.1.5) in the same request. In response to the DHCPREQUEST, the server sends a DHCPACK message to the client assigning the offered IP address (12.10.1.1 in this case).

(iv) **DNS Logs:** Domain systems resolve the name queries raised by end systems to their IP addresses. These servers also keep log information about name resolutions done by different client systems. These logs will be simple and

```
2021 Dec 14 08:05:01 dhcp.abc.com  dhcpd:DHCPDISCOVER  from 00:2a:55:cd:c9:12 via eth0

2021 Dec 14 08:05:02 dhcp.abc.com  dhcpd:DHCPOFFER  on 12.10.1.1 to 00:2a:55:cd:c9:12 via eth0

2021 Dec 14 08:05:03 dhcp.prox.com dhcpd:DHCPREQUEST  for 12.10.1.1(12.10.1.5) from 00:2a:55:cd:c9:12 via eth0

2021 Dec 14 08:05:04 dhcp.prox.com dhcpd:DHCPACK  on 12.10.1.1 to 00:2a:55:cd:c9:12 via eth0
```

Figure 9.10 Sample DHCP server logs

Date and Time	Type	Prot	Dir	Remote IP	R/Q	Flags	Record Domain
01-02-2022 15:01:45	0710 PACKET 01C6F78B	UDP	Rcv	98.137.11.164	Q	[0001 D NOERROR] A	www.xyz.com
01-02-2022 15:01:45	0710 PACKET 01C6F78B	UDP	Snd	98.137.11.163	R Q	[0001 D NOERROR] A	www.spoofmails.com
01-02-2022 15:01:45	0710 PACKET 01C6F78B	UDP	Rcv	98.137.11.162	Q	[0001 D NOERROR] A	www.blacklist.com
01-02-2022 15:01:45	0710 PACKET 01C6F78B	UDP	Snd	98.137.11.161	R Q	[0001 D NOERROR] A	www.google.com
01-02-2022 15:01:45	0710 PACKET 01C6F78B	UDP	Snd	98.137.11.165	R Q	[0001 D NOERROR] A	www.yahoo.com

Figure 9.11 Sample DNS server logs.

contain the details of different domain names that have been queried and the timestamp of the query. These logs also come in handy and help to get the details of which all sites and services the user has accessed. For example, if a user visits a domain which is known to send spoofed emails, the name resolution query generated can be of use here which can indicate that such a domain name has been queried by the system (identified by its IP address).

A set of sample DNS logs are shown in Figure 9.11. The first column/field represents the date and time when a DNS client initiated the DNS query to the DNS server. The following field *Type* has three components Thread ID(0710), Context(Packet), and Internal packet identifier(01C6F78B), respectively. The next column *Proto* tells the layer four protocol (TCP/UDP), and the following field *Dir* indicates the direction of the DNS packet(Recieve/sent by the server). The next in the line is the *Remote IP* field indicating the IP address of the DNS client. The *R/Q* field indicates the message type(Query/Response). The *Flag* field represents various predefined flags. The *Flag* value "[0001 D NOERROR]A" indicates a DNS domain name is mapped to an IP address successfully without error. The field *Record Domain* indicates the domain name queried by the client.

9.2.3 Application Logs

Several applications running as network services also generate a rich set of logs which indicate different events happening within the application. These logs can be used to monitor the health of an application, different kind of errors generated, etc. There are a large number of applications which generate logs. Here we cover two popular application layer protocols as representative examples.

(i) **Hyper Text Transfer Protocol Logs:** Web servers and clients communicate using hyper text transport protocol (HTTP). The web server has the feature of keeping logs. These logs give feedback about the events and performance. The logs indicate the access, source of request, and also include a response code which indicates either success or failure of request.

A set of sample logs generated by Apache webserver is shown in Figure 9.12. Apache Server logs keep a track of visitors on a web server. The default log file is located at /var/ log/apache2/access.log. This log format and log file location can be changed as required. A row in a logfile contains the IP address of the visitor, Client ID (as per RFC 1413 identity), A username (via HTTP authentication),

VISITOR IP	CLIENT ID	USER NAME	TIMESTAMP	URL REQUESTED BY THE CLIENT	HTTP RESPONSE CODE	SIZE OF RETURNED OBJECT
1. 192.168.2.20	-	-	[28/Jan/2022:10:27:10 -0300]	"GET /ABC/ HTTP/1.1" - -	200	3395
2. 93.177.1.20	-	-	[29/Jan/2022:10:27:32 -0300]	"GET /img/t.jpg HTTP/1.1" --	300	
3. 23.23.25.10	-	-	[29/Jan/2022:10:27:35 -0300]	"GET /yer/ HTTP/1.1" --	404	7218
4. 120.11.23.34	-	-	[29/Jan/2022:12:04:05 +0100]	"POST /subm.pl/ HTTP/1.1"--	500	539

Figure 9.12 HTTP server logs.

```
CURRENT-TIME  TRANSFER-TIME  REMOTE-HOST  FILE-SIZE  FILENAME  TRANSFER-TYPE  SPECIAL-ACTION-FLAG
DIRECTION  ACCESS-MODE  USERNAME  SER\XADVICE-NAME  AUTHENTICATION-METHOD  AUTHENTICATED-USER-ID
COMPLETION-STATUS

Fri  Apr 1 09:52:00 2022  50  192.168.20.10  896242   /home/test/file1.tgz  b  _  o  r  uday  ftp  0  *  c
Fri  Apr 1 09:57:16 2022  289  192.168.20.10  8045867  /home/test2.tgz       b  _  o  r  uday  ftp  0  *  c
```

Figure 9.13 Sample FTP logs.

Timestamp, Actual request URL, HTTP Response Code (RFC2616 section 10), size of the object returned to the client, a reference URL and user agent string. A '–' (hyphen) in a log tuple indicates that the information is not available.

(ii) **File Transfer Protocol Logs:** File transfer protocol (FTP) is a client-server protocol used for transferring files over network. A FTP server solicits connections from clients and usually clients are asked to provide credentials using which users are authenticated. FTP defines a range of commands for this operation. Not all FTP servers keep logs and obviously there is no uniformity of details logged. A sample log file generated by ProFTPD which logs in */var/log/xferlog* is shown in Figure 9.13. The first entry indicates that a remote client 192.168.20.10 has downloaded a file /home/test/file1.tgz of 896242 bytes on Fri Apr 1, 2022, at local time 09:52:00, and the total transfer time is 50 seconds. The flag *transfer type* in the entry represents the file type of the transferred file (b=binary, a=ascii). Subsequent to flag *b* the next flag is the *special action flag* (C=Compressed, U=Uncompressed, T= Tarred, = No Action). The Flag *Direction* represents the direction of transfer (o=outgoing/download, i=incoming/upload, d= delete). The next Flag is the *access-mode* representing the access method by which user has logged in(a=anonymous, g=guest, r= real user). The next flag *username* (uday in the first entry) represents an authenticated user. The next field is the *service name* which is ftp in this case. The flag at the end represents the completion status of the transfer (c= complete, i= incomplete)

9.3 Need for Correlation

Although logs are great sources of information, these logs, when seen in isolation, may often not be of much help. Consider a network setup as shown in Figure 9.17. In this network, logs are generated at different levels. For example, consider the flow records generated by network switch shown in Figure 9.14, the first entry is showing a data transfer of 55000 bytes in 500 packets from a host 12.10.1.1 to another host

Date	Flow Start	Duration	Proto	Src IP Addr: Port		Dst IP Addr: Port	Packets	Bytes	Flows
2022-01-09	00:10:00:410	0.005	TCP	12.10.1.1:22	→	190.16.1.2:24801	500	55000	1
2022-01-09	00:10:00:383	0.001	TCP	190.16.1.1:24801	→	12.10.1.1:22	1	82	1
2022-01-09	00:00:00:289	0.001	TCP	19.168.0.2:32801	→	192.168.1.2:32901	1	156	1
2022-01-09	00:00:00:289	0.001	TCP	192.168.0.1:24801	→	192.168.0.2:32801	1	64	1

Figure 9.14 Sample flow records.

190.16.1.2. This record will just indicate some interaction and data exchange between two systems; however, in isolation this will not be good enough to conclude anything meaningful about any suspicious activity.

If the same set of flow records are correlated with logs generated either from the same source or from other sources, it may be leading to some useful conclusion. For example, if the same is viewed along with authentication logs shown in Figure 9.15, there are two entries which show that a remote login using SSH service was done from the IP address 190.16.1.2 using the username ubuntu. Now the login event and a large amount of data transfer as seen in the flow record of Figure 14 are in the vicinity of time. First a user logged in from that IP address and subsequently some data transfer took place. Further the IP address offered to the machine in question (inside the target network) can be found using the logs of the DHCP server as shown in Figure 9.16. The whole sequence of events in chronological order can be summarized as shown below.

1. 2022 Jan 09 00:00:01 - Internal server sends a DHCP DISCOVER message to get an IP address to DHCP server.
2. 2022 Jan 09 00:00:02 - DHCP server offers IP address 12.10.1.1 to internal server which it subsequently configures.
3. 2022 Jan 09 00:08:07 - External user ubuntu connects with a key from 190.16.1.2 which is accepted by the server as seen from *auth.log* file.
4. 2022 Jan 00:08:09 - A new session is opened for user ubuntu.

1. Jan 09 00:08:07 ip-10-77-20-248 sshd[1361]: Accepted publickey for ubuntu from 190.16.1.2 port 22901 ssh2: RSA SHA256:KI8KPGZrTiZ7g4FO1

2. Jan 09 00:08:09 ip-10-77-20-248 systemd-logind[1118]: New session 1 of user ubuntu.

Figure 9.15 Authentication logs.

2022 Jan 09 00:00:01 dhcp.xyz.com dhcpd:DHCPDISCOVER from 00:8a:75:ab:c5:11 via eth0

2022 Jan 09 00:00:01 dhcp.xyz.com dhcpd:DHCPOFFER on 12.10.1.1 to 00:8a:75:ab:c5:11 via eth0

Figure 9.16 DHCP server logs.

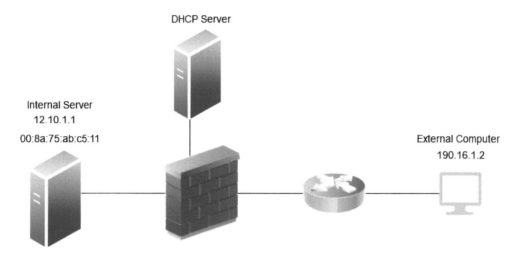

Figure 9.17 Network setup and activity evidence sources.

5. 2022 Jan 09 00:10:00 - A flow start from 12.10.1.1 to 190.16.1.2 lasting 5 seconds and transmitting 55 000 bytes of data in 500 packets.

In addition to the above evidence, if the file transfer is done though the scp command, the same can also be viewed from the history of commands from the target system. Further evidence can also be gathered from other logs and activities on the system and correlated to increase confidence in a hypothesis.

9.4 Correlation Techniques

The activities performed by the users in the network are recorded as events at various places beginning from the end hosts, network applications, security applications, and network elements. In order to investigate cyber security events and incidents, these logs are considered as sources of information and correlated (Qin et al. 2018). As mentioned previously, logs/events from IDS are correlated with other types of security evidence collected from different security components like Zeek (https://zeek.org), NetFlow (https://www.cisco.com/c/en/us/td/docs/ios-xml/ios/fnetflow/configuration/15-mt/fnf-15-mt-book.html), firewalls (https://www.cisco.com/c/en_in/products/security/firewalls/index.html), etc. The correlation can be done in two ways

1. Manually: done with an expert examining the evidence and assigning some meaning to the events as seen in the logs. This is a tedious process and a large number of logs generated will quickly overwhelm the expert.
2. Through SIEM Tools: security incident and event management (SIEM) tools automate the task of correlating the logs. These tools receive the logs from different sources and bring them into a common format which can be used for correlation. Several commercial players have developed SIEM solutions.

SolarWinds Security Event Manager (https://www.solarwinds.com/secu rity-event-manager), Micro Focus ArcSight ESM (https://www.microfocus. com/en-us/cyberres/secops/arcsight-esm), Splunk Enterprise Security (https:// www.splunk.com/en_us/software/enterprise-security.html), LogRhythm Next Gen SIEM (https://logrhythm.com/solutions/security/siem), IBM QRadar (https://www.ibm.com/qradar/security-qradar-siem), McAfee Enterprise Security Manager (https://www.mcafee.com/enterprise/en-in/products/enterprise-secu rity-manager.html) are some popular examples.

A generic view of event correlation as done by SIEM tools is shown in Figure 9.18 where logs collected at different places are taken as input and processed to assign some meaning to the sequence of events. A typical correlation operation has the following three main operations.

(i) **Filtering:** normally log files are large and bulky for processing. Thus the unwanted log information can be safely filtered and only events which are of value can be considered. This filtering operation is dependent on the kind of analysis a forensic expert is carrying out and to a great extent is context dependent. For example, in the event of unauthorized logins and port scans, a security analyst may wish to see the system logs and NetFlow records to identify active connections with the compromised machines in the vicinity of time. The following three generic principles are used for filtering unwanted information.

   1. Events in temporal vicinity: if an event which triggers some suspicion is taken as reference and then other events (from other sources) in the close proximity of time are considered for correlation. This reduces the search space considerably.

   2. Events sharing common attributes: attributes of an activity are considered and logs of other sources are searched for entries sharing common attrib- utes. The ones which do not meet this criteria can be filtered leaving only a handful of logs to correlate.

   3. Hybrid methods: here both methods are used for identifying events which are probably of interest for correlation.

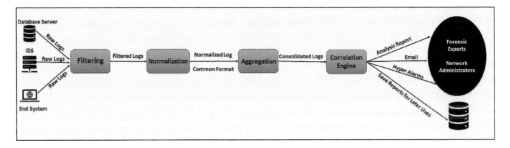

Figure 9.18 Log analysis process flow.

(ii) **Normalization:** the next step in the process is normalization. This is an essential step as security components and devices by different vendors follow different formats for event logging. Normalization takes filtered raw log data as input and parses them to convert log data into a standard format (containing the IP address, username, timestamp, event type, etc.). The normalization process often uses regular expressions to parse log data to extract the fields of interest. For example, it can search for IP addresses in the event log data as it represents the unique identity of devices in the network. To a larger extent, public IP addresses are traceable and can be mapped to reveal the geographical location of the machines communicating in the network. For digital forensics, it is a required field to extract for correlation to identify victim/attacker machines in a security breach. As we know, IP addresses are represented as the dotted-decimal string (for IPV4) xx.xx.xx.xx; the following Perl compatible regular expression (PCRE) will help extract an IP address: /[0-9]{1,3}\.[09]{1,3}\ [0-9].{1,3}\ [0-9].{1,3}/

The above regex catches any string of form xx.xx.xx.xx where x represents a decimal number, but when we talk about IP addresses, we care about only valid IP addresses. The valid IP addresses (public/private) ranges from 0.0.0.0-255.255.255.255. So we need to refine the above regex with additional options to capture valid IP addresses. The following regular expression will help extract a valid IP address:

```
^([01]?\d{0,2}?|2[0-4]\d|25[0-5])\.
([01]?[0-9]{0,2}?|2[0-4]\d|25[0-5])\.
([01]?[0-9]{0,2}?|2[0-4]\d|25[0-5])\.
([01]?[0-9]{0,2}?|2[0-4]\d|25[0-5])$
```

(iii) **Aggregation:** at this stage, repeated logs indicating the same events sharing common attributes are consolidated. This is based on the premise that repeated logs of same attack add nothing extra to the knowledge of understanding the cyber attack methods. For example, logs indicating port scans from the same source do not add any value to the existing understanding.

(iv) **Correlation:** this establishes some relationship between events. These events in our case are recorded in the form of logs. In digital forensics, forensic experts use correlation to uncover the hidden story behind events that happened during a cyber crime. Network administrators and professionals use correlation to discover attack scenarios. In the log analysis process, the correlation engine accepts normalized log records and identifies relationships between the events. The correlation can be done using different methods (Hubballi and Suryanarayanan 2014). Some of the major correlation techniques used for log analysis are described below.

Knowledge-based correlation: this scheme correlates the knowledge base generated from the target network. This knowledge base includes the details of operating systems running on different machines, event database collected from these machines, applications running on hosts and their known vulnerabilities (if any), configuration of the hardware and software of the machine being monitored. This will help to look for relevant information from these systems. For example, suppose a system is suspected of being used for accessing a banking account illegally, knowledge of the operating system running on this system will help to identify other sources of information. If it is a Windows machine the .lnk files can be searched to find all the activities the user has carried out when the user was logged in.

Rule-based correlation: in this case well-known attack patterns are coded as ruleset in the SIEM tools. They can collect logs from security perimeter devices such as firewalls, IDS, IPS, and also from end hosts to gather evidence of a cyber incident. The rules are in the form of *if-then-else* statements and are based on logs generated from different devices. For example, a rule can specify the order of events from a DHCP server, flow record and authentication logs as discussed in Section 9.3. Many commercial SIEM tools like Splunk (https://www.splunk.com/en_us/software/enterprise-security.html) operate using rules for correlation. However, this method requires a rule to be written for every possible correlation. A limitation of this method is that any events for which rules are not written cannot be correlated. Further a strict order among the events and their timing can lead to missed opportunities for possible correlation.

Fusion-based correlation: in fusion-based correlation, multiple layers of correlation are performed for event analysis. After normalization and preprocessing, correlation based on different criteria is performed at each layer creating a hyper alarm. At the initial stage, logs from multiple IDS are fused using spatial behavior, and in the later stages, temporal fusion is done to order logs based on timing information.

Multi-step correlation: this is helpful in modeling complex attacks involving a series of events. Complex attacks can be visualized as a multi-step chain of events, and the logs generated for such events may represent the symptoms of an attack. The assumption is based on the fact that hackers perform a sequence of actions before breaking into the system. For example, consider that an attacker has accessed the email account of some other user using a system. In this case a login event to that system is a prerequisite to the login timing. Such essential relationships among the events are modeled with a *requires/provides* relationship. The next event log will be meaningful if the previous one exists. Several authors (Yu and Frincke 2004) have proposed formal models like Colored-Petri-Nets and LAMBDA (Cuppens and Ortalo 2000) to represent such relationships.

Attack graph based Correlation: these methods (Lallie et al. 2020; Roschke et al. 2011) generate a model of an attack using graphs where each node in the graph represents events/paths/alarms, and the edges represent the relationship between the nodes. It sets a particular target and the goal is to find a sequence of nodes and paths to reach a target. It detects the pattern and the path used by the attacker to carry out the attack. Assume the attacker has set a goal of installing some malicious software like keylogger on a target machine X. One way is for the attacker to directly login to machine X and try installing the malware. This may leave a trace of this attack and can be identified with the previous methods. However, the attacker can use intermediate machines to hide their actions and create confusion in the correlation. Attack graph models build possible paths that an attacker can take to break into a system. It captures all possible paths that an attacker can take to reach a target. An attack is detected and evidence is collected if any of the possible paths can lead to the goal.

Causal relation based correlation: these methods try to identify whether there is some kind of causal relationship among the logs. The causal relationship-based correlation method analyzes a given random set of alarms by creating a directed acyclic graph (DAG). The nodes in the DAG represent logs/events, and the edges represent the relationships. This type of correlation method is helpful in correlating unknown logs to identify novel attack patterns. The relationship is defined using a set of attributes like IP addresses, port numbers, protocol fields, etc.

9.5 Conclusions

Event logs are generated at different places like computer systems, network devices, and applications. These logs capture the digital footprints of a cyber crime. In this chapter, we discussed the sources of logs, their formats, and how they can be used in forensic investigation. Correlation of event logs help further understand the patterns, methods used to commit cyber crime. We discussed the steps involved in correlation and also different correlation techniques using logs generated by different sources.

References

Al Mutawa, N., Bryce, J., Franqueira, V.N., and Marrington, A. (2016). Forensic investigation of cyberstalking cases using behavioural evidence analysis. *Digital Investigation* 16: S96–S103.

Chandola, V., Banerjee, A., and Kumar, V. (2009). Anomaly detection: a survey. *ACM Computing Surveys* 41 (3).

Cuppens, F. and Ortalo, R. (2000). Lambda: a language to model a database for detection of attacks. In: *Recent Advances in Intrusion Detection*.

Cyber Harassment Cases, Bureau of Police Research & Development. https://police.py.gov.in.

https://bugtraq.securityfocus.com/archive.

https://cve.mitre.org.

https://sflow.org.

https://www.cisco.com/c/en/us/td/docs/ios-xml/ios/fnetflow/configuration/15-mt/fnf-15-mt-book.html.

https://www.cisco.com/c/en_in/products/security/firewalls/index.html.

https://www.ibm.com/qradar/security-qradar-siem.

https://www.juniper.net/us/en/search.html.

https://www.mcafee.com/enterprise/en-in/products/enterprise-security-manager.html.

https://www.microfocus.com/en-us/cyberres/secops/arcsight-esm.

https://logrhythm.com/solutions/security/siem.

https://www.pfsense.org.

https://www.snort.org.

https://www.solarwinds.com/security-event-manager.

https://www.splunk.com/en_us/software/enterprise-security.html.

https://www.tcpdump.org.

https://www.wireshark.org.

https://zeek.org.

Hubballi, N. and Suryanarayanan, V. (2014). False alarm minimization techniques in signature-based intrusion detection systems: a survey. *Computer Communications* 49: 1–17.

Lallie, H.S., Debattista, K., and Bal, J. (2020). A review of attack graph and attack tree visual syntax in cyber security. *Computer Science Review* 35: 100219.

Marshall, A.M. (2009). *Digital Forensics: Digital Evidence in Criminal Investigations*, 1e. Wiley Publishing.

Qin, T., Gao, Y., Wei, L. et al. (2018). Potential threats mining methods based on correlation analysis of multi-type logs. *IET Networks* 7: 1–7.

Roesch, M. (1999). Snort - lightweight intrusion detection for networks. In: *LISA '99: Proceedings of the 13th USENIX Conference on System Administration*. USENIX Association, USA, 229–238.

Roschke, S., Cheng, F., and Meinel, C. (2011). A new alert correlation algorithm based on attack graph. In: *CISIS'11: Proceedings of the 4th International Conference on Computational Intelligence in Security for Information Systems*, 58–67.

Spotting the Adversary with Windows Event Log Monitoring, National Security Agency. https://cryptome.org/2014/01/nsa-windows-event.pdf.

Yu, D. and Frincke, D. (2004 January) A novel framework for alert correlation and understanding. In: *International Conference on Applied Cryptography and Network Security*, Springer Verlag.

CHAPTER 10

(Hyper-)graph Analysis and its Application in Forensics

Marcel Worring

Informatics Institute, University of Amsterdam, GH, The Netherlands

10.1 Introduction

Deep learning has changed the analysis of unstructured data sources such as imagery and text in a drastic manner. The accuracy of automatic analysis for basic tasks such as classification of images, speech recognition, or named entity extraction in text has reached human performance and sometimes has even gone beyond it. Forensic tasks are more complex, but also here tremendous progress is being made. Automatic methods have become an important aid to the forensic investigator.

Most of the basic tasks and the well known deep learning methods for addressing them are based on the analysis of individual items such as an image, a document, or a speech fragment of a single person. But in large-scale forensic investigations there are so many more information channels. The evidence of one suspect can have multiple items within one modality or can have multiple modalities with related information. Evidence can also come with contextual information such as time or location leading to groups of items in the same period or region. Suspects can also be part of a criminal network. For forensic investigation we should go beyond single items and pay particular attention to all the possible relations and groupings among the different items.

There are many important examples of potential areas in forensics where relations and groupings are present. Here we consider a number of them.

Social network forensics (Mulazzani et al. 2012) can provide the social footprint of the social network that the suspect is part of. Mulazzani et al. identified a number of forensic questions: 1) What is the social graph of the user, and, in particular with whom are they connected and which friends can be identified? 2) How is the network used for communicating, what method is used for that, and with whom is the user communicating? 3) What pictures and videos were

---

Artificial Intelligence (AI) in Forensic Sciences, First Edition. Edited by Zeno Geradts and Katrin Franke.
© 2024 John Wiley & Sons Ltd. Published 2024 by John Wiley & Sons Ltd.

uploaded by the user, on which other people's pictures are they tagged? 4) When is a specific user connected to the social network, when exactly did a specific activity of interest took place? 5) What apps is the user using, what is their purpose, and what information can be inferred in the social context? Many more examples can be found in the survey given in Karabyiyi et al. (2016). In both papers, relations among items are the core of social network forensics, but also groupings along various dimensions.

As a second example consider cyberattacks as described in Berman et al. (2019). Here deep learning is also coming to the forefront of analysis where the goal is usually to classify a given application as malware or detect an intrusion. The features needed for solving these tasks are only partially embedded in the piece of software used in the attack or exhibited in its direct behaviour. Important information is found in the path the software has taken, the execution graph of the software, or the spreading pattern of the software. All of these require integration of item-based approaches with network analysis.

Predicting communication in an enterprise is a third example. It is especially relevant to find communication that is unexpected. i.e., deviating from the normal communication flows. It can provide valuable forensic evidence (Graus et al. 2014) and form the basis for reconstructing the events in fraud cases such as the well known Enron case. Obviously mere entities are not sufficient as the most relevant information is present in the communication between the entities.

Finally, in fintech forensics defined in Nikkel (2020) as "the application of digital forensic science to financial technologies for the purpose of investigating and reconstructing criminal financial activity" there are also various opportunities for using automatic techniques. Nikkel suggests focusing applied forensic research on the following three activities: 1) understanding the flow and transfer of money, 2) criminal attribution, helping law enforcement identify individuals, 3) anomaly detection, finding technical methods to detect technical fraud in progress, 4) correlating banking infrastructure and transaction logs with criminal activity. What we again see is that the information that is needed to study such types of criminal activity is based on relating items (transactions from one account to the other), relations between channels (infrastructure and logs), and analyzing information in context (criminal attribution).

The basic methods for analyzing networks are based on graph algorithms and social network analysis, see e.g., Tang and Huan (2010). More recently there has been substantial interest in using deep learning-based methods for analyzing graph information. This not only allows incorporation of data-driven relations, but also incorporation of knowledge graphs in a well-founded manner. But graphs are not rich enough to describe the grouping of objects and their relations, so a level up in richness of representation are hypergraphs which are similar to graphs in the sense that they are also comprised of nodes and edges, but every edge can now contain one, two, or more nodes. Clearly a graph is simply a hypergraph where every edge contains exactly two nodes.

So we now have a rich set of new methods for representing data and deep learning methods to use them in various basic relation and group related tasks. They have potential, but forensics poses several specific constraints on the process. We are particularly interested in how to assure fairness, accountability, and transparency for such new methods. This is still a new topic of exciting research, with a lot of promise for visualizations to explain and support the decisions.

The rest of this chapter is organized as follows. We start with a basic survey of different analysis methods for graphs and hypergraphs. After that we consider the explainability and visualization of graphs and hypergraphs. Finally, we consider how we could move forward and bring (hyper-)graph-based analysis to the forensic toolbox.

10.2 Survey of Methods

10.2.1 Preliminaries

A graph is defined as $G(V,E)$ where V is a set of nodes and E the set of edges capturing the relations between the nodes as illustrated in Figure 10.1. In its most general form, both the nodes and the edges can have types and attributes. For example in a social network the nodes can be individuals which can have their name and day of birth as attributes. The edges can then, e.g., correspond to *is-family*, *is-reporting-to*, or *has-communicated-with* relations. In a graph the edges can be undirected or directed. In this chapter we will mostly consider undirected graphs, but most methods generalize to directed graphs as well.

There are two common ways to represent the relations in a graph, namely as an adjacency matrix or as an incidence matrix. An adjacency matrix is square where both dimensions are equal to the number of nodes. A value of 1 means that the

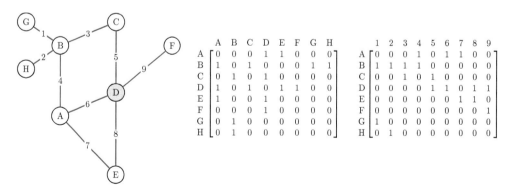

Figure 10.1 Graph representation. Example graph with 8 nodes and 9 edges and its corresponding adjacency and incidence matrices. Note that here we consider the simple case of an unweighted graph. The entries in the matrices could, e.g., also be weights rather than binary values. Source: created by author.

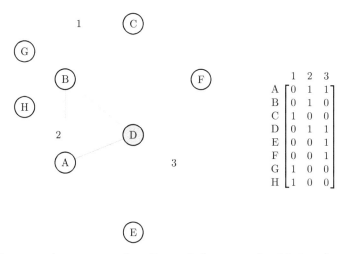

Figure 10.2 Hypergraph representation. Example hypergraph with 8 nodes and 3 hyperedges and its corresponding incidence matrix. Note that in this case we have drawn hyperedges as connected regions but that is not mandatory. Source: created by author.

two corresponding nodes are connected by an edge in the graph, and a value of 0 means they are not. An incidence matrix has the nodes as rows and the edges as columns. In this case a value of 1 indicates that the corresponding node is an endpoint of the corresponding edge and 0 if not.

In modern machine learning methods the core of graph analysis is to use embeddings. The embedding of a node $v_i \in V$ is a low-dimensional vector z_i which incorporates as much structural information of the neighborhood of the node in the graph as possible. Thus, all information in the graph is now represented as a set of $|V|$ vectors.

Hypergraphs (see Figure 10.2) take the notion of relations a step further and allow edges to connect an arbitrary number of nodes instead of restricting it to two.

10.2.2 Tasks

A graph is a complex information structure for which specific methods are needed. But when represented as a set of vectors we can use a wide array of standard techniques to perform the analysis. In particular we can do the following (see Hamilton et al. (2017a)):

- Visualization and pattern discovery: graphs are traditionally visualized as node-link diagrams. The disadvantage of this is that the nodes have an arbitrary position. Embeddings provide an alternative and there are many techniques for mapping a set of vectors to two dimensions so that the whole datasets can be displayed on the screen. Prominent examples of techniques are t-SNE (van der Maaten and Hinton 2008) and UMAP (McInnes et al. 2018). The resulting visualizations can reveal patterns of interest such as communities, outliers, and global structure. One has to be aware, however, that the mapping to two dimensions comes with an inherent information loss so observations have to be verified in the original space.

- Clustering and community detection: automatic clustering techniques can find groups in the data and techniques for doing so are many (Xu and jie Tian 2015). Different techniques find different types of groups and the critical parameter to determine is the number of clusters which can be set manually or automatically, but this always comes with some assumptions.
- Node classification and semi-supervised learning: these are general techniques where you have a limited set of nodes for which you have labels and the classification algorithm is capable of classifying nodes in the graph for which such labels are not available. Clearly the results rely on the assumption that the labels you use for training are representative for the (unknown) set of labels that you need to predict. Especially when using a limited, potentially interactively defined, set of training nodes this comes with a level of uncertainty for the predictions.
- Link prediction: in a similar way as predicting nodes, we can can also predict the existence or attributes of edges. The edges are only implicitly captured in the embedding, but as we will see later they can still be predicted. Again care has to be taken when interpreting the result.

10.2.3 Graph Neural Networks

To get a better understanding of the way we can compute embeddings for graphs, we again follow the excellent survey presented in Hamilton et al. (2017a) where they define a unifying framework to structure existing methods by categorizing them by the choices they make along four dimensions. The framework and corresponding dimensions are illustrated in Figure 10.3.

The general framework to unify existing methods is based on the encoder-decoder framework. In this framework the nodes in the graph are first encoded by mapping them to the lower dimensional embedding which captures information on the node as well as its relations. The decoding step is the reverse step namely going from the embedding to a graph which could aim for a full reconstruction of the graph or specific tasks such as predicting node labels or the neighbors of a node. Given that the embedding is only an approximation of all information in the graph, the graph resulting after decoding is also only an approximation of the original graph. The basic idea of learning a graph representation is that if the decoded graph approximates the information in the original graph well, then the embedding of the graph is also useful for the tasks identified in the previous section.

In the encoding-decoding framework there are four essential functions which determine the characteristics of the method. We will now elaborate on these four dimensions.

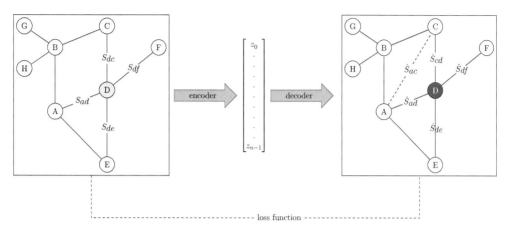

Figure 10.3 Abstract view of different methods to learn graph embedding methods. The similarity function S measures the strength between different nodes in the graph. The encoder computes for a node, as example here D, a latent representation, i.e., an embedding Z capturing as much information on the node D and its neighbors as possible. The decoder reconstructs as much of the information as possible. This leads to new similarities ($\hat{S}$), also between edges previously not connected (dashed line), and updated attributes for the node. The loss function measures the difference between the original data and the reconstructed data. Source: created by author.

1. A **pairwise similarity function** gives a measure of the relation between two nodes. This can be as simple as an indication whether they are connected by an edge (1) or not (0), directly related to the adjacency matrix, but could also be a measure based on their attributes or on their local neighborhoods.
2. An **encoder function** determines how a node is mapped to the embedding, this is typically the function that has parameters that can be optimized to find the best embedding.
3. A **decoder function** reconstructs the graph from its embedding. In most cases the function takes two nodes and gives an approximation of their pairwise similarity. This function in the various methods does not have trainable parameters.
4. A **loss function** measures how well the reconstructed graph, in particular the similarity between nodes, approximates the original graph.

By varying these functions a variety of different methods are possible and Hamilton et al. (2017a) describes many of them. It goes beyond the scope of this chapter to go into the details of all those methods. Here we will focus in particular on neighbor autoencode methods with as prominent examples graph convolutional networks (GCNs) T.N. (Kipf and Welling 2017) and GraphSAGE (Hamilton et al. 2017b).

Both GCNs and GraphSage aggregate local information from the neighborhood of a node to compute the embedding of the node. To do so, they typically employ other information on the node which, e.g., in a graph where nodes correspond to images could be tags associated with the image or a vector capturing the visual features of the image associated with the node, but could also be based on graph characteristics of the node such as the number of neighbors. To aggregate information from a local neighborhood the basic method for doing so is called graph convolutional network. This aggregation is done in an iterative manner and is, hence, similar to what is happening in standard convolutional neural networks where the neighborhood from which information is aggregated is effectively getting larger and larger.

GCNs and GraphSage differ in the way they aggregate the information from the local neighborhood and also how they incorporate information from the previous iteration. GCNs follow, in that respect, an approach that is very similar to what is used in convolutional networks, but instead of using a square neighborhood on a rectangular grid they use the set of connected nodes as neighborhood. GraphSage uses a different function to aggregate information from the local neighborhoods in addition to the simple weighted sum used in GCNs. The method combines information from the previous iteration and the new information in a concatenated representation instead of replacing the old information with a weighted result of the previous and the current information.

The most important advantages of methods like GraphSage over other methods is that they are inductive, they can also say something about nodes which have not been seen during training of the network, while many other methods are transductive only.

Hypergraphs, as a concept, have already been around for a long time (Berge 1973) and methods for learning representations for hypergraphs and using them for various tasks are many (Gao et al. 2020). Several methods see hypergraphs as a special case of graphs. So the typical approach for working with hypergraphs is to develop a method for mapping the nodes and hyperedges in the hypergraph to a graph-based structure and then apply any of the existing graph-based methods. Examples of this are Bai et al. (2021) and Feng et al. (2019) who use clique expansion to convert to a graph while Yadati et al. (2019) extends this with specific nodes acting as mediators.

Seeing hypergraphs as special instances of graphs is conceptually wrong. In fact, it is the other way around. Any regular graph can trivially be modeled as a hypergraph by restricting the number of nodes in every hyperedge to be exactly two. But it is not only conceptually wrong. When mapping the hypergraph to a regular graph essential information on relations between nodes is lost (Arya et al. 2021). Methods are needed that work directly on the hypergraph without requiring graphs as an intermediate representation.

Spectral methods have been developed for directly learning a representation for a hypergraph (Bruna 2014). These methods extend approaches like Kipf and Welling (2017) and have the advantage that they fully leverage the information that is present within the hypergraph. Their major limitation, similar to spectral methods for regular graphs, is that they are restricted to transductive learning, so they can only predict new hyperedges based on the nodes used in learning the representation.

Recently, methods have been proposed that use message passing on hypergraphs, e.g., Arya et al. (2021) and Ding et al. (2020) who are extending upon the same methods as Hamilton et al. (2017b). In particular Arya et al. (2021) define a two level message passing approach (see Figure 10.4). In the first level the vectors of attributes corresponding to each node are aggregated. The simplest aggregation method would be taking the average. As there can be many nodes in a hyperedge we can use adaptive sampling when needed to reduce the computational load. In the second level, for nodes that are part of multiple hyperedges, the aggregated information from the various hyperedges in which such a node is present is combined. By appropriate choices of the aggregation functions information loss is minimized. The reference shows that the generalized means as aggregation function satisfies a number of desired properties while being very versatile. By using the above message passing approach, the full information in the hypergraph is leveraged and at the same time inference on the hypergraphs becomes

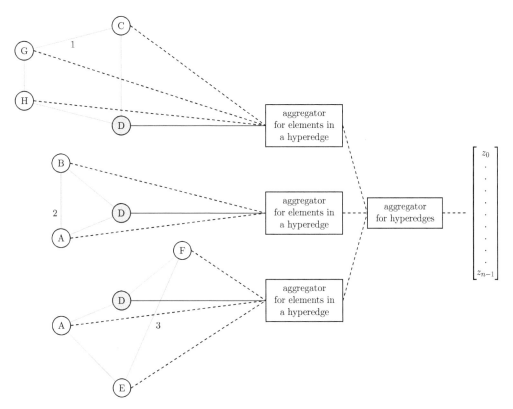

Figure 10.4 Two-level message passing. To learn a representation Z for a node (here D) first messages are propagated between nodes within a hyperedge and subsequently aggregated. Then, at the second level, the information from different hyperedges in which the node is present are aggregated.

inductive and thus can predict nodes and hyperedges even on nodes that have not been seen during training. Message passing on hypergraphs is a promising avenue for working with the large complexity of data in forensics.

10.3 Explainability and Visualization

In any field where critical decisions are made the use of AI methods requires specific care of the decision maker and the system to assure informed final decisions. Forensics is a prototypical example of a field where this is essential. With complex artificial neural network models as the basic machine learning machinery, it is not sufficient to have accurate decisions. The method should also be able to explain how it came to its predictions. It comes at no surprise that explainable AI (XAI) has become a highly active research topic with many methods being developed to support the expert user.

To get a better understanding of what XAI really means, NIST has defined four principles that AI systems should honor before they can be considered XAI (Phillips et al. 2021):

1. Explanation: this principle states that an AI system must supply evidence, support, or reasoning for each decision made by the system.

In forensics this means that the system should be able to explain what decisions are made in every layer of the network from the level of features to the final interpretations. Likelihood ratios (Ramos et al. 2017) are an important tool for reporting the value of the evidence. For neural networks methods have recently been developed that can report LLRs, e.g., for speaker verification (van Leeuwen and Brümmer 2013) and face recognition (Rodriguez et al. 2020). How to compute LLRs for graphs and hypergraphs is still an open challenge.

2. Meaningful: this principle states that the explanation provided by the AI system must be understandable by, and meaningful to, its users. As different groups of users may have different needs and experiences, the explanation provided by the AI system must be fine-tuned to meet the various characteristics and needs of each group.

This is a complex principle as in forensic investigations several stakeholders are involved ranging from the forensic expert to the judge and the defense and in some cases even the general public. Clearly, each of these user groups needs a different level of explanation all of which should be consistent with the evidence the system bases its decisions on.

3. Accuracy: this principle states that the explanation provided by the AI system must reflect accurately the system's processes.

That a system's explanation is meaningful doesn't mean it is accurate. In machine learning there are many different metrics for determining the performance of a system. For forensics it is particularly important that the decision is unbiased not favoring the prosecution or the defense. Again likelihood ratios are a good mechanism to weigh the evidence in an unbiased manner.

4. Knowledge limits: this principle states that AI systems must identify cases that they were not designed to operate in and, therefore, their answers may not be reliable.

This holds for AI systems and experts alike, they both have to know their limits. Yet, every forensic case is different where we have to rely on our knowledge and expertise to make the right decision. AI systems in forensics capable of determining their own limitations are still virtually non-existent.

For general convolutional neural networks an extensive variety of methods have been developed which explain how they come to certain decisions. For image-based networks this mostly results in heatmaps indicating how certain parts of the image contribute to the final class prediction. Several of these methods have now been extended to graph convolutional networks where next to coloring the different nodes in the network, using the equivalent of heatmaps, methods also aim at finding textual descriptions which explain the decision in terms of the relations in the graph. A good survey of different methods is provided in Yuan et al. (2020), providing a taxonomy to structure different methods, generic architectures for the various classes of methods, and a unified open-source implementation of several of the methods. Here we will briefly consider their taxonomy and see how they would apply in forensic investigations.

The taxonomy starts with a major decomposition into instance level and model level explanations. The former give data-dependent explanations and form the bulk of existing methods, the later aim to give a true understanding of the model and only few methods for doing so exist. They both have their use and in future systems we can expect components of both to be present. We will start by going through the different instance-level explanations.

- Gradients/features: this is most common way of explaining decisions. To measure the importance of nodes/edges in the graph, gradients and feature maps in different layers of the network are considered to assess their impact on the final decision by using backpropagation through the network and interpolation to map it to the input.

  These generic methods will be important in several steps of a forensic investigation. In the exploratory phase they can provide guidance in finding relevant areas of the search space giving aggregated indications why such areas could be of potential importance or an informed way of stating that certain areas are not relevant. When the networks have a probabilistic component the instance level visualizations could be given a clear probabilistic interpretation.
- Perturbations: explain the decisions by studying the impact of small changes to the input on the final decision with the aim to identify which parts of the input are essential and which parts can vary without impacting the decision.

For forensics these methods provide a good way to assess the value of the evidence, assuring it is based on robust observations and not on elements which are based on minor changes that would alter the decision. Here, we can make the perturbations probabilistic to study its impact on the decisions. In this case, even when the network itself is not probabilistic, measures of confidence can be created.

- Surrogate: explain decisions by employing a simple model with high explainability and apply it locally around the input for which an explanation is needed assuming that locally the full complexity of the graph convolutional network is not needed.

  With good surrogate models these methods could prove very useful in forensics. As we can separate the analysis model and the explanation model we could design the surrogate model in such a way that it follows sound forensic principles even when the underlying complex model is based on existing architectures over which we have little control.

- Decomposition: explain decisions by decomposing the prediction scores at the top level of the network and follow such decomposition all the way down to the input level.

  When the decomposition leads to meaningful subdivisions of the input and its features these methods are very helpful. They can potentially also be used in conjunction with general hand-crafted feature-based approaches to see whether they align or not.

  The final class of methods are the methods aimed at model-level explanations which are based on

- Generation: given a specific task such as maximizing target prediction, these methods generate the input graphs that would make this happen.

  Although these methods give the best understanding of the model in the network, they might not be the most suitable for forensic investigation. We will often not be optimizing the network for a certain task but using the best available network for the task and are interested in how it works on the specific input that we have.

The survey above gives a good set of methods to work with for graph-based models. To explain hypergraph models there are no such methods, probably because of their versatility and hence inherent complexity. There are, however, a number of visual analytics solutions for analyzing hypergraphs to make working with them easier. The survey in Fischer et al. (2021) gives several methods with Valdivia et al. (2021), Agarwal and Beck (2020), and Fischer et al. (2020) as the best examples. As an example of such a system we elaborate on Fischer et al. (2020) arguably the most comprehensive of the methods described allowing interactive analysis of dynamically evolving hypergraphs. The basis interface of the system is shown in Figure 10.5 for the example of interactively analyzing a text forum. The core of the interface is a matrix-based visualization directly related to the incidence matrix. Dark colors indicate that the user in the specific row is related to the specific forum topic represented

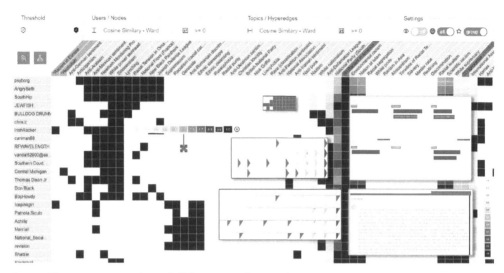

Figure 10.5 Hyper-Matrix. A full hypergraph visualization system (Fischer et al. 2020) in which the expert can visually explore the hypergraph and can interactively ingest knowledge into the analysis. Source: Screendump created by Max Fisher specifically for this paper.

in the columns. There are two elements that make the system special. First, the interface has what is known as semantic zooming. Depending on how many elements are visible the visualization switches from a simple colored square up to a visualization of the number of posts and finally to the actual text of the posts. The second innovation is how an investigator can ingest knowledge into the system. By interactively indicating that a hyperedge is missing, i.e., a relation between a user and a topic, a ripple effect is generated that not only locally affects the results but also has an effect on hyperedges and nodes further away. By interactively updating the hyperedges the investigator can thus more and more steer the final decisions. It goes, of course, without saying, that explicit care has to be taken that decisions remain taken on the basis of genuine evidence and knowledge and that the provenance of the steps taken in the course of the investigations should be carefully kept.

10.4 Conclusion

Forensic case data is shifting more and more to large multimodal collections and with it the importance of relations among items and grouping of those items are needed to understand the full complexity of the evidence. Graphs and hypergraphs are the appropriate way to represent such relations and with the advent of deep learning, a set of interesting tools have become available to analyze large and complex graphs and hypergraphs. But deep learning is more of a blackbox than traditional machine learning methods so making methods explainable is essential, especially in a forensic context. Interactive systems based on deep learned representations which support interactive exploration by forensic experts create the synergy to stay ahead of the complexity of the evidence.

References

Agarwal, S. and Beck, F. (2020). Set streams: visual exploration of dynamic overlapping sets. *Computer Graphics Forum* 39.

Arya, D., Gupta, D.K., Rudinac, S., and Worring, M. (2021). Adaptive neural message passing for inductive learning on hypergraphs. https://arxiv.org/abs/2109.10683 (submitted to IEEE PAMI).

Bai, S., Zhang, F., and Torr, P.H.S. (2021). Hypergraph convolution and hypergraph attention. *Pattern Recognition* 110.

Berge, C. (1973). *Graphs and Hypergraphs*. Amsterdam: North-Holland.

Berman, D.S., Buczak, A.L., Chavis, J.S., and Corbett, C.L. (2019). A survey of deep learning methods for cyber security. *Information* 10 (4).

Bruna, J. (2014). Spectral networks and deep locally connected networks on graphs. In: *International Conference on Learning Representations ICLR*.

Ding, K., Wang, J., Jundong, L. et al. (2020). Be more with less: hypergraph attention networks for inductive text classification. In: *Proceedings of the 2020 Conference on Empirical Methods in Natural Language Processing*.

Dongkuan, X. and Jie Tian, Y. (2015). A comprehensive survey of clustering algorithms. *Annals of Data Science* 2: 165–193.

Feng, Y., You, H., Zhang, Z. et al. (2019). Hypergraph neural networks. *Proceedings of the AAAI Conference on Artificial Intelligence* 33: 3558–3565.

Fischer, M.T., Arya, D., Streeb, D. et al. (2020). Visual analytics for temporal hypergraph model exploration. *IEEE Transactions on Visualization and Computer Graphics* 27 (2).

Fischer, M.T., Frings, A., Keim, D.A., and Seebacher, D. (2021). Towards a survey on static and dynamic hypergraph visualizations. In: *IEEE Visualization conference*.

Fontana, P., Yates, A., Greene, K.K. et al. (2021). Four principles of explainable artificial intelligence. Technical report.

Gao, Y., Zhang, Z., Lin, H. et al. (2020). Hypergraph learning: methods and practices. *IEEE Transactions on Pattern Analysis and Machine Intelligence* 44 (5)PP.

Graus, D., van Dijk, D., Tsagkias, M. et al., (2014). Recipient recommendation in enterprises using communication graphs and email content. In: *Proceedings of the 37th International ACM SIGIR Conference on Research Development in Information Retrieval (SIGIR)*.

Hamilton, L.H., Rex, Y., and Leskovec, J. (2017a). Representation learning on graphs: methods and applications. *IEEE Data Engineering Bulletin* 40 (3).

Hamilton, L.H., Ying, Z., and Leskovec, J. (2017b). Inductive representation learning on large graphs. *Advances in Neural Information Processing Systems* 30.

Karabyiyi, U., Canbaz, M.A., Aksoy, A. et al. (2016). A survey of social network forensics. *Journal of Digital Forensics, Security and Law* 11.

Kipf T.N., M. Welling (2017). Semi-supervised classification with graph convolutional networks. 5th International Conference on Learning Representations.

McInnes, L., Healy, J., Saul, N., and Großberger, L. (2018). Umap: uniform manifold approximation and projection. *Journal of Open Source Software* 3 (29): 861.

Mulazzani, M., Huber, M., and Weippl, E. (2012). Social network forensics: tapping the data pool of social networks. In: *Eighth Annual IFIP WG*.

Nikkel, B. (2020). Fintech forensics: criminal investigation and digital evidence in financial technologies. *Forensic Science International: Digital Investigation* 333.

Philips, P.J. Hahn, C., Fontana, P., Yates, A., Greene, K.K., Broniatowski, D.A., Przybocki, M.A. (2021). Four principles of Explainable Artificial Intelligence. NIST Interagency/Internal Report (NISTIR) - 8312

Ramos, D., Krish, R.P., Fierrez, J., and Meuwly, D. (2017). From biometric scores to forensic likelihood ratios. In: *Handbook of Biometrics for Forensic Science*, 305–327. Springer.

Rodriguez, A.M., Geradts, Z., and Worring, M. (2020). Likelihood ratios for deep neural networks in face comparison*. *Journal of Forensic Sciences* 65: 1169–1183.

Tang, L. and Huan, L. (2010). Graph mining applications to social network analysis. In: *Advances in Database Systems*, 487–513.

Valdivia, P., Buono, P., Plaisant, C. et al. (2021). Analyzing dynamic hypergraphs with parallel aggregated ordered hypergraph visualization. *IEEE Transactions on Visualization and Computer Graphics* 27: 1–13.

van der Maaten, L.J.P. and Hinton, G.E. (2008). Visualizing high-dimensional data using t-SNE. *Journal of Machine Learning Research* 9: 2579–2605.

van Leeuwen, D.A. and Brümmer, N., (2013). The distribution of calibrated likelihood-ratios in speaker recognition. In: *INTERSPEECH*.

Welling, M. and Kipf, T.N. (2017). Semi-supervised classification with graph convolutional networks. In: *International Conference on Learning Representations*.

Yadati, N., Nimishakavi, M., Yadav, P. et al. (2019). HyperGCN: a new method for training graph convolutional networks on hypergraphs. *NIPS'19: Proceedings of the 33rd International Conference on Neural Information Processing Systems*. 1511–1522.

Yuan, H., Haiyang, Y., Gui, S., and Shuiwang, J. (2020). Explainability in graph neural networks: a taxonomic survey. *ArXiv*, abs/2012.15445.

CHAPTER 11

Conclusion

Zeno Geradts[1] and Katrin Franke[2]

[1]*Netherlands Forensic Institute, Laan van Ypenburg 6, GB Den Haag, Netherlands*
[2]*Norwegian Univ of Science & Technology, Høgskoleringen 1,Trondheim, Norway*

In conclusion, artificial intelligence (AI) is rapidly becoming an essential tool in the field of forensic science. It enables forensic scientists to analyze large amounts of data quickly and accurately, making it easier to identify suspects, establish facts, and gather evidence in criminal and civil legal matters. As technology continues to advance, it is likely that we will see even more applications assisting forensic science. The technology allows for faster and more accurate analysis of large amounts of data, which can help to speed up investigations and bring criminals to justice more quickly. As technology continues to advance, it is expected that the use of AI in forensic science will become even more prevalent, providing even more powerful tools to aid in solving cases.

Explainable AI is important in fields such as forensic science, where the decision-making process of an AI system needs to be transparent and understandable to legal authorities, experts, and the public. For example, in forensic image analysis, an explainable AI system would be able to provide an explanation of how it determined that two images are of the same person, such as the specific features that were matched and the confidence level of the match.

There are several techniques that can be used to make an AI system more explainable, such as:

- Rule-based systems, where the decision-making process is based on a set of predefined rules that are easy for humans to understand.
- Decision trees, which provide a visual representation of the decision-making process and allow humans to trace the path of a decision.
- LIME (local interpretable model-agnostic explanations), which can provide explanations for specific instances of a model's decisions.
- SHAP (Shapley additive explanations), which can provide global explanations of a model's decisions by assigning a value to each feature.

Explainable AI is an important aspect of AI development, particularly in fields where transparency and human accountability are critical. With the rise of AI in various fields, explainable AI is becoming a key area of research, and many techniques are being developed to make AI systems. However, if a good mathematical model exists of the patterns (such as with camera identification with Photo Response Non Uniformity) the use of deep learning should only be considered if it works better than the model.

Using the examples provided in this book, we hope to contribute to the good use of AI in forensic science and take care of the ethical and privacy issues.

Index

Note: page numbers in *italics* refer to figures; those in **bold** to tables. Abbreviations used: AIA for Artificial Intelligence Act; ASR for automatic speech recognition; ML for machine learning; NER for named entity recognition; NLP for natural language processing